Forensic Pathology of Asphyxial Deaths

Forensic Pathology of Asphyxial Deaths

Dr. Sudhir K. Gupta
MBBS, MD, DNB, MNAMS, FICS (Chicago)
Professor and Head
Department of Forensic Medicine and Toxicology
All India Institute of Medical Sciences,
New Delhi, India

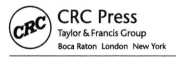

CRC Press
Taylor & Francis Group
Boca Raton London New York

CRC Press is an imprint of the
Taylor & Francis Group, an **informa** business

First edition published 2022
by CRC Press
6000 Broken Sound Parkway NW, Suite 300, Boca Raton, FL 33487-2742

and by CRC Press
4 Park Square, Milton Park, Abingdon, Oxon, OX14 4RN

CRC Press is an imprint of Taylor & Francis Group, LLC

© 2022 Taylor & Francis Group, LLC

ISBN: 978-0-367-13410-5 (hbk)
ISBN: 978-1-032-26448-6 (pbk)
ISBN: 978-0-429-02631-7 (ebk)

DOI: 10.1201/9780429026317

Typeset in Times
by KnowledgeWorks Global Ltd.

Contents

Preface

The respiratory system enables a person to inspire and expire air normally twelve times in a minute by means of expansion of lungs for intake of life-sustaining oxygen and its contraction to remove the carbon dioxide, the byproduct of cellular respiration. The air conduction system or airway extends through nostrils and mouth, pharynx, larynx, trachea and bronchial tree till alveoli. For respiration, this entire airway must remain open from any obstruction from inside or outside during all phases of inspiration and expiration along with a properly functioning supporting musculature, including diaphragm, intercostals muscles and accessory muscles of respiration with an intact rib cage. Asphyxia deaths are caused by the failure of cells to receive or utilize oxygen. In forensic medicine, when we conduct an autopsy, asphyxia is generally obstructive in nature, i.e., some physical barriers exist to prevent access of air to the lungs. Air passages are obstructed by pressure applied over the mouth, nostrils, neck or chest, causing sudden and violent cessation of respiration resulting in asphyxial deaths. In many cases, I have not seen the 'classical' features of asphyxia since the death may have occurred due to syncope immediately and body physiology has no time to develop demonstrable signs of asphyxia. The fear and shock of a homicidal strangulation or the panic of accidental entanglement, sudden entry into an area filled with irrespirable gas, sudden blockage of the air passages or pressure over the neck, may lead to rapid death without any 'classical signs'. These may be due to the release of catecholamines produced during the response to fear, stress or anger which trigger cardiac arrhythmias like ventricular fibrillation resulting in sudden death without any sign of asphyxia. Whereas, when there are ample opportunities to struggle to breathe particularly in partial hanging or manual strangulation cases, these signs of asphyxia are generally seen during autopsy. The traditional signs are not required to be evident to conclude asphyxial death during autopsy whereas it is being concluded by ruling out any other cause of death and assessing reliable circumstantial evidence.

Asphyxial death as a result of fatal pressure on the neck due to hanging, strangulation, smothering, throttling or other methods are accidental/suicidal/suicidal intent/ homicidal and undetermined. Asphyxial deaths amount to almost 50% of unnatural deaths, which is evident from World Health Organization (WHO) demographic details. Suicide is the act of intentionally causing one's own death, and the most common method of suicide all over the world is hanging because the materials used are easily accessible, and it's a feasible and credible method for a rapid and sure painless death. Death by hanging is easily achieved using cheap and easily available materials. Hanging is a mechanical form of asphyxia that is caused by suspension of the body by a ligature that encircles the neck, the constricting force being the weight of body. Death in fatal pressure on

the neck is caused by asphyxia, venous congestion, cerebral anemia, reflex vagal stimulation, fracture dislocation of the cervical vertebrae and sometimes a combination of the above. The highly experienced American pathologist Dr. Lester Adelson has put this caution very well in his excellent textbook *Pathology of Homicide*, in which he calls them the 'obsolete diagnostic quintet', saying: The co-existence of these findings, in themselves does not prove that death resulted from mechanical asphyxia. All these phenomena are non-specific and are in no way peculiar to this mode of death. In as much as they are observed frequently in deaths arising from unquestioned natural disease, they are of no value in proving that death resulted from mechanical asphyxia.

Equivocal deaths due to fatal pressure on the neck provide one of the most complex and controversial areas of 'asphyxia' deaths, as the mechanism is uncertain and the frequency of such deaths makes them a common problem for forensic doctors, police and court. The cases involving asphyxial deaths become a challenge for the investigating officer in taking decision, whether it is suicidal or homicidal, as there are always two sides of the situation and two versions come forward, about mode of death, by the investigation as well as the judiciary. It is suggested that the opinion of forensic medical expert is conventional, mutable and shifting from one expert to another. The determination of suicide, accident or homicide is mandatorily required, which is the gold standard for conducting death investigations. Forensic investigations serve many audiences, but the court is by far the most critical. The likely questions on direct and cross-examination determine how forensic doctors gather and handle evidence and what conclusions they reach.

Medical differentiation often becomes difficult when there is a well-defined ligature mark and injuries of the subcutaneous tissues/structures/glands/bones and cartilages are present in the neck and other parts of the body. The main dilemma is whether it is a case of suicidal hanging or a case where death was initially by other means and subsequently suspended to mimic suicidal hanging or is it a case of strangulation mimicking a case of hanging by ligature or a case of poisoning subsequently hanged or if it is a complex suicide involving multiple methods of suicidal attempts by the deceased. In such a situation, it completely depends on the wisdom of the surgeon conducting autopsy to give a direction for the investigators. The doctors conducting autopsy find the ligature mark externally on the neck, which is a common feature in all manners of traumatic fatal neck pressure asphyxial deaths; however, the internal dissection beneath the skin may be white glistening or bloody with or without fracture of neck thyro-hyoid complex, which gives a clue of suicidal or homicidal but does not have a rule of thumb. The doctor tries to provide answers demanded by the relatives and loved ones, as well as by the investigators, whether it is suicide or homicide. Since the pattern of injury as well as holistic examination by the doctor and the dead body provide vital clues and help to answer the queries, the how and what about the case, without the answer to these questions, the guilty party may go unpunished and the relatives and loved ones will remain throughout in dilemma. Hence, an elaborative aspect of fatal pressure on neck in the form of hanging requires having a detailed, scientific discussion in the interest of law and society. Junior doctors, who start their career in forensic medicine, must understand from the very beginning the delicate emotional aspects of loved ones and family in asphyxial deaths since only a trained doctor conducting autopsy will be able to answer the dilemma as well as put to rest the queries about the manner of death to the aggrieved family. Also, without the answer to these questions, the closure in asphyxial deaths is not possible.

Hence, this is an attempt by the author through this book to resolve the various issues in deciding the mode of death in cases of fatal pressure on neck, by citing various photographs, case reports, types of ligatures, manner of death and point of suspension, etc. This book will deliberate on suicidal and accidental hanging, the injuries and findings of asphyxia, brain ischemia and apoplexy, spinal cord injuries, decapitation as well as on death due to vagal inhibition with findings in cadaver. The author will also include the cases where the circumstances indicate the fact of hanging, but the ligature material is broken or detached, and the deceased is found lying with a ligature around his neck, along with cases of ligature strangulation and the same ligature in situ being used to suspend the corpse to mimic hanging. Further, this book will determine the cause of death in cases of hanging, which may include one or more of the following medical condition of death, e.g., asphyxia (closure of the airway), closure of carotid arteries causing ischemia, closure of the jugular veins, induction of carotid reflex, which reduces heartbeat when the pressure in the carotid arteries is high, causing cardiac arrest (reflex vagal inhibition), breaking of the neck (cervical fracture) causing traumatic spinal cord injury or even decapitation.

When a forensic doctor determines that a suspicious death is a suicide, homicide or accident, the decision virtually becomes incontestable by the investigating police officer and it becomes an issue whether the medical opinion was created with necessary checks and balances on the other probabilities of the case? In this context, I will very briefly discuss a case of self-strangulation. Case history: on 26.03.2009, Sh Philomeenaraj and his daughter Pramila Gandhi travelled by train and she was going to her aunt's house in Bengaluru. After getting down at railway station, Sh Philomeenaraj went to his own work, while Pramila supposedly went to her aunt's home. But, after some time, when he could not connect to her daughter's mobile, she asked her aunt if Pramila had visited them. He was informed that she did not visit their house, and then he lodged a missing complaint at the local police station. On 27.03.09, a dead body of a female, aged about 26 years, was recovered in a secluded place, in between two railway stations, located approximately 40 meters away from the railway track. She was identified as the missing Pramila Gandhi and a case was registered U/s 174 IPC on the complaint of the father of te deceased. The neck of the deceased was found encircled in three rounds by thread (naada) of the chudidaar that she was wearing. One end of the thread was tied to the finger of the right hand and the other end was found in the left hand in a loosened grip (separated from finger). On the body of the deceased, no deep wounds were present. The two hands of the deceased and the two fists were fully tightened and she was holding hairs in her both wrists. Case findings: The post-mortem examination was done on 28.03.2009 at Bangalore Medical College and the findings observed were: The face and sclera were congested, tongue bitten, blood-stained fluid present at nose and mouth while the nail beds were blue in colour. Ligature material is chudidara string; dirty green colour which is in two rows around the neck. Hair strands are entangled in between the ligature material and the ligature mark. There is a horizontal ligature mark in front of neck below the thyroid cartilage, which runs on both sides of neck and back of neck. It measures 31 cm × 1 cm and is situated 6 cm below right ear lobule and 6 cm below left ear lobule and 9 cm below mandible. The ligature mark completely encircles the neck and is in the form of a deep groove and the skin underneath is hard and parchmentised. On dissection, there is extravasation of blood in the tissues of neck all around. The hyoid bone and thyroid cartilage are intact. *Postmortem opinion:* The findings are suggestive of ligature strangulation and self strangulation is ruled out as at a stage of cerebral anoxia, ligature is loosened and death does not occur. The *viscera and vaginal swab* of the deceased were also preserved and sent to the State Forensic Science Laboratory. Viscera report did not reveal any common poison. Semen could not be detected on vaginal swab. From the Forensic Science Laboratory findings, sexual assault was ruled out. Initial investigation was done by the Bengaluru police. After the dissatisfaction by the parents of the deceased into the progress of investigation by Bengaluru police even after 4 years, they filed a writ petition to the Honorable High Court of Karnataka. The court transferred the case to Central Bureau of Investigation (CBI) Chennai on 21.10.2013. The CBI enquired the complainant, relatives, friends, neighbors, colleagues of deceased and people residing near the scene of crime, but no culprit could be traced. The main confusion was whether it was a case of homicidal or suicidal strangulation? Investigation by CBI—Stage II: For more than two and half years, there was no breakthrough in the murder investigation by the CBI. Finally, the CBI requested the Head of Forensic Medicine, AIIMS to give expert opinion to guide in the process of investigation and the observation and opinion were:

1. Strangulation may be homicidal, accidental or suicidal, particularly ligature strangulation. Distinction between homicidal and suicidal strangulation by

ligature is often impossible on the basis of anatomical findings alone, although fractures of the larynx in suicidal strangulation are distinctly unusual. The type of noose and knot as well as the number of turns around neck and circumstances under which the body is found, may suggest the manner of death.

2. Postmortem report as well as Forensic Science Laboratory is negative for any sign of biological evidence of sexual assault, which rules out any sexual assault. Also, there are no signs of struggle or any signs of defence injury over the body, which is seen in cases of self strangulation.

3. The Medical Board also observed that the ligature material was tied in right hand finger and another end was in left hand. As per postmortem report, it was seen that the thyro-hyoid complex was intact. In cases of strangulation by assailant, the thyro-hyoid complex is likely to be broken due to greater force which is applied in case of strangulation by an assailant to ensure death. However, no injury in thyro-hyoid complex suggests light compression force in neck, which could be possible by self-inflicted ligature force.

4. The ligature material, a green coloured cotton cloth naada with metallic safety pin attached to one end was examined by the AIIMS Medical Board. Length of ligature material was 190 cm and its breadth was 1 cm. The use of this ligature material and the body being found in accessible, non-remote place again suggests self-infliction, thus ruling out homicidal angle.

5. The opinion of autopsy surgeon mentions that "Self-strangulation is ruled out as at a stage of cerebral anoxia, ligature is loosened and death does not occur." It is inconceivable that anyone could die from compression of neck by his own hand because loss of consciousness would cause relaxation of the constricting fingers. When a ligature is involved the matter is different, as if the ligature is found in situ suicide is unusual but a distinct possibility.

Final unanimous opinion dated 22.04.2015: The cause of death in this case is Asphyxia as a result of ligature strangulation. It is a case of self-achieved strangulation, which is suicidal in manner. Current status of the case: CBI concurred with the AIIMS Medical Board opinion, that it is a case of suicide without any other possibility, which is speaking in nature with justification and references, totally corroborative with their investigation and CBI submitted closure report to Honorable Court. It is suggested that the opinion of forensic medical expert is conventional, mutable and shifting from one expert to another. The determination of suicide, accident or homicide, is mandatorily required, and the same should be of the gold standard for conducting legal death investigations.

The likely questions on direct and cross-examination determine how forensic doctors gather and handle evidence and what conclusions they reach. The author interacted with the investigative authority and crime scene visit was also done along with perusal of postmortem report, subsequent opinion and crime scene photographs and statements of witness and accused. Further analysis of all relevant scientific documents and opinions of other forensic doctors and forensic scientists involved in these cases was done to arrive at an opinion with scientific justification. Sudden, unnatural death of a human being raises suspicion regarding the manner of death, not only among the family members but in the society too. In many cases of sudden and suspicious deaths, there has been unrest at national and international level to know about the cause and manner of death. Questions are raised about the credibility of investigating agency, government, forensic laboratory as well as the doctor who conducted postmortem examination. In these instances, correct analysis and interpretation of forensic evidence are required to correlate with the circumstantial and investigative findings. There has recently been a case of suicidal hanging of a very famous Indian actor, Sushant Singh Rajput, which was misinterpreted as a homicidal case by some media groups and created a huge unrest in the general public at the international level. All the misinterpretations and misinformation were settled by a Medical Board under the chairmanship of the author. The same case has been discussed in the book. Forensic medical expert opinion must be with professional credibility in which the description of body trauma as evidence and an alleged mechanism of death as the way the deceased died is corroborated with the crime. The analysis of a crime scene and subsequent collection and evaluation of evidence (including physical, circumstantial and photographic) require skill, knowledge and ability to combine the two to come to a definite conclusion. A forensic doctor makes an expert opinion based on all these findings and establishes credibility of his opinion with references. The credibility of forensic doctor's opinion hinges on five principles: Who the medical experts are and what are their experience and credibility? Is the circumstantial evidence taken into account of expert opinion? Is it a speaking opinion with justification? How they eliminated other close options? What are the credible references? There are some cases where the forensic medical opinion has been given devoid of the above principles of credible opinion, which resulted in creating confusion for the CBI and became a hurdle in reaching a logical conclusion for a long time. The author illustrates such cases in which these basic principles were used in making credible forensic medicine expert opinion for investigators and judiciary. The book will further discuss the various types of forensic pathology of asphyxial death.

Acknowledgment

This book *Forensic Pathology of Asphyxial Deaths* is a first-of-its-kind book in medical science and is based on more than 25 years of experience and research in forensic autopsy by the author. The author has seen many cases of sudden and suspicious deaths due to hanging where there has been unrest at national and international levels to know the cause and manner of death. Deaths due to fatal pressure on the neck provide one of the most complex tasks for autopsy surgeons; the mechanism is uncertain and the frequency of such deaths make them a common problem for forensic doctors and police in the court of law. In these instances, correct analysis and interpretation of forensic evidences are required to correlate with the circumstantial and investigative findings. The postmortem report and its opinion must be with professional credibility. The forensic medical expert opinion is credible when the description of body trauma as evidence and an alleged mechanism of death as the way the deceased died are corroborated with the crime.

Several case studies have been added, not only to help readers understand how the principles of forensic medicine are applied practically but also to help the judiciary in judging crimes. Numerous colored photographs and illustrations have been added to support the text and to help readers visualize concepts better, and I dedicate this book to all the deceased whose photographs have become very educative. In this fast-paced era of technology, the field of forensic medicine is also rapidly and constantly evolving. To this end, I have made every effort to fortify this book with new and relevant knowledge, particularly with regard to medico-legal investigations and cause of death in cases of asphyxial deaths. The needs of medical students, autopsy surgeons, forensic fraternity, judicial officers, medical practitioners, criminal lawyers and police officers have been taken into consideration to make this book as a useful source of reference in forensic pathology of asphyxial deaths.

Considering the extensive and highly scientific amount of work that went into bringing out this edition, I am most grateful to Dr. Kulbhushan Prasad, Dr. Abhishek Yadav, Dr. Varun Chandran, Dr. Swati Tyagi and Dr. Abilash S from the Department of Forensic Medicine, AIIMS New Delhi; without their active and whole-hearted contribution and direct participation, it would not have been possible.

I thank my wife Dr. Madhu Gupta who actively contributed to scientific clarification in many issues of asphyxial death in this endeavor. I dedicate this book to my loving parents **Shri Kashi Nath Gupta** and **Kasthuri Devi** and son Keshav Karan.

I would also like to thank the CRC Press for providing the opportunity and also Shivangi Pramanik and Himani Dwivedi for guiding me all along the journey of preparing the manuscript.

Last but not least, I sincerely thank many unnamed persons who have played a direct or indirect role in translating my ideas into the script that has been presented here.

Author's Biography

Dr. Sudhir K. Gupta *MBBS (Gold Medal), MD (BHU), DNB, MNAMS, FICS (Chicago)*

Dr. Sudhir K. Gupta is the Professor and Head of the Department of Forensic Medicine and Toxicology at the All India Institute of Medical Sciences, New Delhi, India. He excelled right from his undergraduate times, securing a Gold Medal in the MBBS examination. He completed his post-graduation, MD Forensic Medicine from the prestigious Banaras Hindu University, Varanasi, India and was awarded Diplomate of National Board. He is a well-known teacher in AIIMS, New Delhi, with over 25 years of experience in teaching undergraduate, postgraduate and PhD students. His outstanding work in the medical profession as a distinguished teacher and researcher was recognized by the Indian Association of Medicolegal Experts along with Windsor University, Canada and he was rewarded a fellowship. He is a four-time member of the prestigious Dean's Committee at AIIMS and has been appointed examiner by numerous universities in India and abroad.

Dr. Gupta has published about 150 articles in national and international medical journals and is on the editorial board of many of them. He has authored chapters for several books, the most recent book was titled, 'Forensic Medicine and Toxicology, 3rd ed'. As an expert in the field of forensic medicine, Dr. Gupta regularly attends scientific meetings abroad. In 2010, Dr. Gupta was conferred the Doctor of the Year award by the Indian Journal of Clinical Practice, and was also awarded fellowship by the International College of Surgeons, Chicago, in 2018.

Some of the important cases of national and international repute handled by Dr. Gupta for the CBI India, referred from the Indian judiciary and other investigating agencies, include the death of Mr. Sushant Singh Rajput, death of Mrs. Sunanda Pushkar, Supreme Court-monitored CBI enquiry in more than a dozen cases of encounter killings in Manipur, death of Indian Cabinet Minister Sh. Gopi Nath Munde, Sheena Bora murder case, Shimla gang rape and custodial death case, suicide by IAS officer DK Ravi, death of Dr. Y. S. Sachan, an accused in NHRM scam, Jessica Lal murder case, Sh. Vidyacharan Shukla death case, Nirupma Pathak case, Uphaar fire tragedy cases, Nitish Katara murder case, BMW Lodhi Road accident case, Shivani Bhatnagar murder case, suicide by Ram Singh, the main accused in Nirbhaya case inside Tihar Jail and many more. With thousands of medico-legal postmortem examinations under his belt, Dr. Gupta is regularly called upon for his forensic expertise in homicide cases investigated by the CBI.

Dr. Gupta's efforts have been instrumental in the establishment of new facilities at AIIMS such as the 24-hour embalming facility, the forensic radiology unit, the modern toxicology laboratory, and most recently, the modular odorless autopsy suite. The institution of a state-of-the-art cadaver organ retrieval facility for therapeutic transplantation was also spearheaded by Dr. Gupta. A virtual autopsy center, called AIIMS-ICMR Center for Advanced Research and Excellence in Virtual Autopsy, at AIIMS, New Delhi, which is the first of its kind in India, was launched under the leadership of Dr. Sudhir K Gupta as the Principal Investigator in collaboration with ICMR in 2020.

1 Forensic Pathophysiology of Asphyxial Death

'Asphyxia' is a condition that results in lack of oxygen in blood, which may be due to mechanical interference in its uptake, transportation or cellular utilization, which means cellular oxidation. In forensic literature, asphyxia is considered as one of the modes of death, the other two being coma and syncope. Death due to asphyxia represents the majority of the case load in almost all centers conducting medico-legal autopsies in India. A similar scenario is seen in countries that share a similar socio-demographic profile. Despite there being no definite classification system and detailed treatises on asphyxial deaths in forensic practice, deaths due to asphyxia are the cases that are routinely seen to involve the maximum ambiguity at each step in medico-legal death investigation. Relatives, neighbors or friends of the decedent, the society at large and even the officers of the investigating agencies involved often raise their eyebrows at the conclusions reached by the autopsy surgeon. Such incidents are seen to occur even after one has conducted the complex autopsy by carefully and systematically documenting and interpreting the postmortem findings. He may have preserved viscera to rule out intoxication and corroborate one's opinion via reliable forensic analysis of any recovered fibers so as to definitely match it to the alleged used material that has been examined by qualified forensic scientists for its tensile properties. All these need to be corroborated while giving due consideration to all circumstantial evidences available for perusal, including statements of all concerned persons and a detailed scene of occurrence examination.

While demonstrable signs in cases of fatal asphyxia are abundant, most are not exclusive for a single cause of death. Thus, a holistic and cautious approach is required in dealing with suspicious asphyxial deaths in order to reach an evidence-based and scientifically valid opinion as to the cause and manner of death. The author has attempted to further elucidate such a conducive approach by citing scenarios from the case pile of medico-legal work he has encountered during last two and half decades. Death due to asphyxial mode can be due to a multitude of causes of which suicidal hanging is the commonest across the globe. Hanging is the most preferred modality of suicide across rural and urban populations. This is presumably due to the easy accessibility of ligature materials and of suspension points, and also a popular belief of hanging being quick and painless. Hanging is a type of mechanical asphyxia where death happens by suspension of the body by a ligature encircling neck with the constricting force being the weight of the whole body or a portion of it. Various factors such as the degree of neck compression, the type of ligature material, the type of noose, the placement of the knot, the weight of the individual acting as constricting force, the position of the individual and the height of the drop determine the possible features seen during autopsy. This entire process being dynamic and interdependent, they need to be considered together holistically rather than individually while analyzing the autopsy features.

'Classic signs' or other identified signs of asphyxial death may not be present in many hanging deaths, which can create confusion for the autopsy surgeon in reaching a conclusion, or may later be utilized as an argument to disprove his opinion during cross examination in a court trial. Another cause of uncertainty are cases of partial hanging, wherein limbs or any body part of the decedent touch the ground, practically raising doubt about the possibility of postmortem suspension in the mind of a common man or even at times in investigating officers. Similarly, the presence of aberrant injuries, atypical ligature marks, peculiar pattern of hypostasis with bleeding petechiae, darkened look of dried and protruded tongue, tache noir over exposed sclera and other bizarre findings that are possible in hanging cases can create serious doubts regarding the manner of death. Cases of postmortem suspension and homicidal hanging, though rare, do exist, further complicating the situation. Ligature strangulation and hanging vary mainly on the nature, placement, direction and the amount of constricting force applied. There are many cases where this line of demarcation between hanging and ligature strangulation is very narrow. Giving an absolute opinion in these borderline cases is considered one of the toughest exercise in routine medico-legal autopsy practice. Deaths occurring due to fatal pressure on the neck are one of the most complex and controversial groups among unnatural deaths as the mechanism is uncertain and the high frequency of such cases makes them a common problem for the public, relatives, forensic doctors, police and court. Taking a definitive decision as to whether the manner is accidental, suicidal or homicidal is difficult both for the autopsy surgeon as well as the investigating team in these cases, which eventually ends up in court as a dilemma for the judiciary and causes unnecessary mental suffering to the decedent's close ones.

DOI: 10.1201/9780429026317-1

Even a pressure abrasion typical of hanging, but with multiple underlying soft tissue and bony injuries in the neck, will always raise the doubt of postmortem suspension after strangulation or throttling of homicidal hanging even though most of these cases will later be proven to be suicidal in manner considering all the circumstantial evidences. When more than one method is adopted for suicide, similar confusions may arise. In such situations, the medical opinion, if scientific, confident and precise, can be helpful to many of the different segments of the people involved. Hence, a detailed scientific discussion and an elaborative approach in cases of fatal pressure over neck due to hanging are required in the best interest of law and society. Huge hue and cry, public unrest and mass movements have happened in relation to many such cases in the past. As an expert witness, a forensic medicine specialist who conducted the autopsy should be confident to formulate his opinion regarding the cause and manner of death in these cases wherever possible, and a systematic approach has been followed in this book to facilitate the same. The concepts of postmortem suspension and homicidal hanging along with their differentiating features are discussed in detail, and other causes of mechanical asphyxia like smothering, throttling, chocking, aspiration, drowning, postural asphyxia, traumatic asphyxia, asphyxia due to muscle relaxants including toxins and many others have been explained along with multiple photographs, pictorial demonstrations and detailed case reports in their respective sections.

Asphyxial deaths include death due to deficiency of oxygen in the respired air, such as cases of sewage tank cleaning accidents and 'ghost well' deaths. Peculiar postmortem findings and analysis of composition of gases obtained from various levels can be useful in reaching a reasonable conclusion about cause and manner of death in these cases. Hypoxia due to high altitude may lead to death of an individual, in whom acclimatization has been not achieved properly. Postmortem findings along with history and other circumstantial evidences will be helpful for the autopsy surgeon to give a scientific opinion for concluding these cases. Inhalation of excess quantity of toxic gases like carbon monoxide, carbon dioxide, hydrogen sulfide, etc. can also result in fatal tissue hypoxia. Carefully and systematically conducted autopsies along with a logical evaluation of the circumstances will be needed in similar cases where the postmortem findings such as the 'typical' color variation of postmortem hypostasis due to different toxic gases are subjective and are hardly even evident in many cases due to the relatively darker complexion of certain races.

Now it is established that even absence of all 'signs' of asphyxia at autopsy is not a hindrance in concluding a death as due to asphyxial means. However, this should be done only after ruling out all other possible causes of death and taking into consideration all the available circumstantial evidences. In common practice, once the autopsy surgeon has opined on the cause and manner of death, that is virtually seen as incontestable by the investigating agency. So it's mandatory for the autopsy surgeon to consider all other

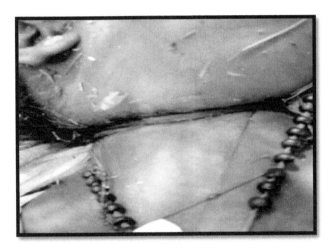

FIGURE 1.1 Ligature material present in situ around the neck of deceased.

possibilities before giving an opinion regarding the cause and manner of such deaths. In this context, the author wishes to discuss one case that was brought to him for expert medical opinion by the Central Bureau of Investigation (CBI) India a few years back.

This case involved a 26-year-old unmarried lady who had been reported missing on her way to her aunt's home and was later found dead at a secluded place with her pajama draw cord (locally termed as naada) seen tied around her neck in three loops (Figure 1.1). One of the free ends was tied to right hand fingers and the other was loosely gripped in her left palm (Figure 1.2). On autopsy, no relevant injury other than a transverse pressure abrasion completely encircling the neck below the thyroid cartilage was found on the body. Signs of asphyxia including cyanosis, facial congestion and edema were present. Neck dissection revealed some hemorrhages in the soft tissues near the ligature mark. The laryngeal cartilages and hyoid bone were intact. The autopsy surgeon had opined this as homicidal

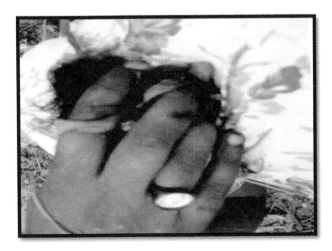

FIGURE 1.2 Ligature material tied to the right hand of the deceased.

ligature strangulation as he believed that sustained pressure could not have been maintained by the deceased herself since cerebral anoxia would likely have made her unconscious and caused the grip to be loosened. Hence, he ruled out the possibilities of suicidal or accidental strangulation. Examination of preserved vaginal swabs and visceral organs did not reveal any trace of semen or any kind of intoxication or poisoning. The local police investigated the 'murder' case and ruled out an offence of that nature. Later, as per court direction, the case was transferred to CBI. Even after investigating the case thoroughly, findings were not suggestive of any homicidal angle, and the investigation team approached a team of forensic doctors headed by the author for a scientific opinion regarding the possible cause and manner of death. All evidences including the ligature material found around the neck of the decedent were available for perusal by the team.

The author's team made note of the following points in this case: (i) no injury suggestive of struggle mark was present, (ii) there were no signs of an attempted theft/robbery, (iii) the characteristics of the pressure abrasion that was present on the neck were not suggestive of any slippage of ligature material, (iv) there were no muscle contusions, (v) no laryngeal injury, (vi) the ligature material had been found tied in three loops around neck, (vii) one end of the ligature material had been tied to the fingers and the other end had been in the palm of the decedent, (viii) no sign of sexual assault was present on the body, (ix) no incapacitating drugs was detected on visceral organ examination, (x) statements of all witness negated the possibility of any likely perpetrator, (xi) the ligature material had been a part of the clothing worn by the decedent, (xii) the cause of death was ligature strangulation. Based on all these facts and findings, the panel of doctors opined that the manner of death in the case could be suicidal. The opinion was consistent with all of the investigation findings of the CBI, and they submitted a closure report to the concerned honorable court stating that it was a case of suicide by ligature strangulation. Such a possibility has been corroborated by Taylor who described four situations where in suicidal ligature strangulation may occur. These are (i) when the constriction is due to multiple turns, with or without a knot, which are sufficient to maintain the pressure (as was seen in the author's case); (ii) tightening of the constricting material is carried out using a rod as a tourniquet; (iii) there is a running noose with a weight attached to its free end; and (iv) one hand is tied to the free end of a running noose.

In the author's view, in all medico-legal opinions furnished by a forensic expert, the following five criteria should be satisfactorily met so to avoid any future embarrassment especially during subsequent reviews by other experts or during trial in a court of law: (i) Is the expert satisfactorily experienced and competent to give a credible medico-legal expert opinion? (ii) Have the available circumstantial evidences been taken into account while reaching the conclusions? (iii) Is it a speaking opinion with reasoning and justifications for all the conclusions arrived? (iv) How did he/she eliminate other close alternative possibilities, and was it explained? (v) Are his/her references credible enough to withstand scientific and logical scrutiny? The author has tried to discuss many illustrative cases from his experience wherein the expert medico-legal opinions were furnished based on these principles and the way in which these helped in solving the mysteries of many unfortunate deaths, thereby enabling the investigators and the judiciary to reach a logical conclusion. There are many instances where the medico-legal opinions given have not been in line with the above stated principles, causing many practical problems for the investigating agencies such as CBI and eventually resulting in collapse of these cases in the court of law.

Opinions regarding the cause and manner of death may be subjected to scrutiny by forensically untrained medical and legal experts at different stages of an investigation and trial. Thus, before giving a final conclusion as the cause and manner of death of a person, the autopsy surgeon has to consider all the available evidences and circumstances of the case to avoid any professional embarrassment in the future. In the above-mentioned case, before reaching a final conclusion, the author got the opportunity to scrutinize the various photographs of the deceased captured at the scene of occurrence as well as during autopsy, forensic science laboratory reports, reports of the initial investigation by the local police and statements of the witnesses and was able to discuss the details of the case with the investigating team. While opining on the cause or manner of death, a forensic expert should be aware of the fact that even though the primary user of his or her report is the court of law, there are many other people who intend to know or understand the report which should be considered before they wish to draw a logical conclusion; these include relatives, friends, investigating agency and by extension the society at large who are keen to know the relevant findings. This is why it is considered good forensic medicine practice that medical opinion in all sudden and unexpected deaths, be they natural, accidental or homicidal, should be given in a clear and unambiguous scientific manner so as to avoid any unwanted speculation. Many cases from national and international scenarios have been cited in this book from author's knowledge where vague medical expert opinions have led to huge public unrest and protest. This mostly occurs when the reports are not based on the existing scientific norms.

Bodies recovered from water provide another challenge in routine forensic medicine practice. Even though drowning is the most common cause of death in this category, occasionally, doubtful situations may arise such as when multiple injuries are found on the body, the body recovered is in a decomposed state, when no signs of drowning are detected and in cases of postmortem immersion. These issues have been discussed in detail in the concerned chapter. The concept of laryngeal spasm, dry and wet drowning, salt and freshwater drowning, drowning in other liquids, the diagnostic value of diatom tests, etc. have also been described in detail.

Beginners in forensic medicine should always be aware of the fact that as long as the queries and concerns of the loved ones and the society remain unanswered, reaching an 'equivocal' conclusion in an asphyxial death is practically not possible in the court of law. In all possible cases, the autopsy surgeon should try to conclude the cause and manner of death unambiguously after giving due consideration to all facts and evidences that have been made available to him or her. In this book, the author has tried to clarify the concepts behind most of the possible circumstances related to the asphyxial mode of death with the help of numerous photographs, illustrated dissection techniques, pictorial demonstrations and case reports from his personal experience in accordance with the latest concepts in current medical literature. Since majority of the cases in this category belong to neck compression and other types of mechanical asphyxia, more importance has been given to this area. All possible atypical scenarios in cases of hanging, like partial hanging, bodies with tied limbs, unconventional ligature materials, hanging in jail, presence of other injuries unrelated to hanging, presence of other neck or other bodily injuries, etc., have been discussed in detail. An entire chapter has been dedicated for discussing issues related to differentiating among ambiguous cases of strangulation, hanging and postmortem suspension by citing cases that had come to the author for his expert medical opinion due to some disputes about the conclusion reached by the autopsy surgeons. The formulation of an opinion regarding the cause and manner of death in all of these cases has been discussed under the relevant heading.

Newer concepts regarding the 'classical' and other signs in asphyxial deaths along with radiological and histological signs have been discussed in detail in the relevant chapter. A deeper understanding of the anatomical structures related to respiration, including the airway, lungs, respiratory centers, involved musculoskeletal elements, their innervations as well as minute details of neck structure, is important in dealing with case of asphyxial deaths. The physiology of respiration and pathophysiology of asphyxial deaths also has to be studied in detail. All these aspects have been covered later in the book. It has been observed that a dedicated work describing all possible scenarios related to asphyxial death will be useful for all practicing forensic doctors, and an attempt has been made in this book to do so for a better conceptual understanding of the subject.

PATHOPHYSIOLOGY OF RESPIRATION

Respiration is a vital function of an individual. A person respires continuously and in a rhythmic manner. This involves expansion and contraction of the lungs for inhalation of the air needed for oxygenation of blood and for expulsion of carbon dioxide produced as a byproduct of cellular metabolism, respectively. This physiological process requires synchronization between the respiratory, musculoskeletal, cardiovascular and nervous systems. The primary objective is to provide oxygen to the tissues and remove

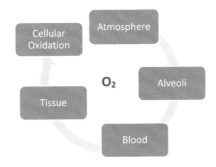

FIGURE 1.3   Direction of flow of oxygen.

carbon dioxide from them. The lack of oxygen at the tissue level, which may either be partial, termed hypoxia, or complete, which is referred to as anoxia, can lead to death. For respiration to occur in an uninterrupted fashion, the respiratory passages, orifices, lung tissue and the supporting musculoskeletal framework should be free from occlusion, obstructions or any external compressive pressures. Though the respiratory system appears to play a major role in the entire respiratory process, the support of other bodily systems is equally important for its effective functioning, and a disturbance in any of these can lead to respiratory failure. The oxygen concentration of normal room air is approximately 21%, but if this drops to about 10–15%, cognitive and motor functioning could be impaired, and if it further falls to less than 10%, then the individual can lose consciousness. Under normal physiological conditions, humans breathe around 12–15 times per minute, exchanging about 500 mL of air with each breath or 6–8 liters each minute.

Respiration is a multi-step process involving a number of steps like (Figures 1.3 and 1.4):

   i. Exchange of gas between atmosphere and alveoli
  ii. Exchange of gas between the alveoli and the blood in pulmonary circulation
 iii. Transport of the gas within the blood stream, i.e., oxygen from lung to tissues and CO_2 from tissues to lung
  iv. Cellular utilization of this oxygen for adenosine triphosphate (ATP) production (cellular oxidation)

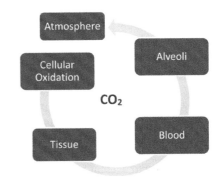

FIGURE 1.4   Direction of flow of carbon dioxide.

MUSCULOSKELETAL SYSTEM SUPPORTING RESPIRATION

The lungs are positioned within the thoracic cavity, protected by the rib cage and supported anteriorly and posteriorly by sternum and spinal column respectively. A number of muscles surrounding the lungs contribute to the process of breathing.

Inspiratory muscles: Inspiration is an active process that involves contraction of the following muscles:

- *Diaphragm:* The diaphragm marks the inferior boundary of the thoracic cavity. It contracts and moves downwards on inspiration, leading to a 75% increase in the intrathoracic volume, and is the primary muscle for inspiration.
- *External intercostal muscles:* The external intercostals are the other important inspiratory muscles. These run obliquely downwards and forwards from rib to rib. The lower ribs get elevated up on their contraction and the sternum moves outward, thereby increasing the antero-posterior diameter of the chest. There is also an increase in the transverse diameter of the thoracic cavity, but to a lesser extent.

Both the diaphragm and the external intercostal muscles individually can maintain the process of breathing at rest.

- *Accessory inspiratory muscles:* The scalenes and sternocleidomastoid muscles in the neck function as accessory muscles of inspiration during deep labored breathing. The scalene muscles elevate the first two ribs and sternocleidomastoid muscle lifts the sternum, thereby causing further increase in the volume of the thoracic cavity.

Expiratory muscles: Normal quiet expiration is a passive process and occurs due to the elastic recoil of the chest wall and lungs when the diaphragm and external intercostal muscles relax. Forced expiration, on the other hand, is an active process involving the contraction of the internal intercostal muscles that depress the ribs and contraction of the muscles of the anterior abdominal wall, especially the recti, which can exert a strong downward pull over the lower ribs.

REGULATION OF RESPIRATION

The regular rhythmic respiration due to contraction of respiratory muscles occurs following regular discharge from the motor neurons supplying them, which in turn is dependent on the primary discharge from the brain. This process can get hampered if the spinal cord gets dissected at a level above/proximal to the origin of phrenic nerve. The electric impulses from the brain that regulate respiration is further affected by alterations in arterial PO_2, PCO_2 and H^+ concentrations, along with multiple non-chemical factors that influence this chemical control of respiration.

Neuronal Control of Respiration

Peripheral/Autonomic Nervous System

It supports the muscles of inspiration and expiration. Respiration is regulated by two different neural mechanisms: the first one is for voluntary control and the second for autonomic control. The cerebral cortex is the seat controlling the voluntary respiratory movements via transmission of regulating impulses through the corticospinal tracts to the respiratory motor neurons. The autonomic control system is orchestrated by a group of pacemaker cells in the medulla oblongata, which activate the motor neurons in cervical and thoracic spinal cord controlling the inspiratory muscles. Phrenic nerve originates from the cervical roots C2–C4 and controls the diaphragm, while external intercostal muscles are controlled by the thoracic nerves of the spinal cord.

Central Control of Respiratory Functions

Medulla and pons contain the central respiratory centers that are responsible for initiating, controlling and maintaining the respiratory pattern. The medullary center consists of a dorsal and a ventral respiratory group, and the pontine center consists of a pneumotaxic center and an apneustic center together forming the pontine respiratory group. The dorsal respiratory neurons initiate the process of inspiration and the ventral group controls expiration. The pneumotaxic center and the apneustic center provide negative and positive feedback to the dorsal respiratory group, respectively, thereby regulating the discharges from this center (Figure 1.5).

Biochemical Control of Respiration

A rise in the P_{CO2} or H^+ concentration of the arterial blood or a drop in its P_{O2} levels causes an increase in the neuronal activity in the medullary respiratory center, while changes in the opposite direction have a slight inhibitory effect. The influence of some dynamic variations of blood chemistry on ventilation are mediated through the respiratory chemoreceptors of the carotid and aortic bodies and a group of cells located in the medulla and elsewhere, which respond to the changes in the chemistry of the blood by producing impulses that stimulate or inhibit the respiratory centers.

PHYSIOLOGICAL FACTORS LEADING TO ASPHYXIA

There are various physiological factors that lead to asphyxia:

1. *Airway obstruction:* Obstruction of airway can decrease the volume of respired air, especially the inhalation of oxygen. The reason for such obstruction may be mechanical or pathological. Mechanical causes include external obstruction through compression of airways as in hanging, strangulation and internal obstruction by foreign bodies such as in choking, gagging, etc. The causes include diseases of the pathway like tumors

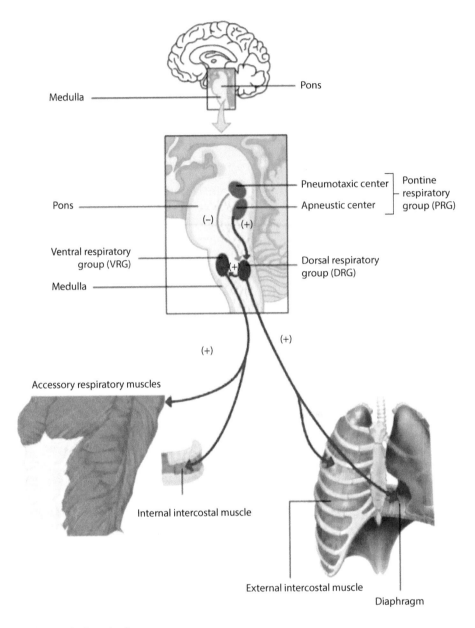

FIGURE 1.5   Neuronal control of respiration.

of larynx, pharynx and trachea, which may also cause obstruction of oxygen inhalation and carbon dioxide exhalation.

2. *Impaired exchange of gases:* Asphyxia or hypoxia can be caused by alteration in oxygen and carbon dioxide exchange at the alveolar level. The reason for such impairment can further be divided into violent and pathological types. The violent type is often due to the inhalation of poisonous gases like carbon monoxide, hydrogen sulfide, phosgene, etc., which tend to interfere with the uptake of O_2 through alveoli by hemoglobin owing to their higher affinity. This condition is also seen in pathologies like pneumonia, alveolar lung disease, pulmonary embolism, systemic lupus erythematosus, sarcoidosis, etc.

3. *Impaired respiratory movements:* The process of respiration involves intercostal muscles, their innervation through the intercostal nerves and blood supply through the internal thoracic artery and intercostal arteries. The thoracic cavity expands during the process of inhalation and relaxes during exhalation. This process can be interfered with by external thoraco-abdominal compression, positional asphyxia and traumatic pneumothorax. Certain pathological conditions can also impair this process of expansion and relaxation such as pathological pneumothorax.

4. *Impaired transportation:* There can be impairment in transportation of oxygen from lungs to the body tissues. This occurs unnaturally in cases of carboxyhemoglobinemia and methemoglobinemia

when certain toxic gases are inhaled. This impaired oxygen transportation affects the metabolic activity of the tissues, which eventually turn ischemic due to anoxia. Pathologically, this situation can also be encountered when the vascular supply to the tissues gets impaired owing to coronary heart disease, circulatory failure, anemia and hemoglobin disorders.

5. *Impaired utilization:* This occurs when there is adequacy of oxygen and a normal functioning respiratory mechanism, but the body tissues are unable to utilize the available oxygen, e.g., cyanide poisoning.

PATHOPHYSIOLOGY OF ASPHYXIA

In fatal asphyxia, the major factor causing death of the individual is the inability of cells or tissues to receive or utilize oxygen. In forensic medicine practice, autopsies in cases of asphyxial deaths due to airway obstruction generally imply the presence of mechanical barrier that prevents access of air from the atmosphere to the lungs. This obstruction to the air passage can be with ligatures or pressure over mouth, nostrils, neck or chest, which causes sudden and violent cessation of respiration, resulting in an asphyxial death. Brain cell death, especially among the neurons of central regulatory centers of the brainstem, leads to cessation of the respiratory and circulatory systems. The energy produced by the brain cells through metabolism is primarily utilized for maintaining the resting membrane potential to enable excitation and conduction of impulses. The energy stores of the brain are limited and a continuous supply of glucose and oxygen is necessary for the uninterrupted production of ATP. Thus, the energy requirement of brain is different from other tissues and organs, which can be much more flexible in adopting their metabolic requirements.

Asphyxia develops when the oxygen perfusion to tissue falls below the necessary level due to any disturbance in respiration. This can be fatal when the levels fall below the threshold level required for sustenance of life, and deprivation of oxygen for even up to 3–5 minutes can cause permanent damage to the brain and cardiovascular system. This starts the vicious cycle of asphyxia, which continues till the person dies. The brain forms 2–3% of the body mass but receives around 20% of the total inspired oxygen as it is required by the neurons for normal brain activity and function. Depletion of oxygen, glucose or ATP causes damage to the neurons (Figure 1.6).

FACTORS CAUSING EARLY SUSCEPTIBILITY OF BRAIN CELLS TO HYPOXIA

When a mechanical obstruction is applied to airways by means such as hanging, strangulation, etc., the respiratory centers of brain continue generating the impulses for rhythmic respiration and muscle contraction against the applied force of obstruction, and there is a significant struggle for a

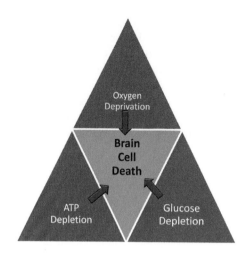

FIGURE 1.6 Factors causing brain cell death.

duration of up to 3–10 minutes between central respiratory impulses and the applied mechanical forces. Eventually, the medullary neurons of respiratory center die owing to the following factors:

- Blood flows to the brain at the rate of 50–60 mL/100 g tissue/min. Brain cell disturbances start when the rate of blood circulation decreases below 20 mL/100 g tissue/min, and at rates below 10 mL/100 g tissue/min, degenerative changes start.
- The amount of oxygenated blood supplied to brain is almost double that required by the brain cells. Thus, oxygen is stored in the brain amounting to about 315 mmol/g, which can sustain brain functions for a period of approximately 8 minutes.
- Neurons are most sensitive to hypoxic disturbances, followed by glial cells and endothelial cells of brain vessels.
- A fall in the partial pressure of oxygen decreases the production of ATP. This leads to cytotoxic edema due to accumulation of intracellular Na^+. Decreased oxygen supplies further causes Ca^{2+} influx, activation of lytic enzymes, mitochondrial dysfunction and finally results in apoptosis of cells due to release of lipases and proteases.
- Further depletion of oxygen and ATP leads to anaerobic metabolism, which causes intracellular acidosis due to production of lactic acid, but the brain only has a limited ability to utilize the anaerobic process to produce ATP.
- The brain stores only small amounts of endogenous fuel. Under normal physiological circumstances, the concentration of the glucose in the brain tissues is around 1–2 μmol/g brain wet weight, which is always lesser than the blood glucose levels of 5–6 μmol/mL blood.
- When the arterial blood supply to the brain is blocked due to compression of the neck as may occur in violent asphyxia or due to other causes, it

interrupts not only oxygen supply to brain tissues, but also hampers glucose supply.

- Medullary neurons form the respiratory center of the brain and function due to the supply of oxygenated blood. Medullary neurons are very sensitive to decreased oxygen supply, and diminished oxygenated blood supply causes their death within minutes. Death of medullary neurons causes failure of function of respiratory system and gradually the cessation of function of the heart, leading to death of the individual. Cells other than brain cells, like skeletal muscles, may survive longer and are among the last to die as per the observed sequence of cellular death. Decreased oxygen supply to the neurons of the medullary respiratory center leads to cell death within 3–5 minutes.

2 Anatomy of Neck and Blood Supply of Brain

ANATOMY OF NECK

The neck is a beautiful and intricate structure with its complex anatomy confined in its deep cervical fascia. The neck is a hollow cylindrical tube which is divided into anterior and posterior triangles by sternocleidomastoid muscle, and it originates from the base of the cranium and inferior border of mandible to the inlet of the thoracic duct. The neck contains important muscles, namely sternocleidomastoid between anterior and posterior triangles of the neck. The anterior triangle originates from inferior border of mandible and descends into the sternum below. The posterior triangle extends backwards to the anterior border of trapezius and inferiorly to the clavicle. The neck is quadrilateral and cylindrical in shape and is bounded anteriorly by anterior median line and posteriorly by the anterior border of trapezius muscle, superiorly by base of mandible and inferiorly by the clavicle.

SURFACE ANATOMY OF NECK

1. Sternocleidomastoid muscle can be seen prominently when neck and chin are turned to the opposite side.
2. External jugular vein is seen crossing the sternocleidomastoid muscle obliquely.
3. The supraclavicular fossa lies above and behind the clavicle and sternum.
4. Behind the auricle, mastoid process is present.

SKIN OF NECK

Lines of greatest tension in the neck are termed 'relaxed skin tension lines'. The next layer is superficial cervical fascia, which consists of the adipose tissue and platysma. The deep cervical fascia surrounds the muscles and other structures of the neck to varying extent. The carotid sheath is a condensed part of deep fascia that encloses the structures like carotid arteries, vagus nerve and internal jugular vein. In health, the tissues within these spaces are either closely applied to each other or are filled with relatively loose connective tissue. However, they offer potential routes by which unchecked infection may spread within head and neck and between the face and the mediastinum.

BLOOD SUPPLY

Facial, occipital, posterior auricular and subclavian arteries mainly supply blood to the skin of the neck.

VENOUS DRAINAGE

Venous drainage of skin drains into jugular and facial veins.

LYMPHATIC DRAINAGE

1. The lymphatic draining of the superficial cervical region occurs into the deep cervical nodes. Some passes over posteriorly to drain into superficial cervical and occipital nodes.
2. Lymphatic from superior region of anterior triangle drains into submandibular and submental nodes.
3. The anterior neck skin below the level of hyoid bone drains to the anterior cervical and anterior jugular nodes and finally to the deep cervical nodes.

BONES OF NECK

The major bones of the neck include the cervical vertebrae and hyoid bone. Laryngeal cartilages consist of thyroid, cricoid, epiglottis, arytenoid, corniculate and cuneiform. They also form an important part of the support system of the neck.

CERVICAL VERTEBRAE

The cervical vertebrae are seven in number, and among them, the third to sixth vertebrae have characteristic features of cervical vertebrae like spinous processes being short and bifid, articular facets being flat and oval, the transverse process containing the foramen transversarium, etc. The first, second and seventh cervical vertebrae are distinct with each one having peculiar features, like the first vertebra is called Atlas and it lacks a spinous process and is more of a ring with anterior and posterior arch. The second vertebra is called Axis; it acts as a pivot on which the skull and the Atlas move, and it also has an odontoid process that forms a joint with Atlas. The seventh vertebra is called Vertebra

DOI: 10.1201/9780429026317-2

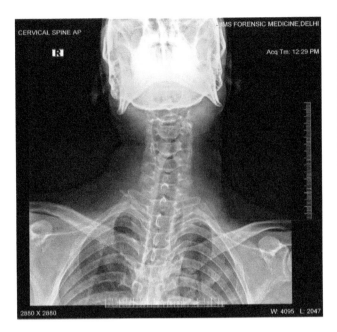

FIGURE 2.1a Antero-posterior view of neck showing the intact airway and neck skeletal structures in PM X-ray.

prominens and has a very long and prominent spinous process, making it easily palpable under the skin. Radiological examination either with X-ray or CT scan is very useful for determination of fracture dislocations of cervical vertebrae which could be fatal (Figures 2.1a–2.2b).

Hyoid Bone

Hyoid bone is classically described as a U-shaped, sesamoid bone (not attached to any bones directly). It consists of five parts, which include a central body; two long projections going backward from the outer borders of the body, called greater cornua; and two smaller conical projections arising from hyoid body or the junction between body and greater cornua, called lesser cornua (Figures 2.3 and 2.4).

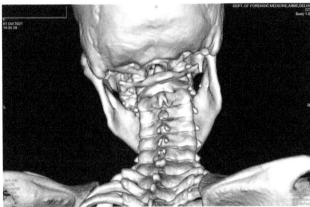

FIGURE 2.1c 3D reconstruction PMCT visualizing the skeletal structures of neck from posterior view.

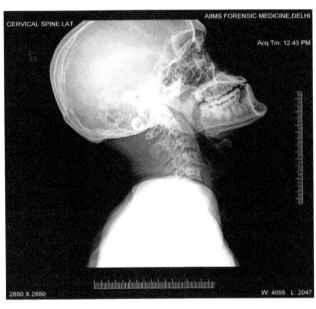

FIGURE 2.2a Lateral view of neck showing intact airway and neck skeletal structures in PM X-ray.

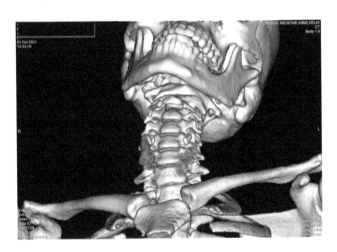

FIGURE 2.1b 3D reconstruction PMCT visualizing the skeletal structures of neck from anterior view.

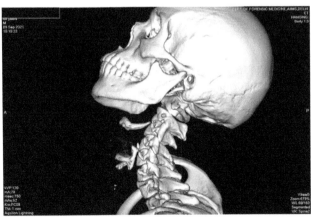

FIGURE 2.2b 3D reconstruction PMCT visualizing the skeletal structures from lateral view.

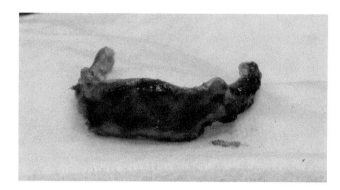

FIGURE 2.3 The hyoid bone after dissection from the dead body.

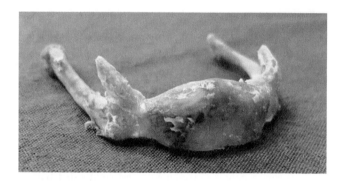

FIGURE 2.4 The hyoid bone after formalin preservation and removal of muscular attachments.

Body

The body is roughly quadrilateral and is elongated side to side. It has four borders (superior, inferior and two lateral) and two surfaces (anterior and posterior). The anterior surface is slightly convex and has depressions. The posterior surface is smooth and concave, and the concavity holds loose areolar tissue and thyrohyoid membrane, which separates the hyoid from the epiglottis.

Greater Cornua

The greater cornua are connected to the body by cartilage in early life, and after middle age, they are usually united by bone. They project upwards and backwards from the lateral ends of the body. They taper posteriorly, ending in a tubercle. When the throat is gripped between finger and thumb above the thyroid cartilage, the greater cornua can be palpated and the bone can be moved from side to side.

Lesser Cornua

The lesser cornua are two small conical projections arising at the junction of the body and greater cornua on their superior border. They are connected to the body by fibrous tissue and sometimes to the greater cornua by a synovial joint, which occasionally becomes ankylosed. Lesser cornua may or may not be ossified, and thus may give the false impression of being absent if only examined using X-ray.

Development and Ossification

The upper body of hyoid and lesser cornua originate from second pharyngeal arch cartilage (Reichert's cartilage). The lower portion of the body and the greater cornua of hyoid are formed by the cartilage of third pharyngeal arch. Although the hyoid body is traditionally believed to have a dual origin from second and third arch mesenchyme, this theory remains controversial. Chondrification of the bone begins in the fifth fetal week in these elements and is completed in the third and fourth months. During infancy, the hyoid is situated anterior to the second and third cervical vertebra. It then descends simultaneously with other functionally relevant structures such as epiglottis and larynx, to ultimately lie at the level of the fourth and fifth cervical vertebra in adulthood at the position of the third molar tooth. Ossification occurs from six centers: a pair in the body and one in each cornu. It begins in the greater cornua towards the end of intrauterine life, in the body shortly before or after birth and in the lesser cornua around puberty. The apices of greater cornua remain cartilaginous until the third decade.

Deviation from normal anatomy of hyoid has been reported to occur in 4–30% of the population. Hyoid anomalies are considered to be either developmental or acquired.

Some of the reported anomalies of hyoid are:

1. *Anomalies in lesser horn:* Elongation of lesser horns (Figures 2.5a–2.12c).
2. *Anomalies of greater horn:* Asymmetry in shape and length of greater cornua; downward curved tips of greater cornua; elongated greater horns (Figures 2.13–2.15).
3. *Anomalies in the body of hyoid:* Presence of one or more median process, or split median process on superior surface of the hyoid body (Figures 2.16–2.18).
4. Presence of a triticeal cartilage in the lateral thyrohyoid ligament.
5. *Anomalies due to ankylosis:* Fusion of hyoid bone with styloid process or thyroid cartilage.
6. Present of almost circumferential hyoid bone.

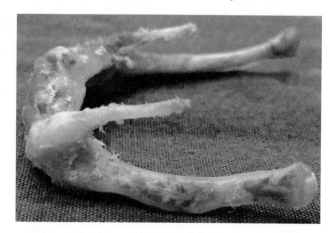

FIGURE 2.5a Hyoid of a 26-year-old female showing elongated bilateral lesser horns, left lateral view.

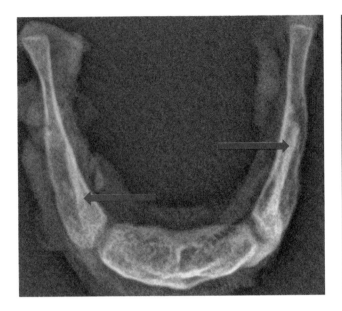

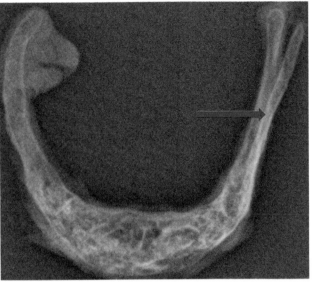

FIGURE 2.5b Plain X-ray, superior view of the same case showing bilateral long lesser horns.

FIGURE 2.6b Plain X-ray, superior view of the same case showing elongated left lesser horn. Also note the asymmetry in the curvature of greater horns.

Some anomalies can be explained by diversion from normal embryology. These are as follows:

1. *Median process or exostosis or lingula:* A small bony projection is seen growing upward from the superior surface of the body of hyoid bone. This has been mentioned by many as median process or exostosis or lingula. This structure demarcates the point where the embryological thyroglossal duct reaches the hyoid bone, and it is believed to be a remnant of thyroglossal duct. However, it is

also believed to mark the first appearance of the hyoid body, and it is hypothesized that this process may be a remnant of a cylindrical-shaped anlage (growth center between left and right-sided bars of second pharyngeal arch cartilage). Instances are reported where there has been presence of two lingula. Its presence has been described in both males and females. However, in author's experience, lingula was found to be more prominent in male subjects. In some cases, this process was

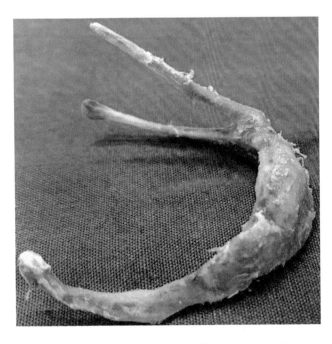

FIGURE 2.6a Hyoid of a 45-year-old male showing elongated lesser horn on the left side, right lateral view. Also note the asymmetry in the curvature of greater horns.

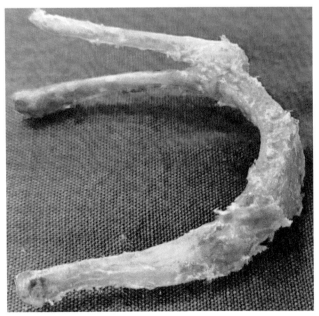

FIGURE 2.7a Hyoid of a 44-year-old male showing elongated lesser horn on the left side, right lateral view.

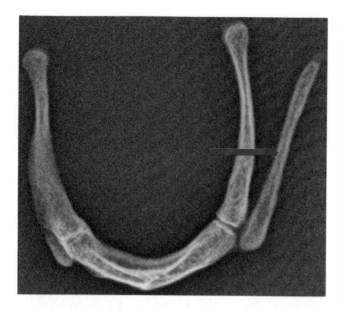

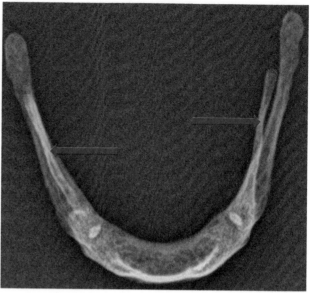

FIGURE 2.7b Plain X-ray, superior view of the same case showing elongated left lesser horn. Note the smaller, ossified lesser horn on the right side.

FIGURE 2.8b Plain X-ray, superior view of the same case showing elongated bilateral lesser horn. Also note the asymmetry in lengths of greater horns.

prominent and found to be grown anteriorly rather than superiorly.

2. *Second pharyngeal arch cartilage anomalies:* Presence of long lesser horn or fusion of styloid process with lesser horn has been found. This is believed to be ossification of stylohyoid ligament. The second pharyngeal arch cartilage persist as cartilaginous bar in stylohyoid ligament, and later it may be either partially or completely ossified. Clinically, elongation of styloid process can give rise to classic Eagle's syndrome or stylocarotid

syndrome. Lesser horns can be bilaterally long and of equal size, bilaterally long but asymmetrical in size, or unilaterally long.

3. *Third pharyngeal arch cartilage anomalies:* It gives rise to any cartilaginous or bony connection between greater cornua of hyoid bone and superior horns of thyroid cartilage (due to ossification of persisting embryological cartilaginous component within lateral thyrohyoid ligament). Most common variation is the presence of triticeal cartilage, which may or may not be ossified. Other anomaly is the complete ossification of this ligament, named as 'congenital hypothyroid bar'.

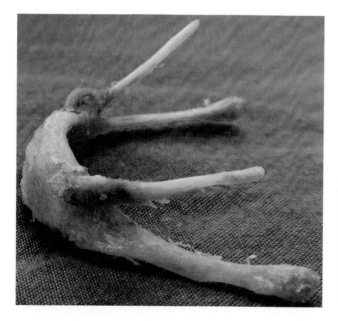

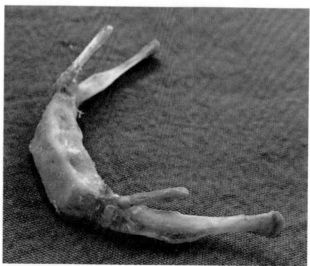

FIGURE 2.8a Hyoid of a 40-year-old male showing bilateral elongated lesser horn, left lateral view.

FIGURE 2.9a Hyoid of a 20-year-old male showing bilateral elongated lesser horns, left lateral view.

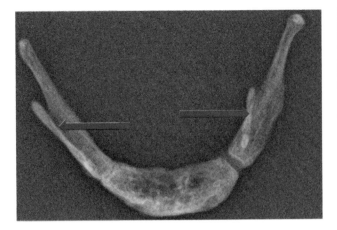

FIGURE 2.9b Plain X-ray, superior view of the same case showing elongated bilateral lesser horns.

Acquired anomalies could be due to osteonecrosis after radiation exposure, or post-surgical after radical neck dissection or mandibular advancement, inflammatory cases or poor oral habits.

Following are the pictures of long lesser horns (because normal length of lesser horn has not been defined, when the lesser horns were equal to or longer than half the length of greater horn, it was considered to be long) and their respective X-rays in superior view after they have been dissected from the body.

There were instances with asymmetrical greater horns showing the following features: where distal part of the greater horns was facing inferiorly (Figure 2.13), where one horn was more curved than the other (Figure 2.14), where one horn lied superiorly to the other (Figure 2.15), where one greater horn was curved upward (Figure 2.14), presence of tongue-shaped lingual (Figures 2.16 and 2.17) or bifurcated lingual (Figure 2.18).

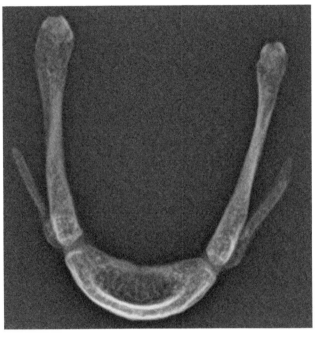

FIGURE 2.10b Plain X-ray, superior view of the same case showing elongated bilateral long lesser horns.

Forensic Relevance

1. Anatomical variants may be related to age, sex and ethnicity. They may be important when using hyoid bone for establishing biological profile.
2. Anatomical variants resembling fractures should be kept in mind when examining the hyoid-larynx complex.
3. Untimely fusion of joints may occur in younger age groups, in which if fractures occur, chances of being missed are high.

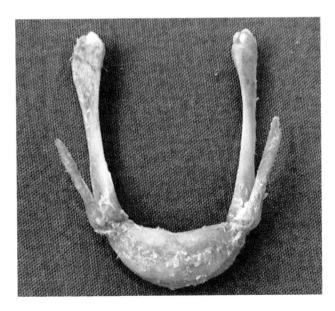

FIGURE 2.10a Hyoid of a 31-year-old male showing bilateral elongated lesser horns, superior view.

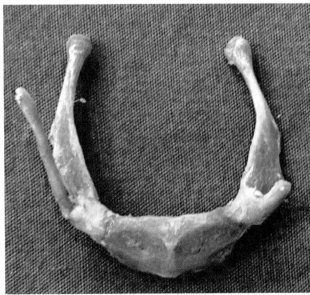

FIGURE 2.11a Hyoid of a 30-year-old male showing elongated right lesser horn, superior view.

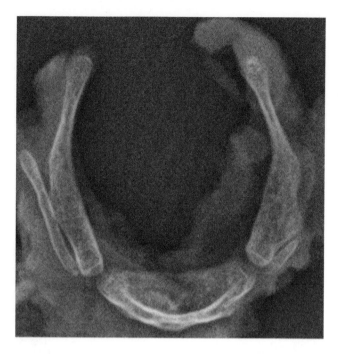

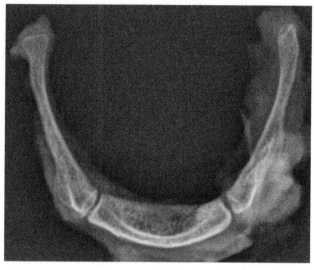

FIGURE 2.11b   Plain X-ray, superior view of the same case showing elongated right lesser horn. Also note the small, ossified left lesser horn.

4. Similarly, fusion in older age groups may not have occurred and, thus, mistaken diagnosis of fracture in case of joint mobility should not be made.
5. Each anomaly may affect the way they are mobilized during neck injuries, which may not always give expected consequences in the autopsy findings.

FIGURE 2.12b   Plain X-ray, superior view of the same case showing absence of elongation of lesser horn (bony shadow) on the right side as it is a cartilaginous extension and has not been ossified.

LARYNGEAL CARTILAGINOUS SKELETON

The laryngeal skeleton consists of nine cartilages, namely:

i. Thyroid cartilage (unpaired)
ii. Cricoid cartilage (unpaired)
iii. Epiglottis (unpaired)
iv. Arytenoid cartilage (paired)
v. Corniculate cartilage (paired)
vi. Cuneiform (paired)

They form the cartilaginous skeleton that protects the larynx. It forms the anterior prominence over the neck referred to as laryngeal prominence or Adam's apple.

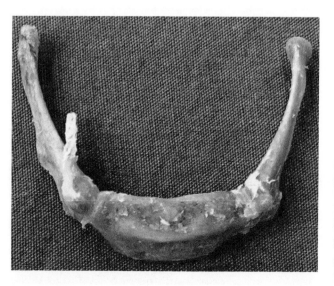

FIGURE 2.12a   Hyoid of a 40-year-old male showing cartilaginous extension of the stylohyoid ligament from the tip of lesser horn on right side, superior view.

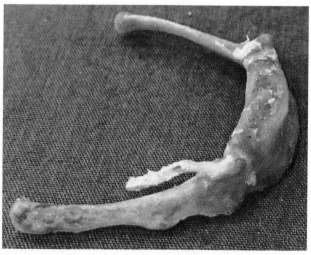

FIGURE 2.12c   Same case as above, right lateral view.

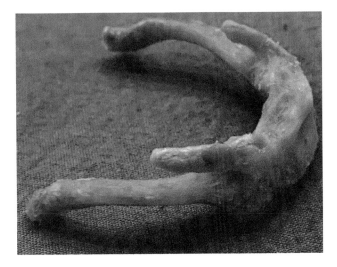

FIGURE 2.13 Bilateral, downward curved greater horns, right lateral view. Also note all the joints are fused.

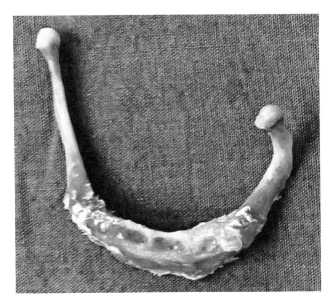

FIGURE 2.14 Asymmetric greater horns, superior view. Left greater horn is curved upwards and shortened.

TRITICEOUS CARTILAGE OF THE LARYNX

The triticeous cartilage is a small cartilaginous or bony part of the laryngeal complex found on the lateral aspect of the thyro-hyoid membrane and is situated between the thyroid cartilage's superior horn on the inferior aspect and superiorly by the hyoid bone's greater cornua. It is made of hyaline cartilage, and later, it sometimes undergoes calcification. The prevalence of triticeous cartilage calcification by both radiological and cadaveric studies is around 5–29%, and the triticeous cartilage prevalence was found to be higher in men. Named for its characteristic shape (from the Latin word triticeous, meaning resembling or shaped like a grain of wheat), this cartilage represents a residual anatomic structure of no known functional significance. A muscular band (musculus triticeoglossus or

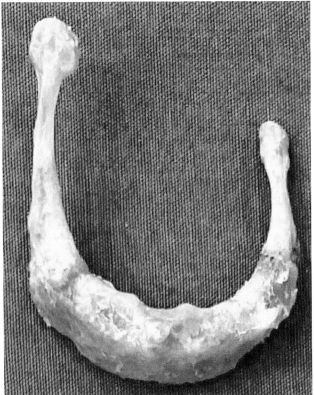

FIGURE 2.15 Asymmetric greater horns. Right greater horn lies at superior level and is longer than left greater horn.

Bochdalek's muscle) has also been described as passing between the tongue's root and triticeous cartilage, but again no functional or pathologic significance has been attributed to such structures. Historically, the triticeous cartilage was thought to be the site of attachment for a 'triticeoglossus muscle (of Bochdalek)'; however, very

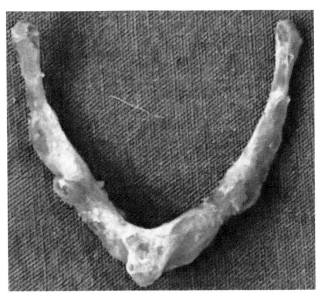

FIGURE 2.16 Tongue-shaped anterior extension of lingual in the median part of hyoid.

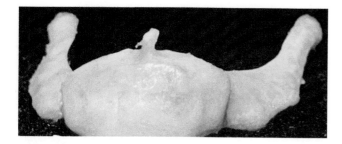

FIGURE 2.17 Lingula present in the median part of body of hyoid bone.

little evidence of the existence of this muscle is available. Few also consider that the role of triticeous cartilage is to strengthen the thyro-hyoid ligament, but no data is available regarding the disadvantage or disability experienced by individuals who lack a triticeous cartilage. From the embryological perspective, cartilages of the laryngeal develop from fourth and sixth pharyngeal arches, and its development starts around the 12th week of gestation. Some consider this cartilage having no function in humans from its functional point of view and the point that its absence in particular does not hamper any function.

The presence of triticeous cartilage is not a constant feature and if present could be either unilateral (Figures 2.19–2.24) or bilateral or in some instances be absent, but if it appears, it will not disappear for the entire lifetime. The pattern of calcification of the laryngeal cartilages is not yet clear, and it is considered that the laryngeal cartilage's extracellular matrix and its contents might have a contributory role.

The presence of triticeous cartilage causes misdiagnosis in the following manner:

1. Radiological examination may cause confusion with the atherosclerosis changes in the common carotid artery seen at the same level of the triticeous cartilage.
2. The triticeous cartilage can be mistaken for fracture of greater cornua of the hyoid bone or of the superior horn of the thyroid cartilage.

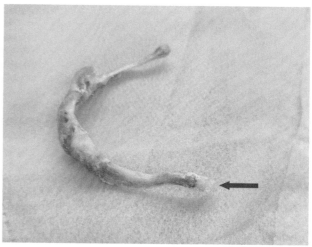

FIGURE 2.19 Lateral view of formalin-preserved debrided hyoid bone showing the triticeous cartilage present unilaterally near the left greater cornua of hyoid bone.

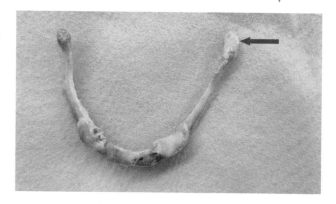

FIGURE 2.20 Superior view of formalin-preserved debrided hyoid bone showing the triticeous cartilage present unilaterally near the left greater cornua of hyoid bone.

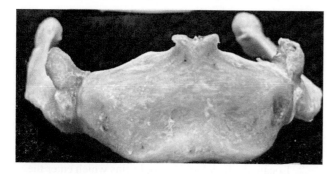

FIGURE 2.18 Split or bifurcated lingula present in the median part of hyoid.

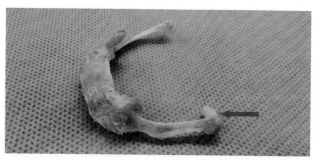

FIGURE 2.21 Triticeous cartilage seen after formalin fixation and debridement of the muscles attached to hyoid bone, near the left greater cornua of the hyoid bone, in this case unilaterally and on the left side.

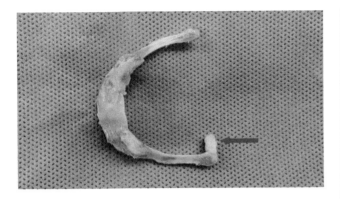

FIGURE 2.22 Superior view of the hyoid bone; triticeous cartilage seen after formalin fixation and debridement of the muscles attached to hyoid bone.

The triticeous cartilage varieties based on degree of calcification are:

1. Cartilaginous
2. Mild calcification
3. Moderate calcification
4. Marked calcification

The triticeous cartilage varieties based on shape are:

1. Round
2. Oval
3. Spindle
4. Elongated
5. Rectangular
6. Teardrop
7. Triangular

Studies show that cartilaginous form of the triticeous cartilage calcification was the highest in the population. This difference might be related to the lifestyle, environment or race. Oval-shaped triticeous cartilage was seen more commonly.

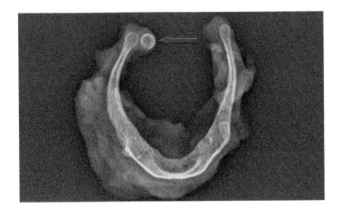

FIGURE 2.23 X-ray of hyoid bone showing presence of triticeous cartilage.

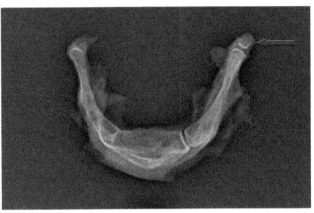

FIGURE 2.24 X-ray of hyoid bone showing presence of triticeous cartilage.

TRIANGLES OF NECK

Anterior Triangle of Neck

- Its anterior border is by the median line of the neck and posterior border is by the anterior end of sternocleidomastoid.
- Base is formed by lower mandible, and apex is at the manubrium sternii.
- It is subdivided into suprahyoid and infrahyoid areas in relation to hyoid bone. It is also divided into digastric, submental, muscular and lateral triangle.

Digastric Triangle

- It is surrounded above by the lower mandible, posteroinferiorly by posterior belly of digastric and by stylohyoid and anteroinferiorly by anterior belly of digastric.
- It is covered by skin, superficial fascia, platysma and deep fascia containing branches of facial and transverse cutaneous cervical nerves.
- Its floor is formed by mylohyoid and hyoglossus.
- Its anterior part contains submandibular gland having facial vein and artery.
- Its posterior part contains lower part of parotid gland.
- External carotid artery curves above the muscle and overlaps its superficial surface as it descends deep into the parotid gland before entering it.
- The internal carotid artery, internal jugular vein and vagus nerve lie deeper and are separated from external carotid artery by styloglossus, stylopharyngeus and glossopharyngeal nerve.

Dissection of Digastric Triangle of Neck

1. Remove the fascia from the area between posterior belly of digastric and superior belly of omohyoid, exposing the internal jugular vein laterally, medially common and internal carotid artery and external carotid artery anteromedial to internal carotid.
2. Locate the facial and lingual veins which enter the internal jugular vein in upper part of triangle and superior thyroid vein entering it in the lower part.

3. Locate the hypoglossal nerve between the vein and internal carotid artery and track it across the external carotid artery.
4. Remove the superficial part of facial carotid sheath that surrounds the internal jugular vein, carotid arteries and vagus nerve.
5. Expose the external carotid artery and its branches. The superior thyroid is the lowest branch in the triangle. The lingual, facial and occipital arteries arise in the upper part of the triangle.
6. Locate the internal laryngeal nerve in thyrohyoid interval. Track it deep to the carotid arteries to the superior laryngeal branch of vagus.
7. Expose the hyoglossus, which is present in the triangle above the hyoid bone. Hypoglossal nerve is present on its surface and lingual artery deep into it.

Dissection of Anterior Triangle of Neck

1. Make an incision in the midline extending from chin to sternum and reflect the skin flap inferolaterally.
2. Reflect the platysma upwards and locate the branches of transverse nerve of the neck as they cross the sternocleidomastoid. Trace them anteriorly till their termination.
3. Find the cervical branch of facial nerve as it leaves the lower border of parotid gland and track it anteroinferiorly.
4. Trace the anterior jugular vein in the midline. Trace it inferiorly till it pierces the deep fascia above the sternum, exposing the deep fascia of the triangle.
5. Then make a transverse incision through the first layer of deep fascia immediately above the sternum and extend the incision about 4 cm upwards along the anterior border of sternocleidomastoid.
6. Then reflect this fascia to open the suprasternal space between first and second layers of fascia.
7. Trace the anterior jugular vein and deep layers of fascia laterally deep into the sternocleidomastoid and follow it upwards till it fuses with the first layer and downwards till it fuses with the back of sternum.

Carotid Triangle

It is bounded by sternocleidomastoid, posterior belly of digastric and superior belly of omohyoid and contains the neurovascular bundle of neck covered by sternocleidomastoid muscle. The medial wall is formed by hyoglossus and thyrohyoid muscles anteriorly and by middle and inferior constrictor muscles posteriorly.

ESOPHAGUS

It is a muscular structure of about 25 cm in length that connects the pharynx to stomach. It arises in the lower border of cricoid cartilage and sixth cervical vertebrae and further descends in front of vertebral column and to superior mediastinum.

TRACHEA

Trachea is about 10–11 cm long, made of cartilage and fibromuscular membrane. It descends from the larynx and extends from the level of sixth cervical vertebrae to the upper border of fifth thoracic vertebrae. It is bifurcated a little towards the right side. It is flat posteriorly. In adults, its diameter is 2 cm in males and 1.5 cm in females. The lumen is 1.2 cm in adults. Anteriorly, the cervical part of trachea is covered by skin, superficial and deep fascia and is crossed by jugular arch and isthmus of thyroid gland.

MUSCLES OF NECK

1. The superficial muscles of neck are platysma, sternocleidomastoid and trapezius.
2. Sternocleidomastoid divides the neck into anterior and lateral parts.
3. The anterior region is further subdivided into many smaller regions called triangles.
4. Muscles in the anterior region are grouped into supra- and infra-hyoid groups.
5. *The muscles that are in the neck are categorized in three groups:* anterior, lateral and posterior.
6. The muscles in these groups lie anterior, lateral or posterior to the cervical vertebrae.
7. The anterior and lateral groups include:
   i. longi colli and capitis;
   ii. recti capitis anterior and lateralis;
   iii. scaleni anterior, medius, posterior and minimi (when present).
8. The posterior group consists of trapezius and levator scapulae.
9. The intrinsic muscles are arranged in superficial and deep layers.
10. The superficial layer contains splenius capitis and cervicis.
11. The deeper layers include the transversospinalis group (semispinalis cervicis and capitis, multifidus and rotatores cervicis), interspinales and intertransversarii, and the suboccipital group (recti capitis posterior major and minor and obliquus capitis superior and inferior).

Platysma

1. Platysma (Figure 2.25) is a superficial broad sheet of muscle covering the upper parts of pectoralis major and deltoid.
2. Its fibers ascend medially in the side of the neck. Anterior fibers interlace across the midline with the fibers of the contralateral muscle.
3. Other fibers attach to the lower border of the mandible or to the lower lip or cross the mandible to attach to skin and subcutaneous tissue of the lower face.

Innervation

Cervical branch of the facial nerve innervates platysma muscle.

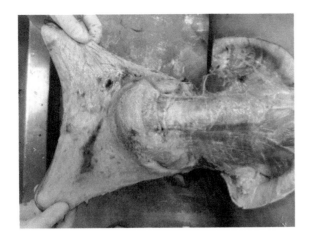

FIGURE 2.25 Reflection of skin of the neck, exposing platysma with subcutaneous tissue and the underlying structures. There is a small hematoma in the platysma and subcutaneous tissue.

Actions

Contraction of platysma helps depressing the mandible, and via its labial can pull the corners of the mouth and lower lip downwards.

Sternocleidomastoid

1. Sternocleidomastoid (Figure 2.26) descends obliquely across the side of the neck and forms a prominent look when contracted.
2. It has a thick central belly and narrow end parts.
3. Inferior aspect of the muscle consists of two heads, clavicular and sternal head.
4. The sternal head is tendinous and rounded; clavicular head is broad and muscular.
5. Superiorly it inserts to the mastoid process.

Innervation

1. Sternocleidomastoid is supplied by the spinal part of the accessory nerve.

Supra-Hyoid Muscles

These include the digastric (Figure 2.27), stylohyoid, geniohyoid and mylohyoid muscles. They are pharyngeal muscles

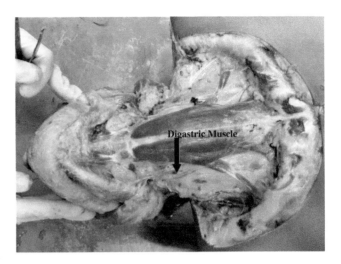

FIGURE 2.27 Digastric muscle.

and play a vital role in the process of swallowing. They have the general action of elevating the hyoid bone and widening the esophageal opening along with their individual different functions.

Infra-Hyoid Muscles

These are also termed as strap muscles (Figures 2.28–2.30), are located over the anterior aspect of the neck and include sternohyoid, sternothyroid, thyrohyoid and omohyoid muscles. They are long and flat muscles with a generic action of lowering the hyoid bone. The hyoid bone can be visualized after layer wise dissection of the supra and infra hyoid muscles (Figures 2.31 and 2.32).

Carotid Sheath Contents

The carotid sheath is a part of the deep cervical fascia of the neck situated on both sides of the neck lateral to the trachea. It contains important structures which include: (i) carotid artery- the common carotid artery (Figure 2.33) below the level of fourth cervical vertebra, internal and external carotid arteries above the level of fourth cervical vertebra, (ii) internal jugular vein (Figure 2.34), (iii) vagus nerve, (iv) part of recurrent laryngeal nerve and (v) deep cervical lymph nodes.

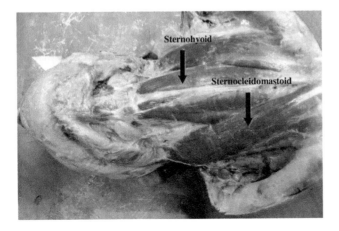

FIGURE 2.26 Sternocleidomastoid and strap muscles after removal of platysma and subcutaneous tissues.

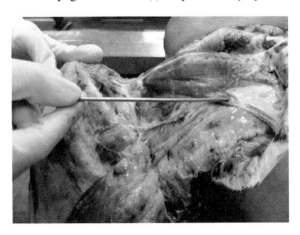

FIGURE 2.28 The superior belly of right digastric muscle terminating into tendon and continuing as inferior belly.

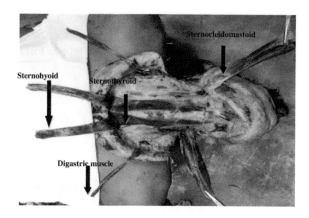

FIGURE 2.29 The sternohyoid muscle and the digastric muscles are separated from their attachments bilaterally, exposing the deeper sternothyroid and thyrohyoid muscles.

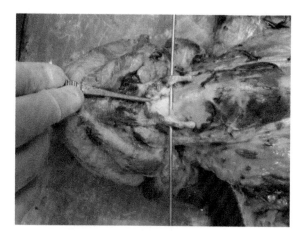

FIGURE 2.32 The thyrohyoid muscles removed to expose the hyoid bone.

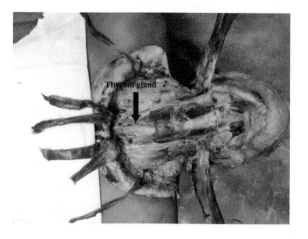

FIGURE 2.30 The thyroid gland is visible after removal of the strap muscles.

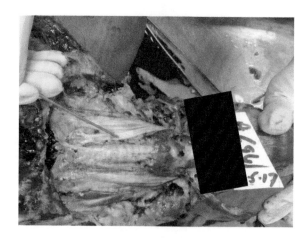

FIGURE 2.33 The common carotid artery.

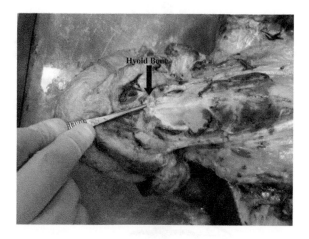

FIGURE 2.31 The hyoid bone seen in situ during the layer-wise dissection.

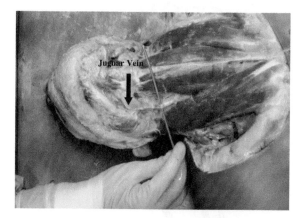

FIGURE 2.34 The internal jugular vein is shown running adjacent to the sternocleidomastoid muscle and then running under it.

BLOOD SUPPLY OF BRAIN

The carotid arterial system and the vertebral arterial system (Figures 2.35 and 2.36) contribute to the arterial blood supply of the brain. Left and right common carotid arteries arise from arch of aorta and brachiocephalic trunk respectively. At the superior border of thyroid cartilage, external and internal carotid arteries arise from the common carotid arteries, with the internal carotid being more medially placed. The internal carotid artery in its intracranial course divides into anterior and middle a cerebral artery which provides the anterior cerebral circulation of brain. The posterior cerebral circulation is mainly by the

Blood supply of Brain

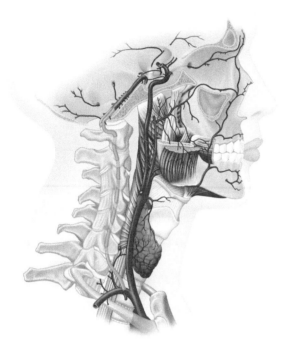

FIGURE 2.35 The right common carotid is seen as a branch from the brachiocephalic trunk arising from the aorta and the vertebral artery is a branch from the subclavian artery on either side.

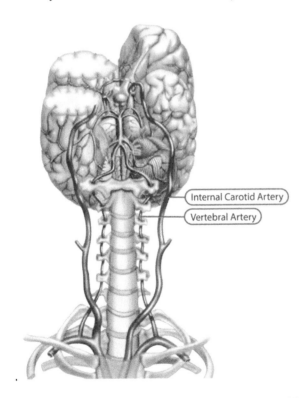

FIGURE 2.36 Right common carotid arises from the brachiocephalic trunk and left common carotid arises directly from the arch of aorta. Vertebral arteries are branches of the subclavian arteries on both sides and travel through foramen transversarium of cervical vertebrae and then enter foramen magnum where they fuse to form basilar artery.

vertebral arteries. Vertebral arteries traverse the foramen transversarium of cervical vertebra and enter the skull through the foramen magnum where they join to form the basilar artery and posterior cerebral arteries are their terminal branches.

ARTERIAL SUPPLY OF BRAIN

The arterial supply to the brain is by two paired arteries, the vertebral arteries and the internal carotid arteries. Circle of Willis is formed at the base of the brain, by both the arterial systems contributing. After entering the foramen magnum, vertebral arteries supply the meninges, cerebellum and spinal branches before converging into a single basilar artery. Basilar artery further continues ascending by supplying the cerebellum and pons. Posterior cerebral arteries are the terminal branches of basilar artery.

The brain requires approximately 3.3 mL of oxygen per 100 g of brain tissue per minute. Cerebral blood flow can increase up to two times the normal value to compensate. Clinical symptoms become evident if this compensation also fails to fulfill the oxygen needs of the brain.

Vertebral artery, unlike the carotids, is deeply located in the neck and has extra protection in the neck from being compressed as it traverses the foramen transversarium of cervical vertebras.

CIRCLE OF WILLIS

Circle of Willis (Figure. 2.37) is an important communicating arterial system which inter-communicates with the

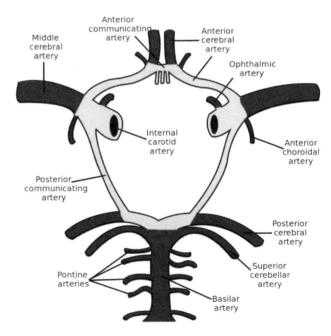

FIGURE 2.37 Circle of Willis (yellow color) present over the base of the brain connecting the two arterial systems supplying the brain. It consists of the posterior cerebral arteries, posterior communicating arteries, internal carotid arteries, anterior cerebral arteries and anterior communicating arteries.

carotid and the vertebral system of arteries supplying the brain. It is formed by:

- Bilateral posterior cerebral arteries
- Bilateral posterior communicating arteries
- Bilateral internal carotid arteries
- Bilateral anterior cerebral arteries
- Anterior communicating arteries

This arterial circle is an important link in maintain the continuous arterial supply to the brain even when one of the feeding arteries, which could be either internal carotid arteries or the vertebral system of artery, is occluded due to internal obstruction or external pressure.

COLLATERAL CIRCULATION

Collateral between Internal Carotid Artery and External Carotid Artery

Occlusion of one side internal carotid artery in the extracranial aspect is compensated by collateral circulation part of external carotid artery supplying blood beyond this point of occlusion (Figure 2.38):

Near the Orbit

Collateral is formed between the ophthalmic artery (a branch of the internal carotid artery) and the middle meningeal artery (a branch of the external carotid artery); or with the deep temporal artery branch of maxillary artery; or the infraorbital artery (a branch of the maxillary artery).

Collateral circulation

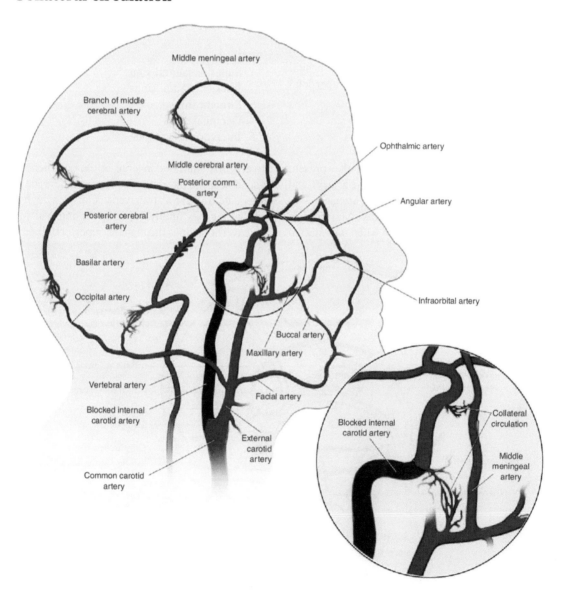

FIGURE 2.38 Collateral circulation is the connection between the different arterial systems supplying the brain, which constitutes the carotid and vertebral system of arteries. This acts as an important connection that can continue to supply blood to the vital brain regions by bypassing any block that can occur in the arterial system at various levels.

Cavernous Sinus

Collateral is formed between the branch called inferolateral trunk, which arises from the internal carotid artery in its cavernous sinus course and which anastomoses with either the middle meningeal artery/deep temporal artery/artery of the foramen rotundum, which are the branches of maxillary artery that originates from the external carotid artery.

Near Ethmoidal Sinuses

Collateral near the ethmoidal sinuses is formed where the anterior and posterior ethmoidal arteries branches of the internal carotid artery anastomoses with the sphenopalatine artery (external carotid artery).

Nose

Collateral is formed between the dorsal nasal artery (internal carotid artery) and the nasal branches of the facial artery (external carotid artery).

Scalp

Collateral is formed between the superior orbital artery branch (internal carotid artery) and the superficial temporal artery (external carotid artery).

Collateral between External Carotid Artery and Vertebral Artery

There are a few collateral pathways that are also present between the occipital artery (external carotid artery) and muscular branches arising from the vertebral arteries.

All these collateral arteries play a very vital role in maintaining the blood supply to the brain when the internal carotid artery occludes due to an external compressing force like a ligature in the neck.

Venous Drainage of Brain

The deoxygenated blood of the brain pours into the dural venous sinuses. All the dural venous sinuses ultimately drain into the internal jugular vein. The dural venous sinuses do not have valves.

There are eleven venous sinuses in total, which are divided into paired and unpaired:

Paired

1. Transverse sinus
2. Sigmoid sinus
3. Superior petrosal sinus
4. Inferior petrosal sinus
5. Cavernous sinus
6. Sphenoparietal sinus

Unpaired

1. Superior sagittal sinus
2. Inferior sagittal sinus
3. Straight sinus
4. Occipital sinus
5. Intercavernous sinus

Most of the sinuses converge at the confluence of sinuses located near the internal occipital protuberance and then on either side traverse as transverse sinuses, which continue as sigmoid sinuses finally forming the internal jugular vein. The cavernous sinus through the superior or inferior petrosal

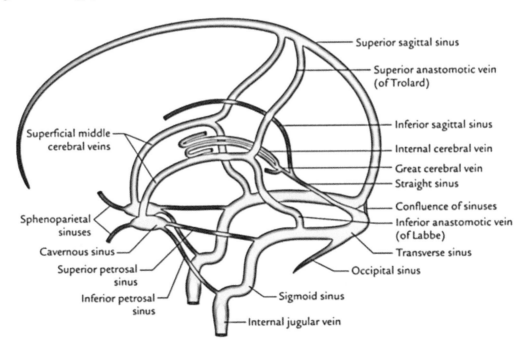

FIGURE 2.39 Venous drainage of the brain, which constitutes both the paired and unpaired venous sinuses draining the brain and most of them converge at the confluence of sinuses near internal occipital protuberance and drain to transverse sinuses on either side, which in turn continues as the sigmoid sinus and the internal jugular vein.

sinuses drains into the internal jugular vein. Internal jugular vein is continuation of sigmoid sinus, and it traverses down through the jugular foramen and enters the carotid sheath in the neck.

BIBLIOGRAPHY

1. Gadkaree SK, Hyppolite CG, Harun A, Sobel RH, Kim Y. An unusual case of bony styloid processes that extend to the hyoid bone. Case Reports in Otolaryngology. 2015 Jun 22:780870.
2. Advenier AS, De La Grandmaison GL, Cavard S, Pyatigorskaya N, Malicier D, Charlier P. Laryngeal anomalies: pitfalls in adult forensic autopsies. Medicine, Science and the Law. 2014 Jan;54(1):1–7.
3. Gnanadev R, Iwanaga J, Loukas M, Tubbs RS. An unusual finding of the hyoid bone. Cureus. 2018 Sep;10(9):e3365.
4. Porrath S. Roentgenologic considerations of the hyoid apparatus. American Journal of Roentgenology. 1969 Jan; 105(1):63–73.
5. Klovning JJ, Yursik BK. A nearly circumferential hyoid bone. American Journal of Otolaryngology. 2007;28(3): 194–5.
6. Inanir NT, Bülent ER, Çetin S, Filiz ER, Gündoğmuş ÜN. Anatomical variation of hyoid bone: a case report. Maedica. 2014 Sep;9(3):272.
7. Singh V, Priya K, Bhagol A, Kirti S, Thepra M. Clicking hyoid: a rare case report and review. National Journal of Maxillofacial Surgery. 2015 Jul;6(2):247.
8. Sittel C, Brochhagen HG, Eckel HE, Michel O. Hyoid bone malformation confirmed by 3-dimensional computed tomography. Archives of Otolaryngology–Head & Neck Surgery. 1998 Jul 1;124(7):799–801.
9. Radunovic M, Vukcevic B, Radojevic N. Asymmetry of the greater cornua of the hyoid bone and the superior thyroid cornua: a case report. Surgical and Radiologic Anatomy. 2018 Aug;40(8):959–61.
10. de Bakker BS, de Bakker HM, Soerdjbalie-Maikoe V, Dikkers FG. Variants of the hyoid-larynx complex, with implications for forensic science and consequence for the diagnosis of Eagle's syndrome. Scientific Reports. 2019 Nov 4;9(1):15950.
11. de Bakker BS, de Bakker HM, Soerdjbalie-Maikoe V, Dikkers FG. The development of the human hyoid-larynx complex revisited. Laryngoscope. 2018 Aug;128(8):1829–34.
12. Parsons FG. The topography and morphology of the human hyoid bone. Journal of Anatomy and Physiology. 1909 Jul; 43(Pt 4):279.
13. Standring S. Gray's Anatomy: The Anatomical Basis of Clinical Practice. 41st ed. 2016. Elsevier; p. 442–74.
14. Nanci A. Ten Cate's Oral Histology: Development, Structure, and Function. 7th ed. St. Louis, MO: Mosby Elsevier; 2008.
15. Carlson BM. Human Embryology and Developmental Biology. 3rd ed. New York: Elsevier; 2004. pp. 317–49.
16. Koebke J. Some observations on the development of the human hyoid bone. Anatomy and Embryology. 1978 Jan 1;153(3):279–86.
17. Fisher E, Austin D, Werner HM, Chuang YJ, Bersu E, Vorperian HK. Hyoid bone fusion and bone density across the lifespan: prediction of age and sex. Forensic Science, Medicine and Pathology. 2016 Jun;12(2):146–57.
18. Ito K, Ando S, Akiba N, Watanabe Y, Okuyama Y, Moriguchi H, Yoshikawa K, Takahashi T, Shimada M. Morphological study of the human hyoid bone with three-dimensional CT images—gender difference and age-related changes. Okajimas Folia Anatomica Japonica. 2012;89(3):83–92.

3 Postmortem Examination in Case of Asphyxial Death

Some cases of asphyxial deaths pose an inherent difficulty in diagnosis due to the lack of specific diagnostic criteria. Most of the features seen in cases of asphyxial deaths are nonspecific. Though most of the asphyxial deaths can be evident at the time of presentation itself, history and presentation of a minor proportion of cases may be misleading to the autopsy surgeon. These cases, if evaluated only on the basis of the provided history and limited circumstances, may lead to faulty deliverance of justice. Hence, in the author's view, all cases of alleged or possible deaths due to asphyxia have to be evaluated by keeping all possibilities open till a clear conclusion regarding the cause and manner of death has been arrived at. Postmortem examination should be holistic and meticulous so that there is no space for any misdiagnosis and no margin for error.

A CASE PRESENTED AS DROWNING, BUT TURNED OUT TO BE LIGATURE STRANGULATION: CASE 1

A 1-year-old girl was brought to the emergency department of All India Institute of Medical Sciences (AIIMS) with a history of found unresponsive in a bucket of water kept in the washroom of her house. Her mother was the only other person who was present at home during the incident. The girl was declared brought dead, and the body was shifted to mortuary for preservation and medico-legal postmortem examination. External examination of autopsy revealed a clear ligature mark (Figures 3.1 and 3.2), and there was no sign of drowning in the airways and lungs. Opinion as to the cause of death was given as asphyxia due to ligature strangulation. In this case, the girl's mother strangled her by using a cloth and presented the case as that of a drowning to the emergency department. The mother confessed the entire event to the police during further investigation. Autopsy surgeons should consider all possibilities while conducting postmortem examination and should not be biased based on the circumstantial findings or narrations of the witnesses.

PRE-AUTOPSY WORK UP: UNDERSTANDING THE BACKGROUND OF THE CASE

Since most of the diagnostic features are non-specific, history of the terminal event possesses great importance while diagnosing cases of asphyxial deaths. Witness credibility needs to be verified, and all statements must be cross-checked with the investigating officer in all possible situations. Alleged scene of incident has to be evaluated. In routine cases, the autopsy surgeon can check the photographs of the scene of crime, made available by the investigating officer. In cases where there is a doubt or the possibility of a future dispute, the autopsy surgeon should take proactive steps to conduct a scene visit before or immediately after the postmortem examination. Procedures of examination of the scene of crime have been discussed under the appropriate heading in this chapter.

All cases brought for a medicolegal autopsy must be accompanied by a formal requisition from the concerned investigating officer. This request usually gives the details of the case in a nutshell. Many supportive documents, including the medicolegal document prepared by the doctor at emergency who received the case (death declaration form), provide a basic idea of the case. Due to heavy workload in emergency departments and their limited awareness regarding wound description, many entries made by the doctors at emergency departments can be misleading, and the autopsy surgeon should be aware of it. The procedures conducted at the emergency department, especially those that can produce artefacts, should be analyzed by studying the emergency notes in detail. For example, endotracheal intubation procedure during the terminal stages at emergency produces mucosal injuries at lips, mouth, pharynx, larynx and esophagus, which can be misinterpreted as injuries of traumatic compression of neck in some instances.

HISTORY OF ANY PRE-EXISTING CONDITIONS

History of any pre-existing illness has to be considered while dealing with cases of asphyxia. Physical incapacitation due to extremes of age or a severe natural illness generally have a correlation with accidental deaths due to smothering, hanging or ligature strangulation. Accidental deaths following drowning or positional asphyxia are also a result of incapacitation of the victim by any debilitating disease or extremes of age. History of drug addiction, alcoholism or any chronic sedative medications should be elicited from relatives or friends. The possibility of acute intoxication has to be evaluated, and the same should be considered while requesting the chemical analysis of the preserved

DOI: 10.1201/9780429026317-3

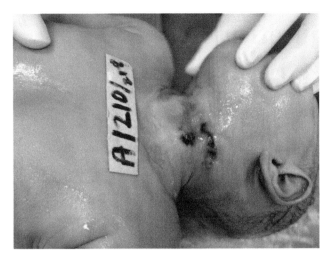

FIGURE 3.1 Ligature mark present in situ in the case of the girl who was brought to the hospital with a history of death following drowning in a bucket full of water. Internal neck dissection showed soft tissue hemorrhages.

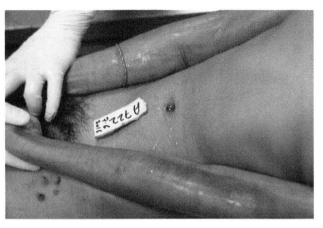

FIGURE 3.3 Multiple old hypopigmented scars of hesitation cuts present over anterior aspect of both forearms showing the tendency of self-harm in the deceased.

viscera. History of any attempt for deliberate self-harm has to be obtained from relatives or friends. Many cases of suicidal hanging reveal multiple parallel hypo/hyper pigmented scars of previous tentative cuts of an attempted deliberate self-harm usually over the forearm (Figure 3.3) or dorsum of foot (Figure 3.4) but can be seen in other accessible places as well. In some cases, attempt to commit suicide by making cuts in their forearm before resorting to the asphyxial mode of death may be appreciated as fresh superficial incised wounds (Figure 3.5). Psychiatric illness history has to be considered very carefully and in detail. The social and family history, such as involvement in criminal activity or being a victim of domestic abuse, must also be elicited from the next of kin.

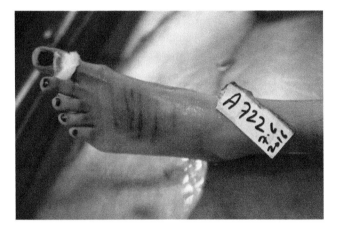

FIGURE 3.4 Multiple old hyperpigmented scars of hesitation cuts present over the dorsum of foot.

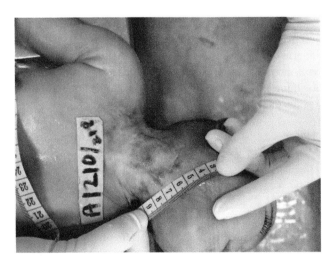

FIGURE 3.2 Ligature mark was present over the front of neck as reddish pressure abrasion, intermittent, having no specific pattern. Folds of neck in children and obese individuals, especially after refrigeration, show artefacts that mimic ligature mark. Possibility of these artifacts should be considered in all cases of suspected asphyxial deaths.

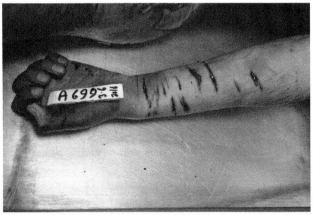

FIGURE 3.5 Multiple superficial hesitation cuts over the forearm, which are fresh and appear to be produced before the deceased attempted his terminal asphyxial mode of death.

INQUEST PAPERS AND STATEMENTS OF WITNESSES

Witness narratives have to be considered in detail. Any possibility of misinformation from the sides of relatives, friends or other witnesses has to be considered in all cases. The possibility of alternative narrations should also be considered. The autopsy surgeon has to read all the supportive documents submitted for his perusal and discuss with the investigating officer about all discrepancies that come to his notice, to get a clear picture of the case. If the autopsy surgeon deems it essential, then pre-autopsy interviews with witnesses, relatives and friends of the deceased have to be done to get more clarification in any case of asphyxial death. The autopsy surgeon should discuss the details of the case with the investigating officer, in all cases that arouse suspicion.

FULL BODY PMCT EVALUATION

In all possible cases and where facilities are available, PMCT examination of the entire body should be done. It is advisable to do the same immediately before conducting the external examination. This order of examination ensures the radiological documentation of the personal belongings and any other foreign bodies present over or along with the body that may become lost or left unnoticed while removing the clothes during external examination. PMCT examination will be useful in identifying any gag in place, any foreign body within the airway and any injury over the face and neck, which are related to asphyxial death. Fracture of hyoid bone, thyroid or other laryngeal cartilages and vertebral column can be easily identified by PMCT. The direction of the distal portions of the fractured structures can be assessed in situ. This will be helpful for the autopsy surgeons to comment on the direction in which force was applied to the neck. PMCT can be done immediately before moving the body to the dissection hall in fully clothed manner to avoid loss of any evidence.

In case PMCT facility is not available, postmortem X-ray (PM X-ray) examination facility can be used to identify the fracture pattern. The bony and cartilaginous structures of the neck can be subjected to radiological examination after removal from the body as well; this technique provides better images due to the absence of the hyper dense vertebral column that is otherwise present. Foreign bodies in the airways can be identified with PM X-ray evaluation in many cases of choking and aspiration. X-ray examination shows the skeletal framework well, including vertebrae, ribs and small bones like hyoid (Figures 3.6, 3.7 and 3.8). Airway can also be appreciated well due to the presence of air (Figure 3.7).

EXAMINATION OF THE SCENE OF INCIDENT

Examination of the scene of incident is very important while establishing and proving the 'corpus delicti'—the essence of crime. It is ideal if the law enforcement agency gets a

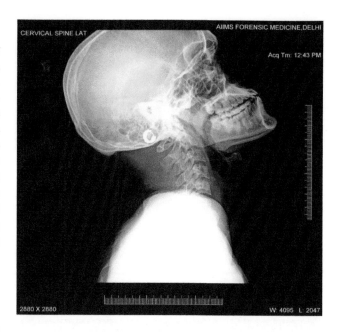

FIGURE 3.6 Lateral view of neck showing the intact airway and neck skeletal structures in PM X-ray.

chance to examine the scene before the victim is removed and transferred to hospital or morgue. Autopsy surgeons rarely get a chance to examine the scene of crime with the dead body still in place. In cases of asphyxial deaths, the injury pattern has to be correlated with the alleged mechanism of causation of injury before concluding the case. It will be easy to identify a staged event if a proper scene of incident/crime examination was done. All possible trace evidences have to be collected from the scene of crime by the concerned forensic scientists. In some cases, the autopsy surgeons can help these scientists to select and collect certain samples that can be vital in the further course of investigation.

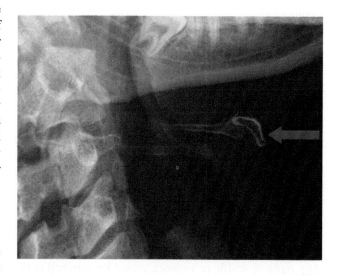

FIGURE 3.7 Intact hyoid bone and airway in PM X-ray.

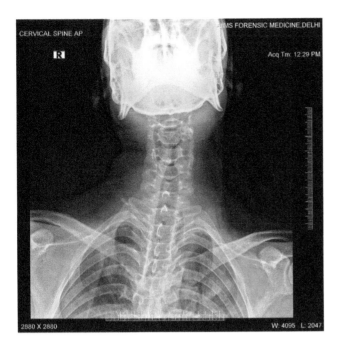

FIGURE 3.8 Antero-posterior view of neck generally will not give a clear idea about laryngeal or hyoid fractures due to the overlapping hyper dense shadow of vertebral column.

Hanging

Usually in suicidal hanging, the scene of incident is a closed space, secured from inside. If the possibility of entry of any perpetrator is ruled out, these cases are considered as hanging. The height of suspension point should be analyzed and compared with the alleged method used for attaining desirable height to hang. Availability of the ligature material for the victim should be assessed. In case of any abnormality found regarding the type of ligature material used, detailed investigation should be done before concluding the case as suicidal hanging. Commonly, the ligature materials used in hanging show tears according to the amount and direction of the pulling force. A simple hand lens will be of immense use when examining the direction of pull by analyzing the pinning pattern of the ligature material. Any stains present over the ligature material should be examined in detail and preserved for further biological and chemical analysis. Pattern of postmortem staining should be photographed at the scene of crime in all possible cases. This will give an idea of the duration of suspension and the presence of any primary pattern of postmortem staining. The posture of lower limbs in cases of partial hanging after the rigor mortis sets in gives a clue regarding the degree of suspension and type of hanging. A rough estimate of the time since death or duration of suspension can be obtained from these observations. If any of these findings show discrepancy, the autopsy surgeon should evaluate the possibility of foul play in detail. Such doubts arise especially in partial hanging cases where legs are in contact with floor and they trigger doubts in the minds of relatives and friends (Figure 3.9). Any signs of scuffle or violence should be searched at the scene of crime. Any foreign material, biological stains

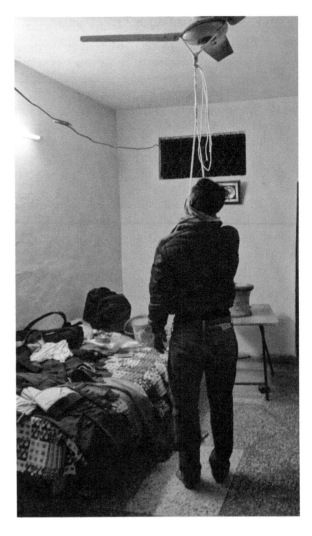

FIGURE 3.9 Hanging in standing position. Partial hanging cases create many queries in the minds of relatives and friends. The possibility of a 'staged' crime scene should be ruled out before reaching a conclusion regarding the cause and manner of death in these cases.

including blood stains, etc. have to be identified and should be sent for further evaluation. In cases of dead bodies found in secluded places, the possibility of postmortem suspension should be ruled out especially when the person is intoxicated (Figure 3.10).

Other Forms of Mechanical Asphyxia

Hanging, smothering and strangulation can be accidental in nature, and such cases can be proven only after considering the circumstances at the scene of incident in detail. Examination of the scene of crime when the body was still in its primary position and posture after death will yield reliable clues regarding the cause and manner of death. In routine practice, autopsy surgeons may not be having access to the scene of crime before the conduction of autopsy. In this situation, the scene of crime photographs or videos recorded by the investigating officer can be used to get an idea regarding the circumstances of the case. The autopsy surgeon can do a scene of crime visit if he

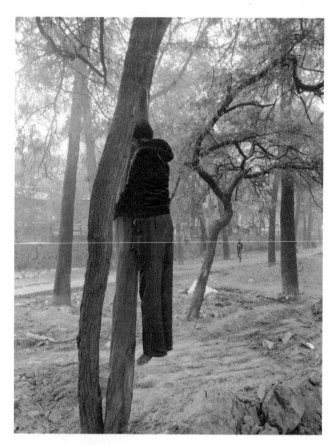

FIGURE 3.10 Complete hanging from a tree, in an open space. In cases where the body is found in a secluded area, all possibilities of postmortem suspension and homicidal hanging should be excluded, especially if the victim has been incapacitated due to intoxication or some other means.

needs clarification regarding any of his findings. Autoerotic asphyxial deaths escape diagnosis and may be concluded as suicidal hanging if a proper scene of incident examination was not done. Choking deaths at home may accompany acute intoxication. Intact or used alcohol bottles, drug remnants, etc. are usually present in the immediate vicinity of the body. In cases of smothering, blood-stained soft broad materials, like a pillow, should be examined in detail for the presence of any blood or salivary stains.

In cases of homicide, signs of scuffle, blood stains, blood-stained finger and footprints and alleged weapon of offence may be found at the scene of crime. Blood spatter pattern will give more idea about the gravity of scuffle that occurred at the scene of crime.

Drowning

Scene of incident examination is important in all cases of drowning where a reliable witness' narration is absent. Injuries present over the body should be evaluated after assessing the scene of incident. The person's ability to swim should be compared with the depth of the water collection and distance from the shore where the drowning happened. Possibility of incapacitation by drugs or alcohol should be assessed by examining the nearby area for proof of use

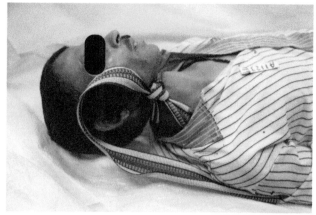

FIGURE 3.11 Ligature material in situ in a case of hanging.

of the same, though chemical examination gives the final verdict regarding the nature and degree of intoxication. In cases of bodies found in shallow waters, on dry land or washed ashore in an open space, the possibility of high tide or heavy raining resulting in temporary collection of water should be considered.

EXAMINATION OF THE LIGATURE MATERIAL

In cases of hanging or ligature strangulation, the ligature material may be brought to the autopsy surgeon in situ around neck (Figures 3.11 and 3.12) or separately. If the material is found around the body, the autopsy surgeon should note down its details including make of the material, color, type and position of knot, presence of any stains over the ligature material, the nature of the ends whether they are fresh cut or not, etc. The knot can be secured first before removing the noose from neck. The portion of the noose placed at maximum distance from the knot should be cut, and both cut ends should be tied together with any string or thread. Total circumference of the noose including the knot should be noted down. Circumference of the ligature

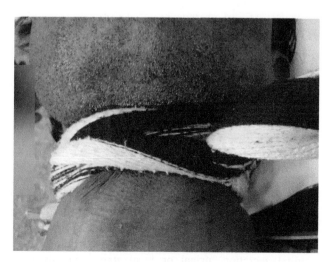

FIGURE 3.12 Ligature material in situ in a case of hanging.

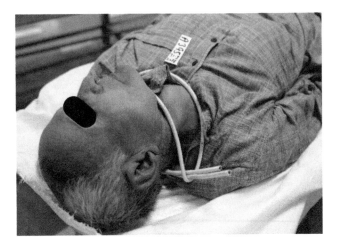

FIGURE 3.13 Ligature material in situ in a case of hanging, but the knot is loosened during transit of the dead body.

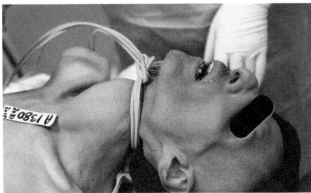

FIGURE 3.14 Wire used as ligature material found in situ in hanging case brought to AIIMS mortuary for medico-legal autopsy. The length of the free limbs needs to be noted for approximating it with the rest of the ligature material.

material in approximation should be measured, which will be useful while comparing the mark with the material for assessment of feasibility. Ligature material can be rope, shawl, saree, kurta, towel, neck tie, leather belt, chain and virtually any object that can encircle the neck and bear the weight of the unsupported portion of body. Ligature material and the corresponding injury correlate in almost all cases. This correlation is very useful in concluding hanging cases. Harder materials produce more prominent ligature marks due to friction and pressure. Very hard and broad materials like leather belt produce friction marks at both borders with an intervening pale pressure band. A specific pattern of ligature material surface gets imprinted at the ligature mark and is more appreciable in oblique illumination. Use of a hand magnifying lens yields better results in imprint pattern identification and correlation. In cases of very soft materials like soft clothes, ligature mark may be absent even after hours of suspension. Ligature material present in situ helps to correlate with circumstantial findings in many cases. In some cases, the ligature could be loosened during transit of the dead especially in running knot or loop (Figure 3.13).

The total length of all the free limbs of the ligature material should be noted. This will be useful while approximating with the remaining piece of ligature material that is brought for examination at a later stage (Figure 3.14). Measurement of length of the ligature material is useful in proving the feasibility of the alleged manner of death especially in different types of hanging cases.

EXAMINATION OF CLOTHES AND OTHER PERSONAL BELONGINGS

Clothes of the deceased should be examined with a focused approach to identify relevant findings, such as pattern of blood stain (Figures 3.15 and 3.16), pattern of salivary stains, other discharges including seminal (Figure 3.17), vaginal secretion, urinal or fecal stains (Figure 3.18). Every step and finding should be photographed for future

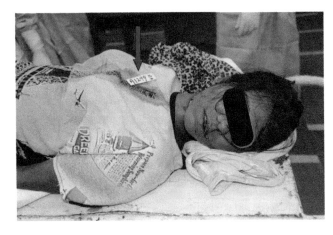

FIGURE 3.15 Blood stain over the clothes of the deceased in a case of hanging.

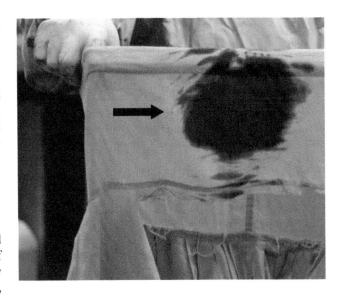

FIGURE 3.16 Fresh blood stains over the salwar/lower of the deceased.

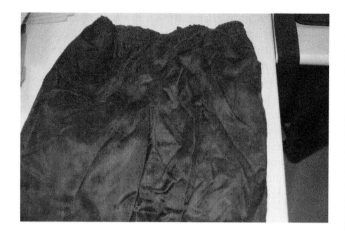

FIGURE 3.17 Seminal stains over the underwear in a case of hanging.

reference. Pattern of tears on the clothes and their placement should be assessed and documented.

Clothes should be thoroughly examined for possible contents like suicide note, phone numbers written on papers, mobile phones, drugs or any other personal belongings like identity cards/driving license, etc., which could help in identification of the deceased (if not identified by the time). Such evidence might also point towards a perpetrator, especially in cases where there was abetment of suicide. All the belongings, including clothes, should be removed, dried, photographed and handed over to the investigating officer in sealed condition on request.

SUICIDE NOTE

Presence of a suicide note is very important in determining the legal outcome of cases of unnatural deaths due to asphyxia. Generally, if a suicide note is present at the scene of incident, the death is considered a suicide. Suicide intent can be expressed in many ways. It can be written on a paper or in a personal diary. This is the most common type of expressing the intention to end one's own life. The scene of incidence has to be searched for the presence of the same

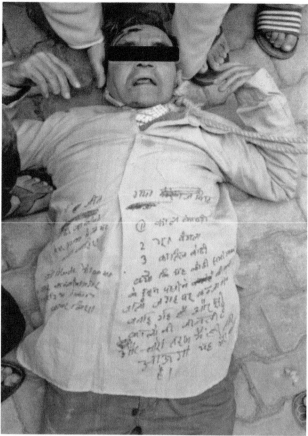

FIGURE 3.19 Suicide note written in detail over the shirt.

in all cases of alleged suicides by asphyxial means. Many unique ways of expressing the wish to commit suicide were noted during the three decades of forensic practice by the author. In some cases, the deceased wrote suicide note over his/her own clothes (Figure 3.19). In some cases, the suicide notes were written over the palm of the non-dominant hands (Figures 3.20 and 3.21), while in other cases, the author came across suicide notes written over the walls of the room or in personal notebooks (Figure 3.22).

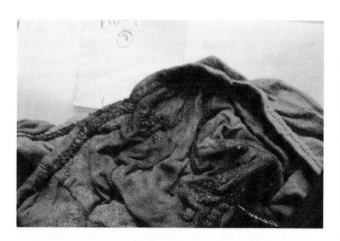

FIGURE 3.18 Fecal and blood stain over the underwear.

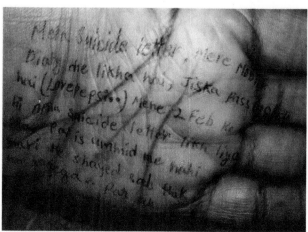

FIGURE 3.20 Suicide note over palm of the non-dominant hand with legible handwriting.

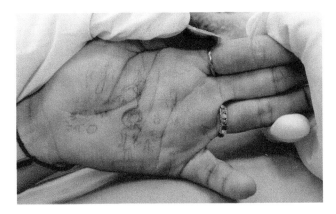

FIGURE 3.21 Suicide note with pictorial demonstration of hanging.

Law enforcement agencies generally scrutinize the content of these writings to find if there is any criminal involvement behind the death. The autopsy surgeon has to examine all belongings of the deceased brought to him. Clothes should be examined in detail. In some cases, the author noted that suicide notes were kept well folded inside pockets.

Though the investigating officer or relatives are informed about the presence of a suicide note, the autopsy surgeon should always consider the possibility of foul play and forging. The authenticity of the note will be finalized in legal

point of view only after getting a positive match of calligraphic comparative evaluation by a forensic handwriting expert. Suicide note in electronic format is an emerging issue and under-researched phenomenon. It is necessary to understand the newer electronic death notes in all their formats. It is not uncommon nowadays to create fake suicide notes for malicious intentions. Suicide notes can be written by a person other than the victim to make a death appear to be suicide. As the trend of using readily available technologies to express suicidal emotions grows, a thorough knowledge of the subject along with a vigilant approach by the law-enforcing agencies is the need of the hour.

AUTOPSY PHOTOGRAPHY

Photography during autopsy is an important part of forensic imaging and is essential for the documentation of autopsy findings. Though similar to medical photography, here the main consideration is that the images are taken primarily for legal purposes; therefore, the results must be accurate, detailed and useful in court. A good photograph clearly demonstrates the required information and minimizes distortion. It includes proper identification, backgrounds, lighting, color, scale, perspective, orientation and cropping. Multiple photographs that focus on various aspects must be taken in order to cover the entire body surface, which should include photographs of the overall view of the area where a finding/injury is found and close-range photographs of that particular finding/injury. An overall view gives us a complete summary of the case, while a close-range photograph gives us a detailed information of a particular finding/injury. In case of asphyxial death, a particular sequence is to be followed so as not to miss any specific finding. The order includes first the preliminary external photographs followed by the detailed postmortem examination findings, including the findings of internal dissection. The preliminary photographs include the photos of scene of death (usually submitted by the investigating officer), ligature in situ along with position of knot, ligature material, clothing, suicide note, etc.

During postmortem examination, the following sequence is to be followed, which starts from anterior, posterior and lateral aspects of head, face and neck followed by eyes, including photographs of inner and outer aspects of upper and lower eyelids, corneas, conjunctivae and sclera. External and internal aspect of both nostrils is to be carefully examined for any injuries, bleeding or fracture. Photographs of outer and inner aspects of upper and lower lip, tongue, teeth, gums and oral cavity are to be taken carefully to avoid missing any finding. Dribbling of saliva, if present, should be photographed in order to obtain a clear idea of location and direction. Ears, including ear lobule and external auditory canal, are to be examined and photographed for any concealed injury. Anterior, posterior and lateral aspects of trunk and limbs along with hands and nails are to be photographed. Any discharge in the form of urine, semen, stool or vaginal discharge should

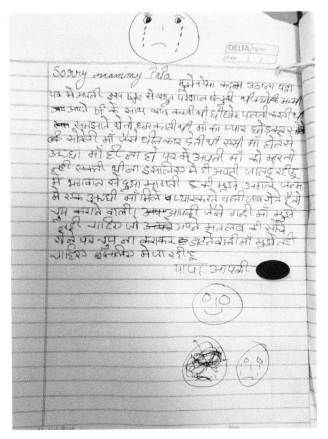

FIGURE 3.22 Suicide note by an adolescent written in her notebook.

be photographed. For internal dissection of the neck, bloodless field is a prime requirement for good photographs to avoid misinterpretation of the possible artefacts. Any positive internal finding is to be photographed in situ as well as after its excision or removal with a clear and bloodless background.

EVIDENCE COLLECTION

All the samples that can be collected from the exterior of the body should be collected before or during the removal of clothes. In all suspected homicide cases, the clothing in its entirety and all personal belongings have to be preserved intact and have to be handed over to the investigating officer.

Swabs for detection of traces like foreign DNA or any other trace evidence have to be collected as early as possible to avoid possible contamination. Sample collection, preservation, sealing and transportation to the Forensic Science Lab should follow the accepted standard protocols, and documentation of the same should be done properly to avoid any possible dispute regarding improper maintenance of chain of custody. These samples include nasal swabs, oral swabs, penile/vaginal swabs, anal swabs or swabs from any part of the body where there is any suspected stain. The autopsy surgeon should exercise maximum caution to avoid contamination of the samples preserved. Other common samples include blood samples for DNA profiling, plucked or cut scalp or body hairs and fingernail clippings or scrapings.

In cases of asphyxial deaths, trace evidences of the ligature material (fibers of the cloth in most cases) can be seen over the ligature mark. Naked eye examination is sufficient for gross detection of ligature fibers which can be identified by magnifying lens examination (Figure 3.23).

There fibers can be lifted by using adhesive transparent tapes, and the same can be transferred to slides or overhead projector (OHP) sheets. This test, if positive, gives a

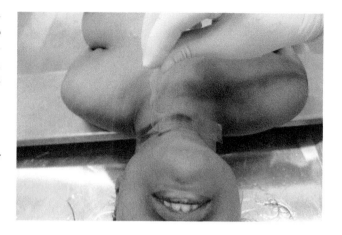

FIGURE 3.24 Cellophane tape lifting of fibers from the ligature mark.

correlation between the ligature material used and the ligature mark. It is advisable that in all cases of mechanical compression of neck, cellophane tape lifts (Figure 3.24) from the ligature mark be preserved for comparison with the fibers of alleged ligature material.

If the ligature material is present in situ, the autopsy surgeon gets a chance to correlate the pattern of the compressing surface of the ligature material and the imprint patterns of the ligature mark. After in-situ evaluation, the ligature material can be removed by securing the knot with a thread. Cut the ligature material exactly opposite to the position of the knot and fix the cut ends with a thread. Then the ligature can be removed and examined in detail, then preserved, sealed and handed over to the investigating officer.

In all suspected cases of homicide or any involvement of a second person, fingernail clippings should be preserved for detection of foreign DNA and further cross matching. In cases of suspected murder following sexual violence, all possible samples should be collected as per the current sexual assault victim autopsy protocols.

EXTERNAL EXAMINATION

Systematic head-to-foot examination should be done in all cases of asphyxial deaths.

Scalp

Scalp hairs should be checked for any stains or breakage. Scalp should be palpated for any hidden injuries. If needed, doubtful areas should be shaved for better visualization of the scalp injuries.

Face

Face should be examined carefully. The entire face should be examined for pallor, congestion, petechiae, edema and cyanosis. All these findings can be present in asphyxial deaths, to variable extent. Congestion and petechiae (Figure 3.25) are present over the face, extending up to the ears. Examination of the neck is the most crucial exercise in cases of asphyxial death.

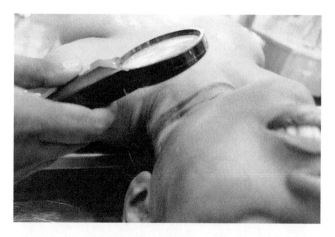

FIGURE 3.23 Examination for fibers over ligature mark by magnifying lens fitted with LED lamp. These lenses are useful in identifying the minute imprint pattern of meshes as well as fibers of cloth material of the ligature mark.

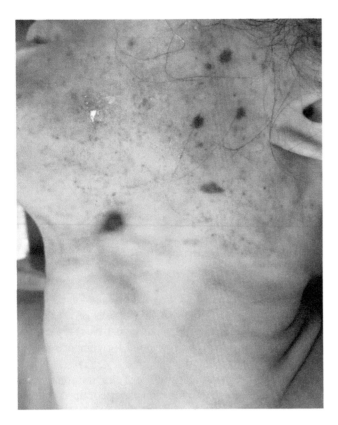

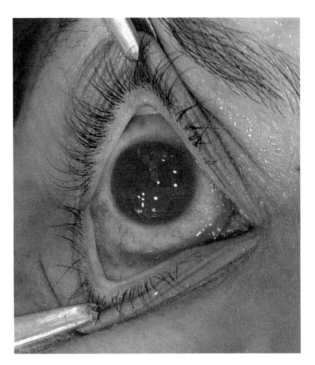

FIGURE 3.26   Examination of palpebral and bulbar conjunctiva using non-toothed forceps.

FIGURE 3.25   Petechiae present over the face.

Eyes

Bulbar and palpebral conjunctivae give variable signs in different asphyxial deaths. Careful examination of the eyes and correlation with other signs will give a better idea in understanding the cause, manner and mechanism behind each asphyxial death. Palpebral conjunctivae can be examined by everting the free margin of the eyelid using non-toothed forceps (Figure 3.26). Sclera and the bulbar conjunctivas can be exposed to the maximum by universal eye speculum. If the eye is found partially open during autopsy, color changes following prolonged exposure and drying of the area (tache noir) should be anticipated. The author has seen cases in which untrained autopsy surgeons have noted this postmortem feature as subconjunctival hemorrhage. Subconjunctival hemorrhage (Figure 3.27), subconjunctival petechiae (Figure 3.28) and internal hemorrhages have to be identified and noted in all cases of suspected asphyxial deaths. Bulging of eyeballs is common in violent asphyxial deaths due to edema and hemorrhages in the retro-orbital soft tissues as a result of asphyxia and congestion; bulging of eyeballs due to decomposition has to be ruled out in this situation by comparing with the other changes of decomposition. In cases of drowning in big water collections, the possibility of postmortem aquatic animal activity resulting in loss of tissues has to be considered at the soft tissues around the orbit and eye lids, sometimes resulting in complete absence of the eyeballs. Few inexperienced autopsy surgeons misinterpret these injuries as ante-mortem injuries, resulting in erroneous opinion formation.

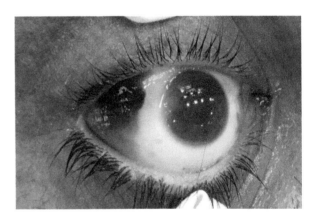

FIGURE 3.27   Subconjunctival hemorrhage is seen in many violent asphyxial deaths.

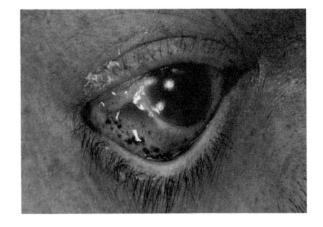

FIGURE 3.28   Subconjunctival petechiae are common in asphyxial death with a congestive mechanism contributing to death.

Findings

Position of the eyelids should be noted, whether they are closed or open. Bulbar and palpebral conjunctivas should be examined for paleness, congestion, petechiae or intense subconjunctival hemorrhages. Corneas should be examined for transparency, and inner eyeball hemorrhages should be assessed using an ophthalmoscope. Tache noir, the color change over the exposed conjunctiva, should not be misinterpreted as hemorrhage or any other lesion.

Nose

Examination Technique

Externally, bridge of nose, alae of nose and the adjacent cheeks have to be examined in detail in all cases of asphyxial deaths. Injuries of soft tissues are common in cases of smothering. Bridge of nose may show fractures in rare instances. Abrasions, contusions and laceration can be visualized in many cases of smothering. Visual external examination should follow palpation to avoid misdiagnosis of nasal bone fractures. Inner aspect of the nostrils has to be examined in detail preferably with a nasal speculum for better visualization. Nasal hemorrhages, mucosal injuries, etc. can be demonstrated by this examination. The nose is palpated to detect any abnormal movement suggestive of a fracture. A nasal speculum is inserted into the nostrils and is then released to visualize the interior of the nose.

Findings

Alae and bridge of nose should be examined for any possible injuries. As a routine practice, nasal bridge should be examined by palpation. Nostrils should be evaluated in detail using nasal speculum. Mucosal injuries have to be evaluated in cases of suspected smothering. Blood stains (Figure 3.29), frothy fluids, regurgitated stomach contents, any foreign bodies, etc. have to be identified and documented. Adjacent cheeks have to be evaluated for any injuries externally.

Mouth

External examination of the lips has to be conducted in detail in all cases of asphyxial deaths. Inner aspect of lips can be examined by inverting the same using non-toothed forceps. Inner aspect of cheeks, gums, teeth, tongue, hard and soft palates, tonsils and tonsil beds can be examined if the rigor across temporomandibular joints is forcefully broken. Injuries are common at these structures especially in smothering and other violent asphyxial deaths. Inner aspect of lips and mouth can be explored further by reflecting the facial skin flap, which is discussed in detail at the end of this chapter. In this method, the facial flap can be made as a continuation of the upper skin flap of the V-shaped neck incision. The flap can be elevated till the tip of the nose without disfiguring the face. This method of facial dissection gives a clearer view of facial soft tissue injuries including those of inner aspect of lips. Temporomandibular joints can be accessed and, if required, disarticulated by

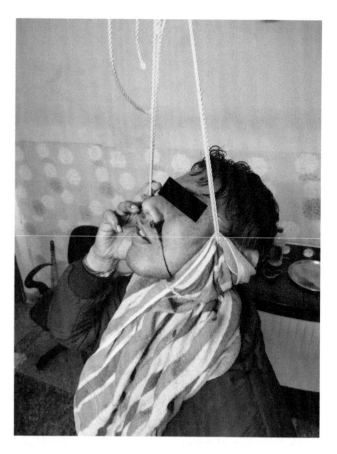

FIGURE 3.29 Blood stain from nose, in a partial hanging case. Note the position of right upper limb. The fingertip was entangled between the rope and the face of the deceased during his failed terminal attempt to remove or loosen the ligature.

dissecting the fibers of masseter muscle. This will help in disarticulation of mandible, which gives more access to the oral cavity and the protected upper airway, i.e., the nasopharynx and oropharynx. This dissection method is useful in dealing with cases of asphyxia especially of choking and gagging. In this method, injuries of the soft tissues around pharynx, mouth and tongue can be demonstrated vividly.

Examination Technique

Both the lips are held by non-toothed forceps and everted to visualize the gums, frenulum and teeth (Figure 3.30) and whether the tongue is protruding out and clenched between the teeth (Figure 3.31). Oral cavity is to be examined as far as possible. Due to rigor mortis, opening of the mouth will be difficult. Rigor can be overcome by cutting the masseter muscle so that rigor will be released and visibility is enhanced.

Findings

Outer and inner aspects of upper and lower lips should be examined in all cases of asphyxial deaths. Mucosal congestion, cyanosis and injuries in the form of abrasions, contusions and lacerations should be identified and documented. These injuries are common in homicidal cases and may be the only positive findings that can suggest the manner of

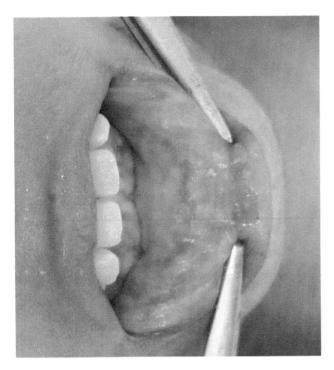

FIGURE 3.30 Non-toothed forceps for everting the lips to visualize injuries over the mucosal aspects. This will avoid artifact injuries at inner aspect of lips.

death. Frenulum of both upper and lower lips should also be examined and documented in all cases of asphyxial deaths. If injuries are present over the inner aspects of lips, they should be correlated with the sharp pointing edges of the teeth (Figure 3.32). Oral cavity hygiene, discoloration of gums and teeth, signs of infection, presence of fluid discharge or pus are also to be noted. Tongue protrusion

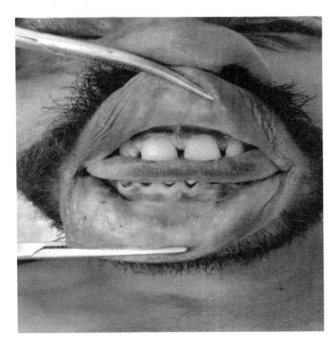

FIGURE 3.31 Examination of mouth with tongue protruding out and clenched between the teeth.

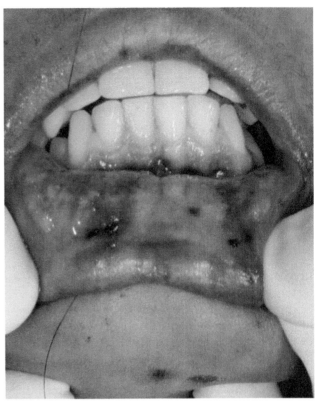

FIGURE 3.32 Injuries present over the inner aspect of lip corresponding with the sharp margins of teeth. These injuries are commonly seen in cases of homicidal smothering.

should be checked in cases of hanging, but it is not mandatory to be found in all cases. Drying of the exposed portions of lips and tongue causes dark reddish or blackish discoloration of the exposed areas (Figure 3.33). This may confuse inexperienced autopsy surgeons and may be misinterpreted as ante-mortem lip or tongue injuries.

Chin

The chin is to be examined for the presence of external injuries, i.e., abrasions, contusions, nail marks or any other form of injury. Placement of the knot near the chin is seen in cases of hanging; the knot marks are generally seen as isolated pressure abrasions (Figures 3.34, 3.35 and 3.36). The autopsy surgeon has to correlate the entire ligature mark pattern and examine the ligature material before committing on the manner of causation of these lesions.

Dribbling of Saliva

Generally, signs of excessive salivation are seen in hanging cases. The saliva dribbles out of the mouth usually from the angle of the mouth that is present at the lower level due to possible tilt of head (Figure 3.37). It is postulated that this occurs due to direct pressure and stimulation over the sub-mandibular salivary glands due to the compressive force from the ligature noose. Dried dribble mark of excessive salivary discharge is commonly seen starting from the angle of mouth that was at lower level during hanging

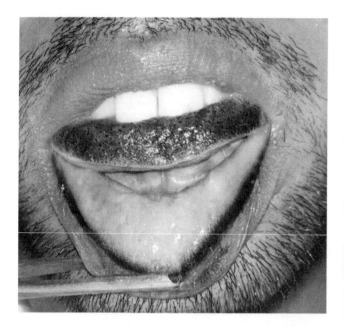

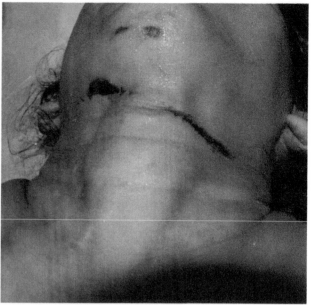

FIGURE 3.33 Protuded tongue in a case of hanging. Note the reddish discolouration of the mucocutaneous junction and over the exposed areas of tongue due to postmortem drying. These artefacts are commonly mistaken as injuries in cases of hanging by inexperienced autopsy surgeons.

FIGURE 3.35 Ligature mark with another distinct injury at the chin. In these situations, the possible mechanism of such injuries has to be explored in detail; in this case, it was due to knot over chin.

(Figure 3.38). The autopsy surgeon should evaluate the direction of ligature mark and make sure that the course of salivary dribble mark follows the laws of gravity and anatomy. The pattern of drying should be consistent with the postmortem duration. The autopsy surgeon should be aware of the possibility of staging by artificially implanting

dried stains resembling salivary trickle marks. In this situation, swabs can be taken from the suspected mark and can be sent for analysis like amylase test. DNA cross matching is also possible with salivary stains. In many cases, these trickle marks extend to the front of trunk and can be seen over the floor immediately beneath the body. Direction and placement of these marks can be analyzed holistically before reaching a conclusion.

Intense pulmonary edema, mucosal congestion, etc. can result in postmortem collection of fluid in pharynx, mouth

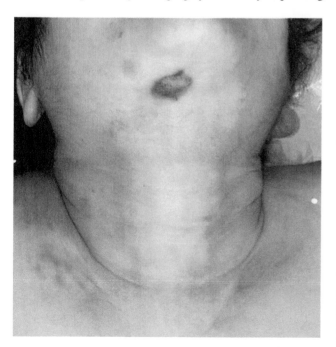

FIGURE 3.34 Pressure abrasion over the chin without any other visible ligature mark is not rare in case of hanging. This is common when a soft material is used as the ligature material and the knot is at the front of the neck.

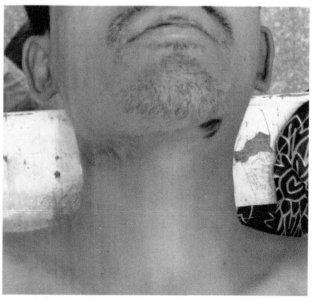

FIGURE 3.36 Faint ligature mark with prominent knot mark over the chin seen in this case.

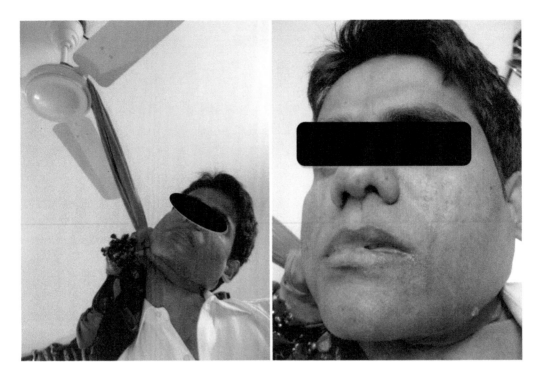

FIGURE 3.37   Dribbling of saliva seen from the lower angle of the mouth due to stimulation of the salivary gland by the ligature compressing the neck.

and nostrils. These fluids can trickle out through the mouth during transport or other manipulation of the body. These wet or dry fluid trickle marks are rarely misinterpreted as salivary dribble marks. In such cases, the trickling is almost horizontal in direction (Figure 3.39). The author is of the opinion that the direction of the salivary marks should be analyzed in all cases of alleged or suspected deaths following hanging before reaching a conclusion. In case of any doubt, the stains should be collected and sent for further forensic evaluation.

Ears

Otoscope can be used for detailed examination of the external auditory meatus, tympanic membrane and middle ear in cases of ruptured tympanic membrane. Otoscope can also be used for capturing photographs of these findings. The anterior and posterior aspects of ear lobules should be

examined for the presence of any injuries. External auditory meatus has to be examined for any injuries or hemorrhages. Tympanic membrane can also be examined as many cases of mechanical asphyxia can show tympanic hemorrhages, but these are considered as a nonspecific finding by many authors.

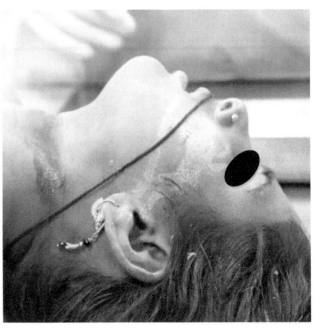

FIGURE 3.39   Dried stains over face in case of hanging. The direction of the stains suggests a postmortem oozing of the fluid that can be due to manipulation of the body during transport or shifting.

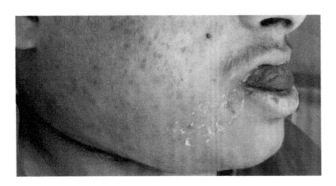

FIGURE 3.38   Dried salivary stains seen at the angle of the mouth due to dribbling of saliva in a case of hanging.

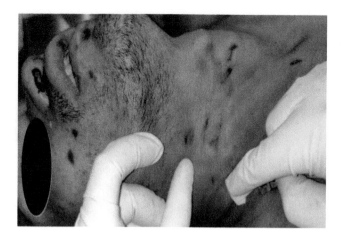

FIGURE 3.40 Fingernail abrasion and surrounding dermal contusions in a case of manual strangulation.

Neck

The neck is the most important region of the body to be examined in all cases of asphyxial deaths. Neck should be extended to the maximum by placing a wooden slab, block or neck rest under the shoulder. Neck should be examined for abnormal mobility due to fracture of vertebral column. Any injury over the neck following traumatic neck compression should be described in detail with regards to their type, size, shape, location and direction. Vivid descriptions of the ligature mark, fingernail marks (Figure 3.40 and 3.41), finger pad contusions (Figure 3.42), hesitations cuts by sharp weapons, defense wounds and injuries suggestive of final struggle for life or attempt to escape, etc. should be made. The same should be captured by appropriate photographs. Magnifying hand lenses, hand torches, infra-red or

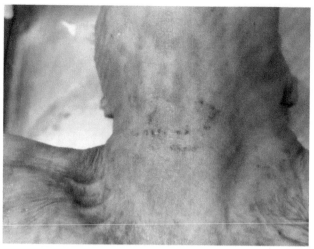

FIGURE 3.42 Minimal dermal contusions over the neck in a case of strangulation. If the victim is incapacitated, external injuries may be minimal.

ultra-violet photography can be useful for further evaluation of the ligature marks.

Ligature Mark

Color of the ligature mark is relevant since generally, marks of postmortem suspension are less dark and yellowish. Zones of erythema above and below the level of the ligature marks should be identified and documented. One of the most important characteristics of a ligature mark is its direction. Though there are a few exceptions, hanging marks inevitably show an obliquity due to the downward pull by gravitational drag of the body (Figure 3.43). Neck injuries of manual strangulation, ligature strangulation, palmar strangulation and other forms of mechanical compression of the neck are variable. These injuries range from an intact skin to obvious abrasions, contusions and/

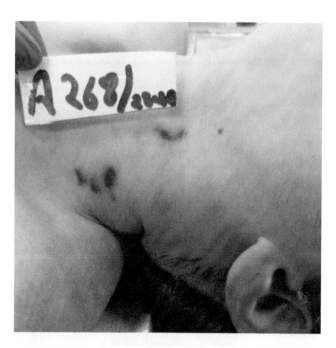

FIGURE 3.41 Contused abrasions over the front of the neck. These injuries are common in cases of manual strangulation.

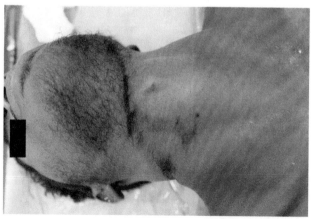

FIGURE 3.43 Ligature mark over the anterior and lateral aspects of the neck. The slippage mark of the ligature is visible as reddish abrasion at the right side of the neck. These injuries should not be misinterpreted as injuries of assault over the neck. They can be described as extension of the ligature mark.

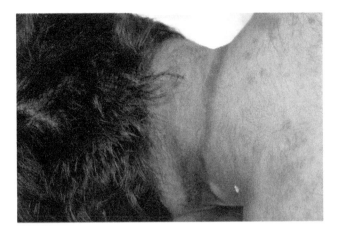

FIGURE 3.44 Continous ligature marks below hairline are seen in cases of hanging when the knot is at the front of the neck.

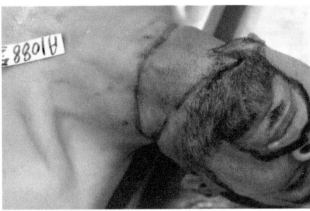

FIGURE 3.46 Two separate ligature marks found in a suicidal hanging case. Two loops of the ligature were found around the neck.

or lacerations. Ligature mark should be examined in detail regarding its course, continuity either on anterior, sides or posterior aspect of neck (Figure 3.44), multiple ligature marks due to multiple loops (Figures 3.45 and 3.46), pattern (Figure 3.47), measurements, physical appearance either broad (Figure 3.48) or thin, texture, associated injuries like blisters (Figure 3.49), abrasions, etc. Width of the ligature mark at different regions of the neck should be noted with respect to anatomical landmarks. Total length of the ligature mark should be mentioned in the report. Total neck circumference of the neck has to be mentioned in all cases of asphyxial death for future comparison and correlation with the alleged ligature material. If any evident pattern of ligature mark is identifiable, the same has to be mentioned in the postmortem report and has to be captured photographically.

Upper Limb

Inner aspect of arms and forearms has to be examined in all cases of asphyxial deaths. Finger pad 'six penny' contusions suggest the involvement of another person who grasped the

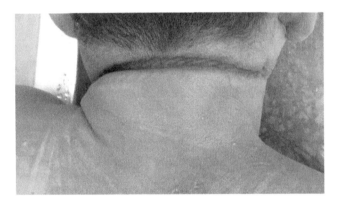

FIGURE 3.47 Patterned ligature mark with visible imprint pattern of the ligature material.

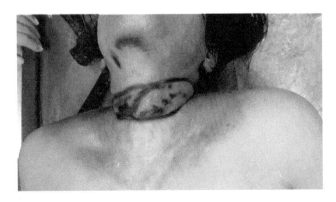

FIGURE 3.45 When the noose of the ligature material consists of multiple loops, the pattern of the ligature mark may confuse the autopsy surgeon. But comparative assessment of the ligature mark with the ligature material can be done to clear doubts in this regard.

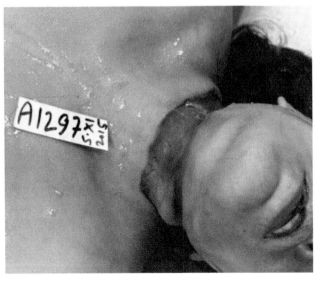

FIGURE 3.48 Broad ligature mark present over the neck.

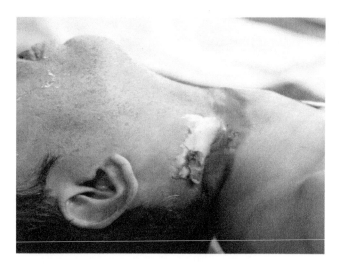

FIGURE 3.49 Pressure blister formation and rupture of the same resulting in a peeled area of skin is not rare in cases of hanging. The autopsy surgeon should be careful while interpreting these injuries.

upper limb of the deceased when he/she was alive. These injuries should be interpreted with care, since these can be produced in the agonal period during rescue.

Hesitation Cuts

Fresh, transverse parallel cuts on the anterior and inner aspect of the forearm of the non-dominant upper limb depicts the classic picture of hesitation cuts (Figures 3.50 and 3.51). These injuries also need proper documentation and interpretation. Multiple linear, transverse, hypo-pigmented scars also suggest suicidal ideation or deliberate self-harm in the past. Progressively narrowing and ending as a pointed tip, the 'tailing' is commonly seen over the medial aspects of these superficial or even deeper incised wounds. In the author's experience, razor blades are the most common weapon used to make these injuries, and counter injuries are seen over the inner aspects of the first

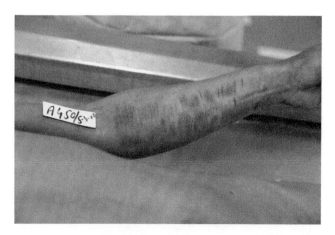

FIGURE 3.50 Multiple fresh, parallel transverse linear abrasions and superficial incised wounds present at the front of non-dominant forearm, suggestive of suicidal ideation.

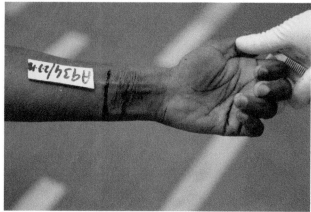

FIGURE 3.51 Multiple hesitation cuts present over the ventral aspect of lower third of forearm.

two or three fingers of the dominant hand, which occur due to holding of the razor blade. These injuries are generally very shallow, oblique incised wounds, at the thumb and index fingers of the right hand. The pattern of these injuries has to be analyzed keeping in mind the possibility of staging of hesitation cuts by an intelligent perpetrator. The investigating officer should be informed about these injuries, and the weapon can be examined by experts. Many cases of suicidal hanging show multiple hypo-pigmented transverse scars at the front of non-dominant forearm. Many of them are suggestive of previous failed attempts of deliberate self-harm.

Examination of Hands and Fingers

Any injuries present on the hands should be noted in all cases of asphyxial deaths, and the autopsy surgeon should evaluate the possible mechanisms behind them. Any possible defense wound should be examined and must be mentioned in detail in postmortem report for possible future expert evaluation. A possible hint for any other cause of death like that of electric entry burns, etc. should be looked for in the hands in all cases of alleged or suspected asphyxial deaths, keeping in mind the possibility of postmortem suspension and staging. Rigor mortis prevents the opening of the hands completely and thereby hampers the examination. For proper and complete examination, flexor tendons present on the anterior aspect of the wrist joint are to be cut for proper extension of palm and fingers as shown in Figure 3.52.

Fingernail Beds and Cyanosis

In living persons, 'cyanosis' represents increased concentration of reduced or deoxy hemoglobin in blood. It is observed as bluish discoloration of the mucosa of lips and at the peripheries like tips of fingers and toes. This bluish discoloration is appreciable when the concentration of the reduced hemoglobin concentration goes above 5g/100ml of fluid blood. The total amount of hemoglobin is not relevant in appearance of cyanosis. Oxygen utilization happens at tissue level even after somatic death. So the 'cyanosis'

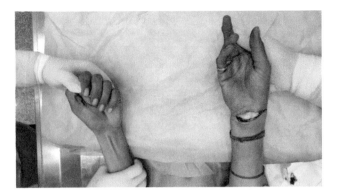

FIGURE 3.52 Incising the flexor tendons over the anterior aspect of the wrist to release the rigor of the hand for detailed examination of inner aspect of palm.

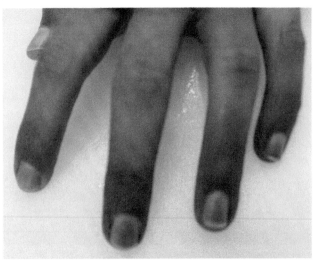

FIGURE 3.53 Bluish discoloration of fingernail beds.

present at the mucosa and fingertips may not represent the exact oxygenation status of hemoglobin at the moment of death. But it is observed that asphyxial deaths show evident cyanosis in most instances. Since nails are transparent, discoloration of the fingernails will be appreciable during autopsy (Figures 3.53 and 3.54). Examination of fingernails is an integral part of asphyxial deaths. Freshly broken nail tips suggest some kind of scuffle immediately before death and the broken pieces have to be preserved for detection of foreign trace evidences, including foreign DNA.

Discharges

Discharge of Urine

Violent asphyxial deaths commonly show involuntary discharge of urine during the terminal phases of struggle. Loss of muscular coordination during the convulsive phase or other terminal phases could be the reason for the same. Some authors are of the opinion that the discharge could be due to postmortem primary relaxation of the sphincters too.

In some cases of asphyxial deaths, urine discharge may be seen. Clothes should be examined for such discharges, and in cases of hanging, the stains over the floor also can be collected and sent for examination.

Discharge of Semen

The early stages of cerebral hypoxia are associated with elevated sexual arousal. This is considered as the reason for many bizarre autoerotic practices. Many cases of asphyxial deaths, especially hanging cases, show discharged seminal fluid over the undergarments and at tip of penis. Many authors consider it as a sign of asphyxial mode of death. Seminal discharges can be collected over a slide and examined if needed. Another possible mechanism postulated for this seminal discharge is expulsive force generated as a result of rigor mortis of muscles of seminal vesicles. In the author's experience, seminal discharge is more commonly

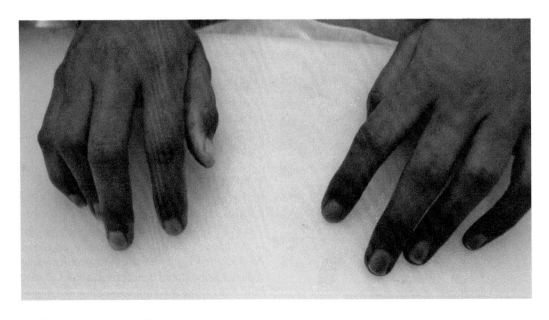

FIGURE 3.54 Bluish discoloration of fingernail beds.

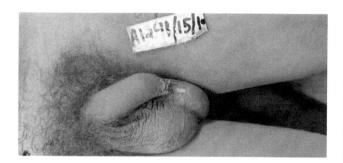

FIGURE 3.55 Seminal discharge seen at the tip of penis. This finding is common in asphyxial deaths, including cases of hanging.

seen in hanging cases and has a correlation with asphyxial mode of death (Figure 3.55). Examination, testing and documentation of the same have to be done in all cases where the discharge is present.

Discharge of Fecal Matter

Soiling of underwear or cloth with fecal matter is commonly seen in asphyxial deaths. It should be examined and documented whenever present. Discharge of fecal material is possible in many other causes of death and is inevitably seen in cases where the gas collection due to decomposition has started within the body cavities and intestinal loops.

Bloody Discharge from Vagina

In menstrual phase of endometrium, blood stains can be seen at undergarments or sanitary pads of the victim. These stains can be identified as menstrual blood in microscopy. Intense congestion due to gravitational hypostatic phenomenon causes bloody discharge from vagina in many cases of hanging. This finding should be noted in all cases of asphyxial deaths. If blood-stained discharge is present, the possibility of forceful vaginal penetration has to be ruled out by making sure that there are no injuries present over the genitalia or within the genital tract.

Lower Limbs

In cases of hanging, prolonged suspension after death produces intense hypostatic discoloration over the inferior aspect of lower limbs in a 'stocking' pattern (Figure 3.56). The more the duration of suspension, the more intense will be the hypostasis. In many cases of hanging, hypostatic postmortem petechiae are visible at lower limbs, and in rare cases, these petechiae burst and give a mimicking ante-mortem hemorrhages. Meticulous and focused external examination clears doubt in this regard. Soles of feet show bluish discolorations in cases of prolonged suspension. This should be separated from contusions of soles of feet in custodial torture by methods like falanga.

Genitalia

External genitalia need special attention in cases of homicides. Forceful sexual penetration or manipulation of the genitalia produces signature injuries that should be

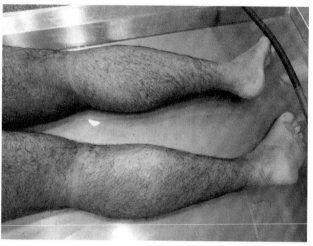

FIGURE 3.56 Intense postmortem staining at lower limb in 'stocking' pattern in a case of a suicidal hanging with prolonged suspension. Note the hypostatic petechiae over both limbs.

evaluated and interpreted. In case a recent sexual intercourse is suspected, all swabs and samples of pubic hair should be preserved. Postmortem drying of scrotal skin resembling an abrasion is a common postmortem artifact seen especially in cases of hanging. In case of prolonged suspension, the scrotum appears more congested due to the passive pooling of blood and resembles a contusion (Figure 3.57). Fecal, urinal and seminal stains have to be checked and noted. Anal sphincter has to be examined, and if needed, swabs have to be preserved.

Neck Dissection

Anterior Neck Dissection

Many cases of asphyxial deaths, including deaths following hanging, show intense congestion at face and neck. Dissection of neck structures in this congested field is notorious to produce artefacts that could be misinterpreted as ante-mortem injuries. To avoid hemorrhagic artefacts while

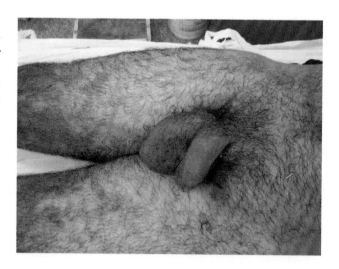

FIGURE 3.57 In cases of prolonged suspension, there is deep congestion of the scrotum due to postmortem staining and drying.

doing neck dissection in a congested field, a separate technique has been adopted for neck dissection in all cases of suspected deaths with possibility of traumatic compression of neck. The first requirement in this method is removal of brain and dura mater to decongest the neck. Similarly, thoracic block should also be removed. After the release of neck congestion by removal of cranial and thoracic structures, the neck should be kept untouched for some time before dissection, for complete draining of blood.

The upper trunk should be elevated by using supportive block. Then the neck can be examined by layer-wise examination. Chin to suprasternal notch – 'I'-shaped neck incision is sufficient to give a reasonable view of anterior neck structures in most of the cases. Many autopsy surgeons follow this incision for neck dissection due to ease while dissecting and approximation while suturing. Another neck incision is the 'V'-shaped mastoid to suprasternal notch incisions of both sides of neck. The incision runs just along the posterior margins of both sternocleidomastoid muscles. This incision gives a better view of posterolateral neck structures.

Some autopsy surgeons prefer to dissect platysma as a separate layer, but the same is not warranted in all cases since the injury at that layer can be visualized in the skin flap if examined from its inner aspect.

Layer-wise dissection of neck structures involves the following steps (Figures 3.58a–3.58i):

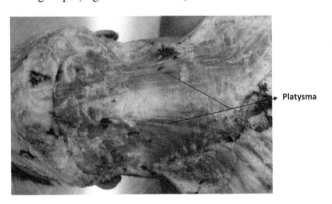

FIGURE 3.58a Reflection of skin flap with intact platysma muscle in layer 1 dissection of neck.

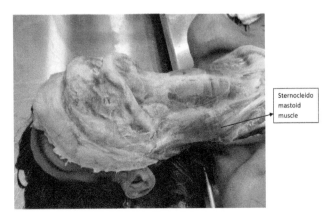

FIGURE 3.58b Reflection of skin flap along with platysma during layer 2 dissection of neck.

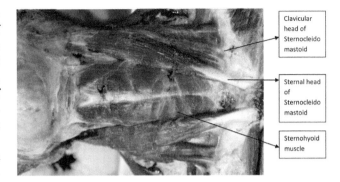

FIGURE 3.58c Sternocleidomastoid muscles and sternohyoid muscles of both sides are visible.

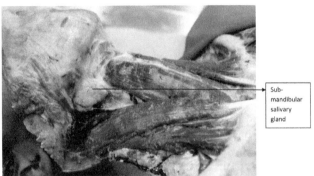

FIGURE 3.58d Submandibular salivary gland visible during dissection of neck.

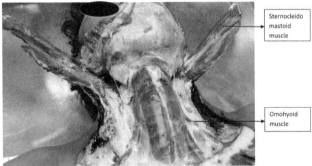

FIGURE 3.58e Reflected sternocleidomastoid and omohyoid muscles in situ.

Layer 1

The skin and superficial tissues of the neck are reflected by extending the incision, which exposes the underlying tissues that have to be examined. The subcutaneous tissues under the ligature mark appear dry, pale, hard and glistening due to excess force exerted on the tissues, which causes only pressure abrasion. In cases of other forms of neck compression, like ligature or manual strangulation, many signature dermal injuries can be appreciated by examining this layer.

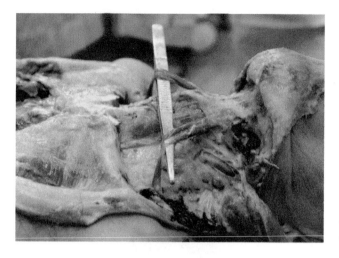

FIGURE 3.58f   Reflected omohyoid muscles.

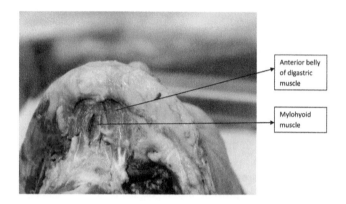

FIGURE 3.58g   Mylohyoid muscle and anterior belly of digastric muscle of floor of mouth.

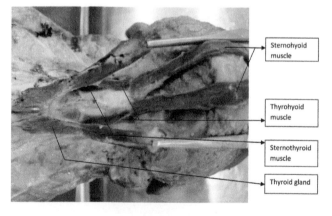

FIGURE 3.58h   Reflected sternohyoid and sternothyroid muscle. Thyrohyoid muscles can be seen in picture.

Layer 2

Inspection of platysma should be done for any contusion. Many autopsy surgeons take this layer along with the skin layer itself due to the difficulty and time consumption for separating out this thin layer of muscle fibers.

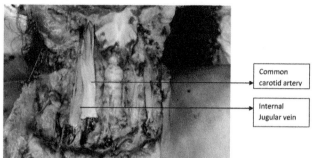

FIGURE 3.58i   Common carotid artery and internal jugular vein are opened in situ. Branching point of common carotid artery is visible. Internal jugular vein is seen parallel to the opened right common carotid artery.

Layer 3

Sternocleidomastoid muscles should be incised at their sternal and clavicular head origins and reflected towards their insertion at mastoid. Origin of these muscles show hemorrhages in most of the cases of hanging and is considered a sign of vitality by many authors. Muscle fibers should be dissected to look for any concealed hemorrhages.

Layer 4

After the reflection of sternocleidomastoid muscle, the superior belly of omohyoid muscle can be examined for any hemorrhages and the same can be reflected.

Layer 5

In the next step, three paired muscles of the anterior neck can be examined one by one. The outermost sternohyoid muscle can be examined first, followed by sternothyroid and thyrohyoid muscles. Any injuries at these muscles have to be identified and documented.

After the removal of all these muscles, the carotid sheath structures can be examined. Carotid canal structures including common carotid artery with initial portions of its branches, internal jugular vein and vagal nerve can be examined in situ itself. These structures can also be removed and dissection can be done along with that of neck block.

Thyroid glands can be examined and removed when the neck block is in situ itself, or it can be examined after taking out the block.

Laryngeal cartilages (Figures 3.59 and 3.60) and hyoid bone (Figure 3.61) can be examined for fractures in the removed neck block. For removal of the neck block, muscles of floor of mouth have to be dissected close to the inner margin of mandible. Then the tongue has to be pushed back into the pharynx. Soft tissue attachments of the neck blocks should be released, and the block can be removed. For routine practice, dissection can be done immediately after removal of the block. After the removal of neck

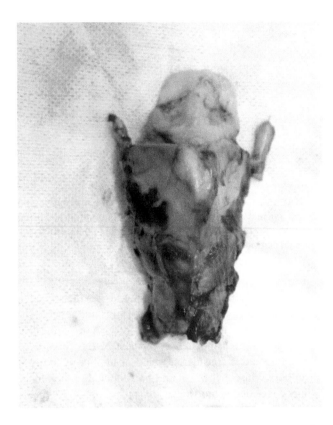

FIGURE 3.59 Entire laryngeal complex and upper trachea after dissection of the neck block.

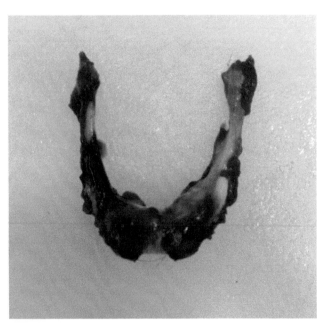

FIGURE 3.61 Fracture of hyoid bone with surrounding infiltration.

structures, the neck block can be fixed in formalin for one day, which will give a clear picture of ante-mortem infiltrations (Figure 3.62). This method can be used for cases that need more clarity of the findings or in cases where some injuries are anticipated.

While dissection, esophagus can be dissected first. Thyrohyoid membrane should be dissected to release the connection between hyoid bone and the larynx. Soft tissues adherent to the hyoid bone and the laryngeal cartilages have to be removed for proper visualization of hemorrhages around fracture site. In case of any need of microscopic evaluation, the portion has to be subjected to histological examination. Some authors suggest a radiological

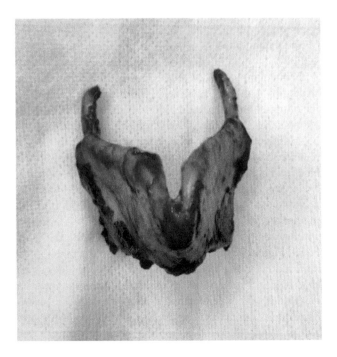

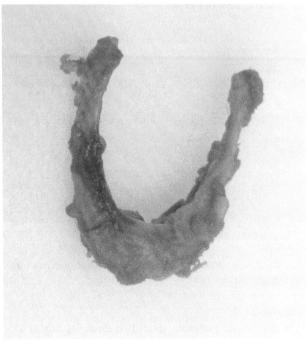

FIGURE 3.62 The same fracture mentioned in the above figure after fixation in formalin. Note the visible infiltration, a sign of vitality.

FIGURE 3.60 Dissected out intact thyroid cartilage.

examination of the eviscerated neck block in order to better appreciate the bony structures for evidence of any injury; the vertebral column hinders proper visualization when radiological examination like X-ray is done in an in-situ position of the neck.

The underlying tissues have to be examined by hand or using a non-toothed forceps to avoid postmortem artefacts. In cases of hanging, there will be presence of minimal hemorrhage or no bleeding in the underlying tissues, except in some cases where the bleeding may be seen in the **muscles** of the neck, if considerable force is applied.

In microscopic examination, the intima of **carotid artery** may show tears and hemorrhage due to the horizontal pressure exerted by the ligature and vertical pressure caused by the high pressure of blood column of the carotid artery, which tries to pass through the obstructed lumen due to ligature to supply blood to the brain.

Posterior Neck Dissection

Posterior neck dissection is not conducted routinely in all cases of asphyxial deaths. It is mainly intended to examine the injuries, hemorrhages in ligaments of the upper neck, subcutis and muscles of posterior aspect of neck. Prior to dissection, the body should be placed in prone and elevated position (elevating the chest such that the neck appears slightly flexed). Prior autopsy is usually adequate to decompress the veins of the posterior neck. Posterior neck dissection can be done after all other dissection procedures over the front of the body have been completed.

Technique: An inverted "T"-shaped incision is used with a vertical part along the nape of the neck and a horizontal part in the scapular region (Figures 3.63 and 3.64); the extent of horizontal incision is till the level of tip of acromion on both sides. The vertical portion of the inverted "T"-shaped incision extends in the midline up to the occiput.

The skin is reflected laterally creating two large flaps, exposing the underlying trapezius muscles (Figure 3.65). Numerous muscles are present on the posterior aspect of neck. Layer-wise elevation of the superficial and deeper muscles can be done (Figure 3.66). The dissection area should be as wide as possible so as to get a clear view of the deeper structures.

Once the superficial and intermediate muscles are elevated, the deep paraspinal muscle on the posterior surface of the cervical spine will remain, along with the deep sub-occipital muscles. Dissect the deep para-spinal and sub-occipital muscles by cutting the muscles from the surface of the vertebrae to check for any vertebral fractures (Figure 3.67).

Further dissection will reveal the deep cervical spinal ligaments, cervical vertebrae and extra cranial portion of vertebral artery. Integrity of the atlanto-occipital and atlanto-axial ligaments can be easily identified and assessed. Hemorrhage as a result of any injury can also be easily assessed. En bloc excision or segmental excision of vertebral artery is done if required.

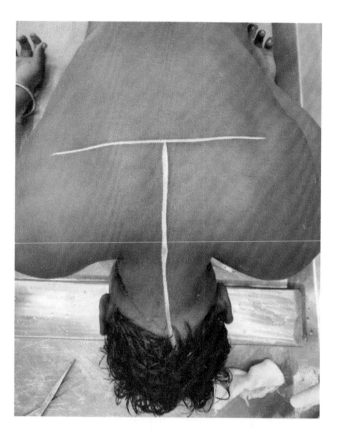

FIGURE 3.63 An inverted "T"-shaped skin incision is made with the vertical limb over posterior aspect of neck and the horizontal incision in the scapular region.

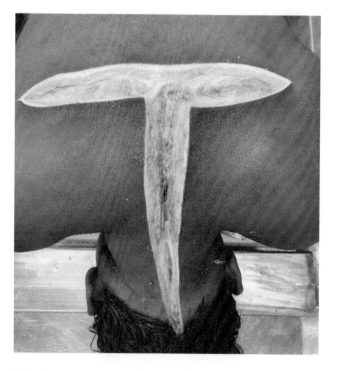

FIGURE 3.64 Extending the inverted "T"-shaped incision into deeper plane of subcutaneous tissue until muscular fascia is reached.

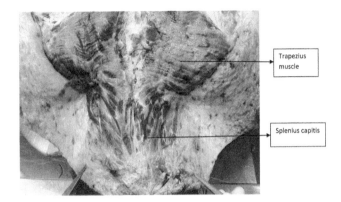

FIGURE 3.65 Bilateral skin flaps are raised and underlying trapezius and splenius capitis muscles are visible.

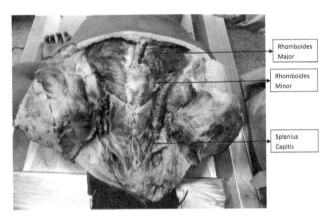

FIGURE 3.66 Layer-wise dissection of the superficial and deep muscle layers. This layer is after the reflection of trapezius muscle. Underlying splenius capitis and rhomboids muscles are clearly visible.

Each layer of the posterior neck dissection should be photographed in the same plane, including orientation and close-up images. Injuries should be photographed with a scale.

EXAMINATION OF FACE AND ORAL CAVITY DURING DISSECTION

The upper skin flap of the V-incision of neck can be further reflected beyond margins of jaw bone if the autopsy surgeon needs a better visualization of the tongue, mouth cavity

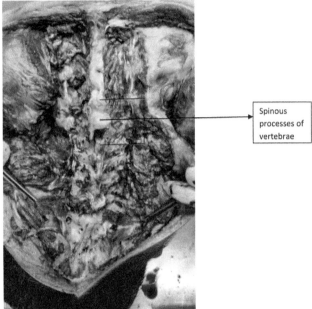

FIGURE 3.67 Deep dissection revealing the spinous processes of cervical vertebrae.

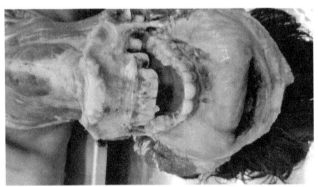

FIGURE 3.68 Face-flap is reflected for better appreciation of the injuries at the inner aspect of lips and cheeks.

and lip injuries (Figure 3.68). During this step, the masseter muscles can be dissected and the Temporo-mandibular joint released. This will give the surgeon a better picture of tongue, hard and soft palates, nasopharynx and oropharynx. Injuries of the inner aspect of the lips and cheeks can be visualized better with this method.

4 Fatal Pressure Over Neck by Hanging

Hanging is the most common modality of suicide presumably due to the easy accessibility of the requisite logistics, its high success rate and the popular belief of it being swift and painless. With very few exceptions, hanging is almost always suicidal in manner and should be presumed to be so unless proven otherwise. It has been seen that for the constriction of neck to be fatal and cause death by asphyxia, a weight of approximately 5 kg or even less is sufficient. In some cases, even just the weight of head (Figure 4.1) has been sufficient to cause death.

CONSEQUENCES OF BRAIN HYPOXIA IN ASPHYXIAL DEATH

In cases of hanging, constriction of neck due to the gravitational pull of the body causes asphyxiation, leading to death of the individual. The progressive lack of oxygen in asphyxiation causes a series of reactions in the body, and five stages of asphyxia have been identified in relation to these. A few authors have studied these stages by analyzing video recordings of the victims during the act, while other studies have been based on scrutinizing the reactions of volunteers by subjecting them to controlled cerebral hypoxia using pressure cuffs around neck.

Cerebral hypoxia in cases of hanging occurs mainly due to the complete obstruction of the upper airway due to the upward and backward displacement of the tissues of the floor of mouth and anterior upper neck. This will result in approximation of the displaced antero-inferior wall of

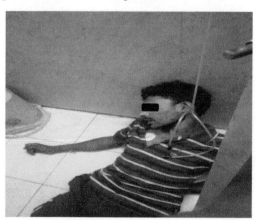

FIGURE 4.1 A case of fatal hanging wherein the only constricting force is the weight of the head.

oro-pharynx with its postero-superior wall. Along with this airway obstruction, arterial and venous occlusions at the level of the constriction play some role in determining the pace of appearance of these stages.

Brain stem regulatory centers, including vital medullary centers, are prone to hypoxic injury leading to rapid cellular dysfunction if the supply of oxygen is cut for a minimum of 3 minutes. But this duration has been observed to be highly variable and may reach up to 10 minutes in many cases. Position of the noose around the neck, the magnitude of compression, the degree of suspension, the nature and width of the ligature material, whether or not there is slippage of ligature during the course of hanging, the position of knot and the height of drop are some of the factors determining the duration of time required for complete cerebral dysfunction culminating in the final apnea and death.

These stages of asphyxiation are described below.

1. **Stage of dyspnea:** Loss of consciousness generally happens within the first 10 seconds of hanging. This stage shows laborious respiratory movements as the victim struggles to breathe. These violent breathing efforts are termed as 'air hunger'. All the accessory muscles of respiration are actively engaged during this stage. The heart rate increases and the blood pressure of the victim shoots up. Facial cyanosis also develops during this stage of asphyxia. There may be an involuntary protective action to remove the ligature, which can cause some injuries over the neck apart from those by the ligature (Figure 4.2). Similar injuries may also occur during rescue of the victim where the rescuer forcibly tries to remove the ligature and may unknowingly cause injuries over neck or chin (Figure 4.3).

2. **Stage of convulsions:** After the dyspneic phase, the victim enters the stage of convulsions. Here, tonic clonic convulsions are commonly seen due to hypoxic injury to neurons of the cerebral cortex. Generally, this stage does not continue for more than 2 minutes. Consciousness will be completely lost at this stage, and the convulsions may cause limb and trunk injuries due to forceful contact with nearby structures. During this stage, the pupils dilate and the blood pressure and heart rate shoot

DOI: 10.1201/9780429026317-4

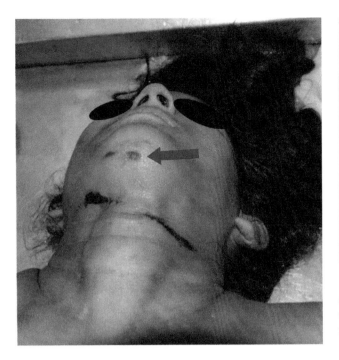

FIGURE 4.2 The victims of suicidal hanging may attempt to pull away the ligature as a reflex action to preserve life, thus inflicting nail marks on the neck near chin or around the ligature. Rarely, such injuries can also be seen over the chin.

up further. In some cases, involuntary release of urine and feces also happens during this stage.

During the convulsive stage, the person usually suffers multiple injuries due to contact with rough surfaces in the vicinity. The author himself has come across several cases with injuries over the body parts in contact with the ground or wall at the scene of occurrence. One such case has been illustrated, wherein a middle-aged man was found in a partially hung position inside his house and had injuries over dorsum of foot and toes in addition to the ligature mark. This was confirmed with crime scene photos (Figures 4.4 and 4.5).

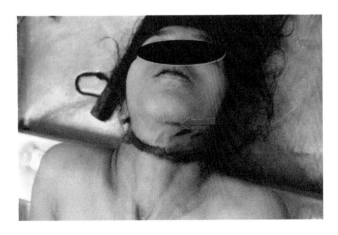

FIGURE 4.3 In attempted rescue, nail marks can also be produced by the rescuer while trying to remove the ligature.

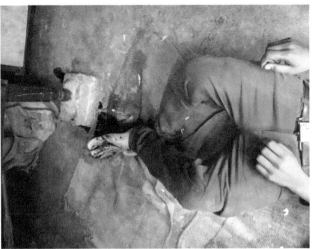

FIGURE 4.4 Crime scene photo with injuries found on the dorsum of the foot and toes in a case of suicidal partial hanging with the legs fixed in semi-flexed position and further development of rigor mortis in that position.

These injuries may be misinterpreted as injuries of criminal involvement and can cause doubts in the minds of relatives, investigating officers and even the autopsy surgeons. In case of doubt, scene of occurrence examination has to be done to get clarity about such injuries.

3. **Stage of pre-terminal apnea:** This is a stage of temporary apnea that may last up to 1 minute in duration. Here the respiratory movements stop for the first time and blood pressure also starts decreasing. An increased cardiac rate is seen as in the preceding stages.

4. **Stage of terminal agonal respiration:** These are irregular and disorganized movements of respiration seen in the agonal period. There are respiratory movements during this phase, but these are

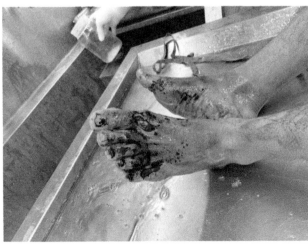

FIGURE 4.5 Injuries noted over the dorsum of foot in the case of partial hanging where the violent movement of legs in convulsive phase caused multiple lacerations and abrasions.

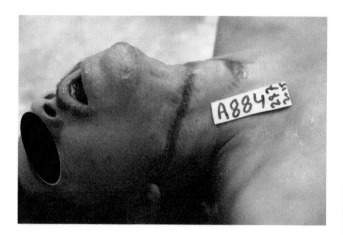

FIGURE 4.6 A double ligature mark over the neck with both showing significant parchmentization, indicating that the ligature was in both positions for considerable periods of time.

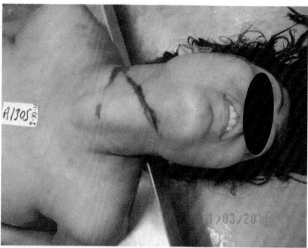

FIGURE 4.7 A double ligature mark over the neck with both showing significant parchmentization, indicating that the ligature was in both positions for considerable periods of time.

not synchronized. The duration of this stage is variable and lasts for approximately 1–4 minutes in most cases. The muscles of neck become rigid during this phase.

5. **Stage of apnea:** This is the final stage of asphyxiation. Here the individual slips into an irreversible stage of apnea. The medullary centers as well as other brain stem centers go into complete hypoxic paralysis. Hypoxia of the vagal center results in the release of cardiac inhibitory signals, which may result in tachycardia in some cases. Though the respiratory movements stop, the heart may continue to beat for up to 20 minutes. The time interval between the initiation of hanging and death is 3–10 minutes, and it varies with the position and type of ligature material, force of suspension and the final constriction of the airway. In some cases, it is seen that there is a primary ligature mark and another is above, which causes constriction of upper airway by means of asphyxia. The author has conducted autopsies of multiple cases of this nature and has observed that significant parchmentization and abrasions are seen in both the positions, indicating that the ligature material was in that position for considerable time (Figures 4.6 and 4.7).

COMPLETE HANGING

Hanging is called complete when the complete body weight works as the constricting force around the neck through a noose. Complete suspension means 'foot is off the ground' or off any object. Generally, complete hanging results in sudden complete occlusion of all arteries and veins. Depending upon the position of the knot, complete obstruction of the airway also happens in many of these cases. Sudden stoppage of arterial supply results in facial pallor in almost every case of complete suspension. Sudden increase in pressure over the carotid sinuses may result in reflex

cardiac arrest in some of these cases. Complete hanging results in early loss of consciousness and causes death due to complete stoppage of cerebral perfusion. Judicial hanging methods always ensure complete suspension. Complete hanging is generally achieved by the use of a stool or a chair or a table when suspension point is high and cannot be accessed by the individual using his or her own height. Hence the point of suspension is reached with the help of some platform that may be kicked off by the deceased after putting the ligature (Figures 4.8 and 4.9).

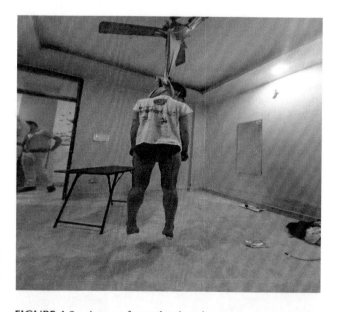

FIGURE 4.8 A case of complete hanging autopsy conducted by the author at his center [All India Institute of Medical Sciences (AIIMS), New Delhi, a premier institute under the Government of India]. The examination at the crime scene shows that the table was used to reach the desired height so as to commit hanging. The foot is off the ground, hence fulfilling the criteria for complete hanging.

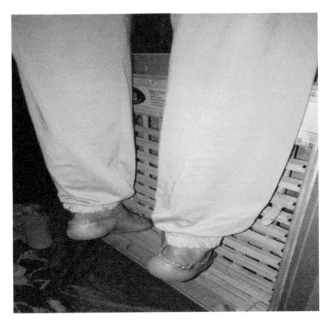

FIGURE 4.9 In this case, the deceased committed hanging by using an air cooler to reach the desired height so as to tie the ligature to the suspension point to commit suicide.

Discussion on a Case of Suicidal Hanging of a Senior Civil Servant at His Residence During Office Hours

Soon after a senior IAS officer's suicide, several organizations and the public held protests (Figure 4.10) demanding a CBI inquiry into his death. He was described as an intense person who was highly sensitive, impulsive and aggressive on problems that would affect the common public. The investigation showed that the deceased was found to be under constant work pressure and had a tendency of getting physically exhausted after the day's work. It was also reported that he was in a state of depression after his posting was changed from a place where he worked for some time, and the refusal of a woman IAS officer to pick his call

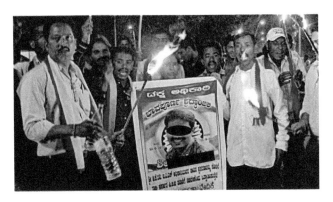

FIGURE 4.10 The protest by public and several organizations who were denying the fact of suicidal hanging by a senior civil servant and demanded enquiry by the Central Bureau of Investigation (CBI); the picture shows banners in Kannada (local language) showering condolences to the deceased.

acted as a last trigger factor that made him commit suicide. He also used to get frustrated on facing failures and would always like to see that his viewpoint gets the acceptance. On the fateful day, this senior civil servant, when on duty, left office in his official vehicle to home at about 11.30 AM. Since he was not responding to calls, his wife and father-in-law were anxious and reached the flat where he was residing. The house was locked, but they opened it using a spare key. The officer was found dead, hanging from a fan by using a sari (silk type yellow and orange with maroon border) as ligature material; it was a complete hanging and the deceased had used a chair to reach the desired height for tying the ligature in position.

A team of Forensic Science Laboratory, Bangalore, visited the scene of incidence and collected samples. They collected fingerprints of the deceased and checked for presence of any foreign fingerprints in the crime scene and did not find anything suggestive of foul play in the death of the deceased.

A board of three senior forensic doctors conducted the autopsy at the state government hospital. Based on the autopsy examination findings, the board members concluded the cause of death as, 'Asphyxia as a result of Hanging'.

Viscera were preserved during autopsy, and the investigating agency of the state government forwarded the viscera to three different forensic science laboratories in Bengaluru, Hyderabad and New Delhi for examination for the presence of any poison or any other toxicological agent. Viscera analysis gave negative tests for the presence of common poisons, and cellophane tape lift from the ligature mark gave identical fibers of the ligature material used. The forensic science team who visited the crime scene also gave an opinion that the hanging was suicidal in nature.

The public and some organizations were not satisfied with the opinion and alleged the involvement of state government in not providing justice to the deceased. They demanded the case to be transferred to a higher investigative agency for providing justice. The case was transferred to the CBI for enquiry, and an expert medico-legal opinion was requested from AIIMS, New Delhi as there were a lot of organizations protesting on the need for higher authority to take over the investigation for a fair outcome. A Medical Board headed by the author was constituted at AIIMS, New Delhi. The Medical Board members visited the alleged scene of occurrence and also interacted with the initial team of forensic doctors who had conducted the postmortem examination. The Medical Board studied all the submitted documents related to the case, photographs and videos of the crime scene examination and postmortem procedures. The Medical Board observed the following facts:

Crime Scene Study

The forensic science team noted the deceased hanging from the ceiling fan and it was a complete hanging with foot above the ground (Figure 4.11). The team also checked for the presence of any foreign fingerprints in the crime scene and measured the height of the individual and possibility to reach the fan with the help of chair for fixing the ligature

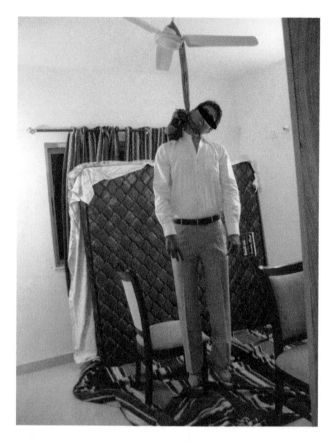

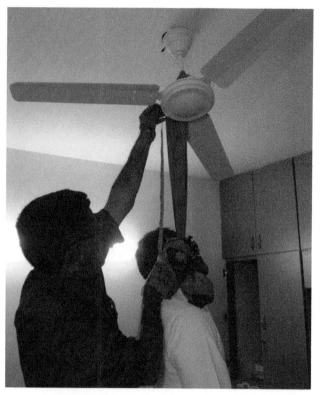

FIGURE 4.11 Crime scene examination revealed that the deceased used a chair to reach the desired height to fix the ligature material from the suspension point (which is fan here) and after fixation and tying the ligature around the neck suspended for committing suicide by complete hanging. The tilting of the fan is seen due to suspension and weight of the deceased.

material and committing suicide. The main motive was to assess the crime scene if it was primary crime scene and was not staged, and it was opined as primary crime scene (Figures 4.12 and 4.13).

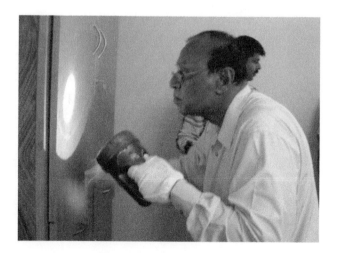

FIGURE 4.12 Crime scene examination by the forensic team for the presence of any foreign fingerprints and ruling out possibility of the crime scene being staged.

FIGURE 4.13 Forensic team examining the ligature in-situ and measuring the length of the deceased, the length of the ligature material from the suspension point on fan, dimensions of the knot and checking if the deceased could reach the desired height for fixing the ligature.

The ligature material was a sari that was yellow orange with maroon border made of silk material, which was suspended from the ceiling fan. The knot was a slip knot present on the right side of the neck, below the right ear and just behind the right angle of the mandible (Figure 4.14). This position of the knot made the head tilt to the left.

The dead body was brought down by the forensic team with precautions such as cutting the ligature material far from the knot along with support given to the deceased to avoid any injuries by sudden drop (Figure 4.15). Precautions were also taken to avoid disturbance to the knot and the ligature surrounding the neck, and the dead body was shifted to a state government hospital for autopsy with precautions of not causing any postmortem injuries due to transportation.

Clothes Examination

Clothes worn by the deceased at the time of incidence were intact, undisturbed and did not show any signs of tear due to struggle (Figure 4.16). There was a stain observed on the front-left side of the pants, which was analyzed later by the forensic team and was found to be seminal stain (Figure 4.17). The stain was analyzed for DNA, which matched with the DNA profile of the deceased. The stain was due to the seminal discharge from the deceased during hanging. No other stains were seen over the clothes or the dead body.

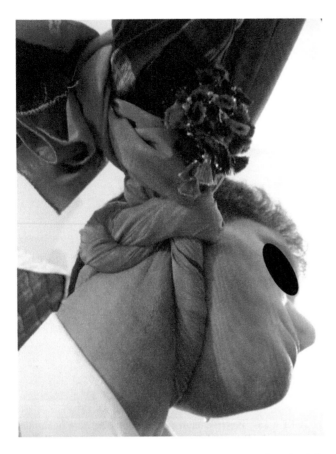

FIGURE 4.14   The knot is a slip knot positioned below the right ear and near the mastoid and behind the right angle of mandible, thus causing the tilting of the head to the left.

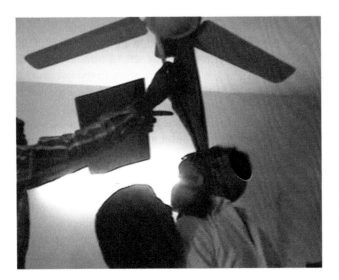

FIGURE 4.15   Precautions to be taken to remove the dead body in hanging cases where the dead body has to be supported and the ligature material should be cut as far as possible from the knot and the ligature material should be left in situ for examination at autopsy.

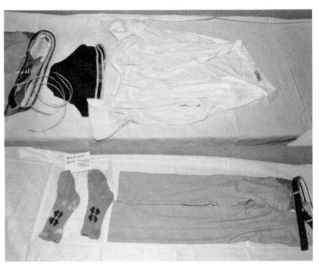

FIGURE 4.16   Shows the clothes of the deceased worn at the time of hanging. No tears or disturbance due to struggle are seen in the clothes as would be expected in cases of homicide.

Autopsy Observations

General examination of the dead body showed the ligature material in situ. Face was seen to show *Le Facie Sympathique* appearance, which is seen in cases of hanging, especially complete hanging, as was this case and is caused when the ligature knot compresses cervical sympathetic ganglion causing the eye on the same side to be open and that of the opposite side to be closed, which was noted; face was noted to be without much congestion (Figure 4.18). Dribbling of saliva was seen on the left side, which was the lower aspect due to tilting of the head to the left and the secretion of saliva due to the stimulation of the salivary glands caused by compression by the ligature material over

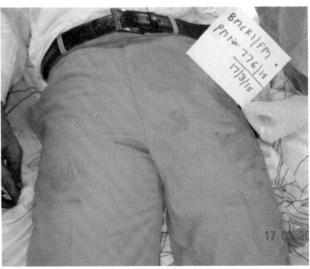

FIGURE 4.17   The stain present over the pant on the left side was sent for analysis and was found to be seminal stain, and DNA analysis proved that it belonged to the deceased.

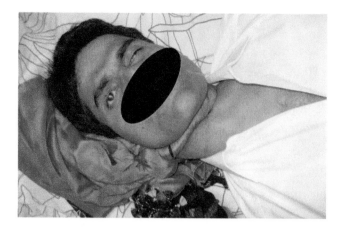

FIGURE 4.18 *Le Facie Sympathique* appearance caused when the ligature knot compresses cervical sympathetic ganglion. The eye on the same side is open and that of the opposite side is closed.

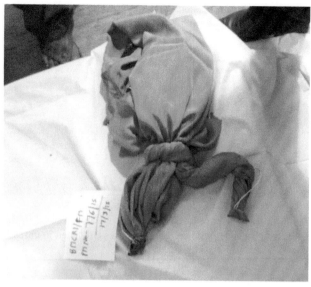

the neck and the base of the head. Tip of the tongue was seen protruding through the rows of teeth (Figure 4.19).

The ligature material present in situ was removed with precaution by cutting the noose away from the knot and before cutting the ligature on either side of the site of cut was secured using thread. The ligature material was checked for

FIGURE 4.20 Ligature material during removal from the neck of the deceased, with precaution taken to preserve the knot by cutting the noose away from the knot and securing the cut ends with a string/thread.

the presence of any stains or any other marks, tears or cuts, which were absent (Figure 4.20).

Livor mortis was present in glove and stock pattern. Petechial hemorrhages were present in both lower limbs due to prolonged hypostasis or postmortem lividity (Figure 4.21). Tip of the tongue was slightly protruded and bitten. Cyanosis was present over nail beds, which was due to the asphyxial nature of the death (Figure 4.22). Dribbling of saliva from the mouth was seen on the left side, which co-related with the position of the head during suspension. Discharge of semen was observed in this case, which

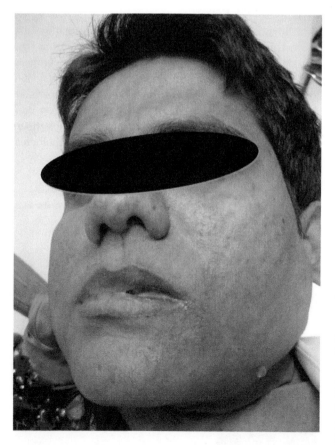

FIGURE 4.19 Dribbling of saliva from the angle of the mouth is due to stimulation of the salivary gland by the ligature compressing the neck; this is more in cases of complete hanging as the pressure is more, as seen in this case. Tip of the tongue was seen protruding between the teeth.

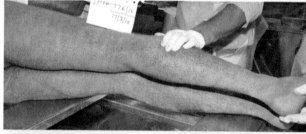

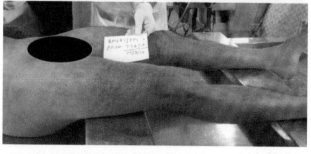

FIGURE 4.21 Hypostatic petechiae in the dependent parts of the lower limbs due to suspension and part of the glove and stock hypostasis seen in hanging due to prolonged period of suspension.

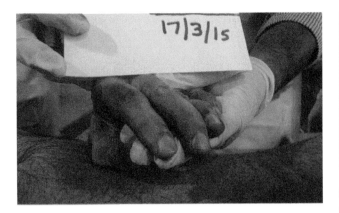

FIGURE 4.22 Cyanosis of the nail beds was observed in this case, which is due to deoxyhemoglobin usually seen in cases of hanging because of asphyxia.

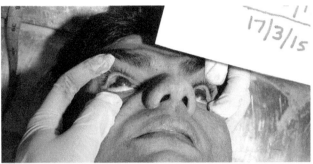

FIGURE 4.24 Examination of conjunctiva in crime scene showed pale appearance of the conjunctivae; the face also does not show any features of congestion. During autopsy, it showed tache noir.

is seen in many cases of hanging, usually due to the rigor mortis of the muscle lining the seminal vesicles, and it is also considered by a few as due to the central nervous system stimulation in asphyxial deaths (Figure 4.23). Seminal discharge was present from penis, which also caused a stain over the pants and was confirmed by the cytology report, stain analysis and DNA matching with the deceased. The internal viscera were congested. Petechiae were present in lungs.

Examination of the eyes showed that the conjunctivae were pale, and the first examination in the crime scene did not show any tache noir but the same examination during autopsy revealed the presence of tache noir as the eyes were partially open on both sides (Figure 4.24). Examination of the nostrils, skin over the cheeks and skin surrounding the mouth did not reveal the presence of any injury (Figure 4.25). Mouth was examined, which showed that the tongue was bitten and oral mucosa and the inner surface of both upper and lower lips were pale and without any injuries (Figure 4.26).

Ligature mark was observed over the neck and was clear, higher up in position above the thyroid cartilage, obliquely placed and incompletely encircling the neck, with no other

surrounding injuries seen over the neck (Figures 4.27–4.29). Brain and lungs showed congestion and a few petechial hemorrhages (Figures 4.30 and 4.31).

On bloodless neck dissection of the neck, the base of the ligature mark was dry, hard and parchment like. The muscles, thyro-hyoid complex and vertebrae with its ligaments were intact. No other injuries were observed over the neck (Figures 4.32–4.34).

Histopathology Report

Skin bit was sent for histopathological examination, and microscopy showed: 'Multiple sections studied from ligature site show breaking up of the epidermis with compression and wrinkling. The dermis shows compressed deviated adnexal structures with no congestion and hemorrhage. At the periphery of the ligature mark there are few congested blood vessels. The subcutaneous and muscle fibers appear unremarkable. Impression of the histopathological

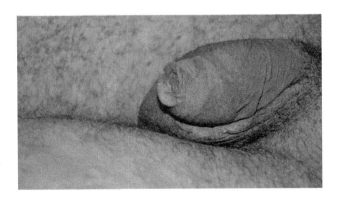

FIGURE 4.23 Discharge of semen was observed in this case, which is seen in many cases of hanging, usually due to the rigor mortis of the muscle lining the seminal vesicles, also considered by a few due to CNS stimulation in asphyxial deaths.

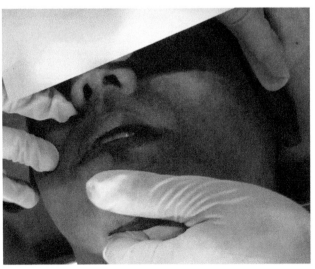

FIGURE 4.25 Examination of the nostrils, skin around the nostrils and mouth shows absence of any injuries, blood stains and bleeding from nose, ruling out the possibility of obstruction to airway by means of smothering.

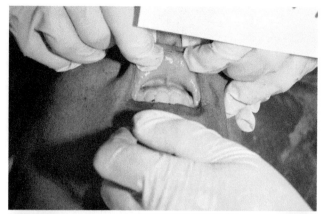

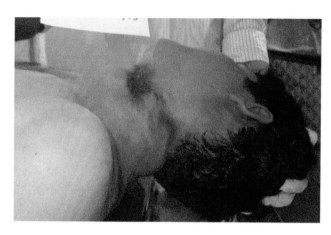

FIGURE 4.28 Shows the pressure abrasion due to ligature positioned above the level of thyroid cartilage and running obliquely upwards towards the posterior hairline. No other injuries are seen over the neck.

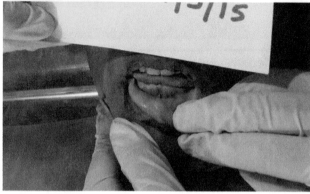

FIGURE 4.26 Oral mucosa on examination shows pale appearance with no injuries and congestion, practically ruling out the possibility of smothering in a conscious man who is well built.

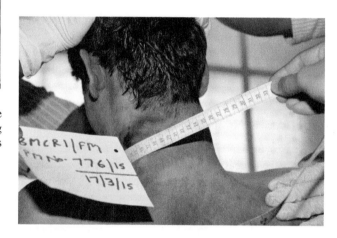

FIGURE 4.29 Shows the pressure abrasion due to ligature running obliquely and upwards and over the posterior aspect of the neck; the ligature mark is merging with the posterior hairline at the nape of the neck. No other injuries are seen over the neck.

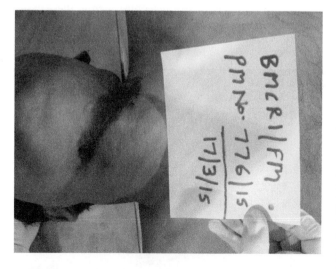

FIGURE 4.27 Neck shows ligature mark running obliquely and upwards and to the right side, above the level of the thyroid cartilage and is incomplete on the right side where the suspension point of the ligature was present. No other injuries are seen over the neck.

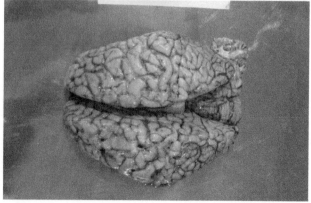

FIGURE 4.30 Shows brain with congestion, which is usually seen in cases of hanging.

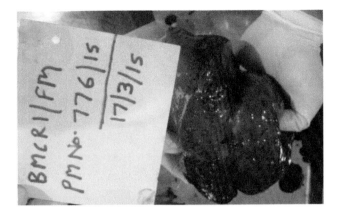

FIGURE 4.31 Lungs showed features of congestion and few petechial hemorrhages in the interlobar fissure.

examination of the ligature mark was, 'Possibility of ante-mortem injury needs to be considered'.

The Medical Board, after perusal of the previous crime scene report, postmortem report, viscera analysis reports, histopathology report, crime scene visit and checking the photos and videos of the crime scene examination and autopsy, came to the logical conclusion of death due to **suicidal hanging** in the case after ruling out all other possibilities.

PARTIAL HANGING

The cases of hanging in which feet or any other part of body of the deceased touches the ground or any object are referred to as 'incomplete or partial hanging'. In these cases, the constricting force through the noose is the gravitational

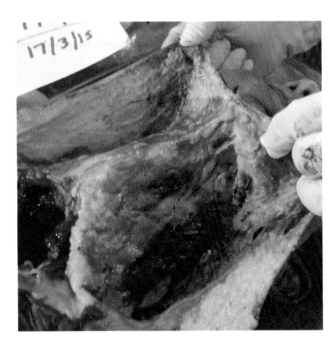

FIGURE 4.32 Bloodless internal dissection of the neck shows parchmentization of the skin at the place of ligature mark; no other injuries or hemorrhages are seen in the neck.

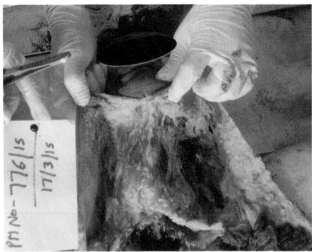

FIGURE 4.33 Bloodless internal dissection of the neck shows parchmentization of the skin at the place of ligature mark; no other injuries or hemorrhages are seen in the neck.

pull due to the weight of only a 'part' of the body, resulting in vital structure compression and death. Partial hanging deaths can happen in different body positions like standing, kneeling, sitting or lying down (Figure 4.35). The degree of compression of vital structures of the neck varies with the weight transmitted to these through the noose. The mechanisms of death and postmortem signs also vary accordingly. Minor constricting forces compress only the veins of the neck, while the deeper, more muscular arteries continue transporting oxygenated blood to the brain. This results in obstruction and severe congestion above the level of constriction. This venous congestion eventually results in cerebral hypoxia and death due to the pooling of deoxygenated blood. Generally, these deaths are easily diagnosable due to intense facial congestion, cyanosis, oedema and presence of multiple sub-conjunctival petechiae seen in these cases. Congestive petechiae may be seen at other sites above

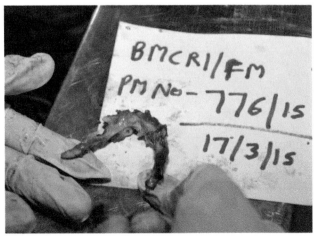

FIGURE 4.34 Shows the hyoid bone intact without any surrounding muscular contusions, hemorrhages or fractures.

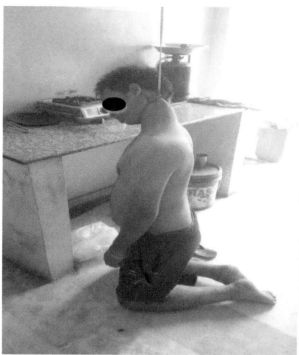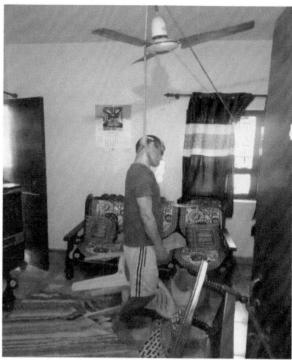

FIGURE 4.35 Cases of partial hanging where part of the body of the deceased is in contact with the ground. Left photo shows knee in contact with the ground. Right photo shows feet in contact with the ground (with cloth inside the mouth to avoid shout or cry to be heard outside).

the level of constriction such as the skin over the eyelids, cheeks, back of auricles and mucosa of mouth and pharynx.

The fact that a person can die of hanging when a portion of the body is touching the ground may not be easily digestible for a non-forensic person. Controversies, litigations and re-investigations have happened in many partial hanging cases, either due to doubts of relatives or due to wrong interpretations of forensic surgeons. A few such cases of partial hanging are discussed below, which caused confusion to the autopsy surgeons and they opined it to be a homicide or inconclusive, but on further deliberation by experienced doctors, it was opined as a case of suicide.

Discussion on a Case of Partial Hanging of a 14-Year-Old School Girl in Her Dormitory of Boarding School

The death of a 14-year-old girl in a boarding school in Imphal resulted in a lot of hue and cry due to public outrage (Figure 4.36). Though initially it had been opined to be a case of suicide, her family members were alleging murder, arguing that a suicide could not have been possible in a dormitory with 37 other boarders. They refused to take the dead body back, and her body had been lying at the morgue of the government-owned Jawaharlal Nehru Institute of Medical Sciences (JNIMS). Thus far, two post-mortems have been conducted, and in both the reports, the cause of death was given to be hanging, even when one of the board members included a doctor chosen by the Joint

Action Committee (JAC) and her family. A 24-hour shutdown was called for by the public seeking justice in this case, and following pressure from various organizations, including the All Manipur Students' Union, the two hostel wardens were taken into custody and sent for 14-day judicial remand. While the wardens were arrested after a local court refused to grant them anticipatory bail, the principal and the administrator were let out on interim bail. The state government and the honorable court handed the investigation over to the CBI, and the CBI requested an expert medico-legal opinion from the Forensic Medicine Department of AIIMS, New Delhi.

This Medical Board constituted at AIIMS led by the author observed that the decedent had been found dead in partial hanging posture in her dormitory bunk bed by a synthetic rope (Figure 4.37a). There was no sign of any scuffle or forced entry by an outsider in the room. Postmortem staining showed a fixed glove and stocking pattern, and rigor mortis was fully developed in all the limbs and fixed in the same body posture of partial hanging. The ligature mark was an incomplete, discontinuous, dark brown pressure abrasion running obliquely around and placed higher up on the neck. Tongue was seen protruding out and bitten with drooling of saliva from the angle of the mouth and corresponding salivary stains on the T-shirt worn by the deceased (Figure 4.37b). There were no other ante-mortem injuries anywhere except for a partially healed, superficial, linear, horizontally placed incised wound at the front of her lower forearm with tailing towards the inner aspect.

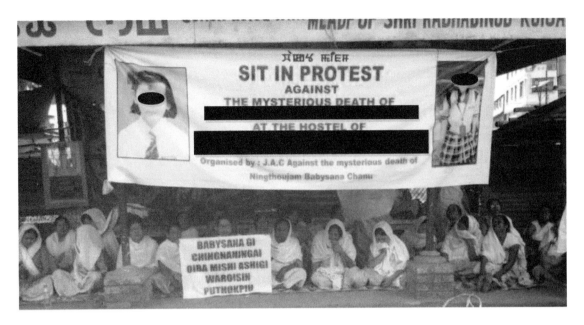

FIGURE 4.36 Deceased found in partial hanging position with a synthetic rope as the ligature material and suspended from the dormitory bunk bed.

No physical or laboratory evidence of sexual violence was present. The team also visited the scene of crime, discussed the case with the concerned forensic doctors who had conducted the previous two autopsies and studied every aspect of the case through the materials submitted to them for perusal. These included the postmortem report with videos and photographs of the autopsy procedures, videos of the scene of occurrence, Forensic Science Laboratory reports and statements of all the people concerned obtained by the CBI officials. The Medical Board concluded it as a case of partial hanging of suicidal manner.

Parents and the society at large usually feel suspicious about these kind of suicidal hangings at a young age. The author has noticed that the allegation of homicidal hanging or postmortem suspension usually arises in such cases, especially when the body is found in partial hanging position. The forensic pathologists dealing with these cases should take a systematic approach as far as possible to avoid

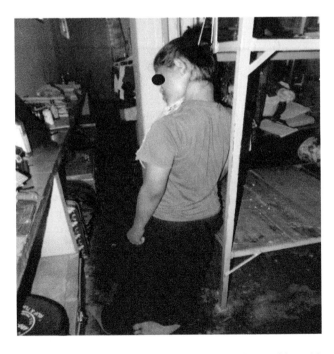

FIGURE 4.37a Deceased found in partial hanging position with a synthetic rope as the ligature material and suspended from the dormitory bunk bed.

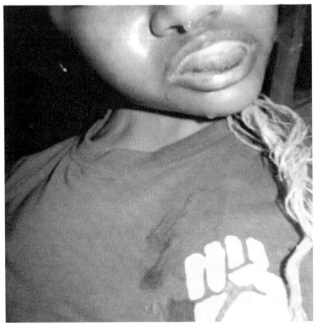

FIGURE 4.37b Tongue is seen protruding out and bitten with drooling of saliva from the angle of the mouth and corresponding salivary stains on the T-shirt worn by the deceased.

any future controversies and collect all possible specimens for future forensic examination. In such cases, the minimum samples that have to be collected include the ligature material with the knot undisturbed, cellophane lifts from the ligature mark site, hand swabs or fingernail clippings and swabs to rule out recent sexual acts.

DISCUSSION ON A CASE OF PARTIAL HANGING FROM SHIMLA, WHICH WAS HIGHLY CONTESTED BY PARENTS AS HOMICIDE DEATH IN 2011

Reaching a definitive cause and manner of death is the main target of any investigation. Detailed investigation and meticulous postmortem examination are key for reaching this objective. This is one such case where the same postmortem findings were interpreted by multiple Medical Boards but were unable to scientifically lead the investigating team to a logical conclusion and address the concern of the parents regarding a few of the autopsy findings.

A 21-year-old female had married her lover against her parents' wish. Two years into her marriage, she was found lying dead on the bed. A call regarding a suicide was made to the police station by an unidentified caller, and when police officers reached the place, they found the dead body of the deceased lying on the bed (Figure 4.38). An FIR was registered at the nearest police station by the mother of the deceased regarding the mysterious death of her daughter, and the dead body was shifted for the postmortem examination.

Postmortem was conducted at ESI Dispensary, Nalagarh, District Solan, which mentioned the following facts: 'A young lady who was of average built with no external injuries. Ligature mark which was yellowish brown in color 'V' shaped, with apex of the V on the left side. Ligature mark encircled the entire neck except for the left side below the left ear. It was present above the level of thyroid cartilage between the larynx and the chin. All internal dissection findings were reported as normal'.

The cause of death was opined as asphyxia due to antemortem hanging, and postmortem interval was given as 24 hours. Viscera analysis revealed no poison; the opinion on the wound on the left jaw seen in the photograph of the deceased was of an old burn wound from hot liquid and on the left cheek of the face was of acne vulgaris (Figure 4.39).

As this opinion was not satisfactory and explanatory for the family members of the deceased, they approached the court to get an opinion from a medical board. After considering a few unexplained facts, the Honorable High Court directed IGMC Shimla to give the opinion on 19.08.2009.

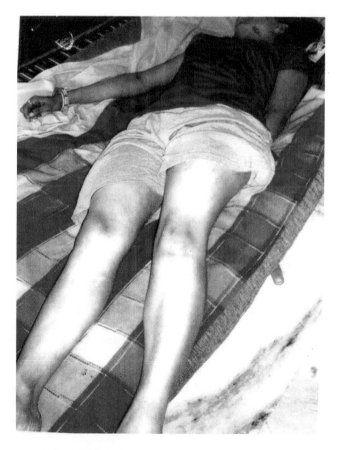

FIGURE 4.38 The deceased female was found lying dead on the bed when the police reached the place after receiving a call of someone committing a suicide.

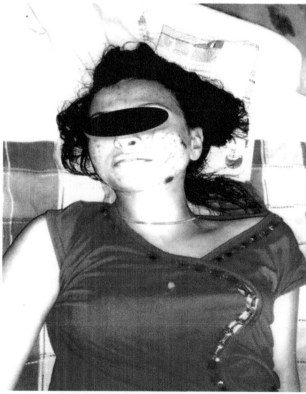

FIGURE 4.39 The deceased female was found lying dead on the bed with an injury over the left jaw and acne vulgaris over her left cheek.

Reason for the Medical Board Opinion

After dissatisfactory initial investigation by the police, the chief investigating authority constituted a board. Postmortem report and a few lacunas in the investigation created doubt among the family members of the deceased, which had to be resolved before reaching a conclusion. Major lacunae were:

- No magistrate inquest as per 176 CrPC was conducted even though victim was only 21 years old and death occurred within 7 years of marriage.
- Why was the postmortem initially not conducted by board of doctors?
- No request was made for preservation of hair and nail sample.
- Description of the postmortem report was not self-explanatory.

First Medical Board Opinion from IGMC Shimla

A board of six doctors, including five members and a chairman, reviewed all the documents given to them for their perusal, and after going through them, the board was of the opinion that from the available records, it was not possible to give the exact cause of death due to want of complete records and partial findings; however, there was nothing to suggest about the possibility of strangulation in the absence of the struggle mark, poisoning and any other factors contributing to the cause of death.

The Honorable High Court was not happy with the opinion given by the board and raised a few questions that were not systematically explained in a view that the court could understand. The court objected that the doctors could not explain the multiple injuries present on the face of the girl as per photographs in the records. Similarly, the reasons for some of the facts were not clearly explained to the court, i.e., if it's a case of hanging, why the neck was not found stretched and elongated? The eyes are closed or partially open? No dribbling of saliva is present in this case. Do they think it's a sure sign of hanging? In the present case, none of the findings suggesting hanging were found. So the court thinks that these signs were overlooked by the doctors. Considering the above facts, the court rejected the medical board's opinion.

Further, in view of the case, the honorable court asked for another medical board opinion with special mention that the report must be self-speaking based on the evidence brought on record till date, including Postmortem report, Forensic Science Laboratory report, photographs and connecting evidences.

Second Medical Board Opinion from AIIMS, New Delhi

The honorable court asked the Director AIIMS to constitute a medical board for the opinion. For the same, a board of three doctors was constituted, and the final opinion given was as follows:

After careful perusal of the inquest papers provided, photographs of the deceased, finding as mentioned in PM report, FSL report, examination of the exhibits and opinion of the medical board of IGMC Shimla, we are of the considered opinion that:

- The cause of death in this case is Asphyxia due to Antemortem Hanging by Ligature.
- In absence of signs of struggle and FSL report negative for common poisons, the hanging in this case could be suicidal in nature.
- Dribbling of saliva is considered to be the surest sign of antemortem hanging whenever it is present but it is not seen in all the cases of hanging.
- Neck is not necessarily found stretched and elongated in case of hanging.
- The faint ligature mark as mentioned in postmortem report could be possible by the dupatta/chadar as mentioned. But the ligature mark is unlikely to be caused by the cable wire.
- The photograph show acne vulgaris on the face with slight bleeding on the left cheek as well as impression of the ligature on left side chin near the angle of mandible. The bleeding from the acne could have occurred during the process of hanging and is unlikely to be because of injury.

Even after a detailed, clear and self-explanatory opinion, the honorable court rejected the same as giving the fact that the main purpose of the report from AIIMS was an **independent opinion wholly uninfluenced by the earlier report from IGMC**. As this opinion was influenced by the earlier report, it was rejected. So an order for a third medical board from Lady Harding Medical College, New Delhi for an independent opinion was passed.

Third Medical Board Opinion from LHMC New Delhi

After two consequent rejections of medical board opinions, the court ordered the Medical Superintendent, LHMC for opinion. After considering all the facts, the third medical board observed lacunae in the description of scene of crime, inquest papers, about the investigation and proceedings by investigating officer (IO), PM report and photographs. After that, it was opined as: "It is not possible for us to give the exact opinion regarding the cause of death from the supplied material and it is further asked that the investigating agency submit few more detailed photographs, reports of blood stains on the ligature material and stains over the t-shirt and dupatta.'

The medical board of LHMC was of the opinion that the **"Possibility of death of deceased as a result of Asphyxia due to Hanging cannot be ruled out. There is nothing on the record to suggest that death could have been occurred due to strangulation."**

As the opinions by different medical boards were not given with certainty, which hampers the path of law, for reaching a particular conclusion, a definitive opinion based on the facts is required, which can stand in the court of law. Now, the honorable court transferred the case to the CBI for an independent, unbiased opinion.

CBI Opinion from AIIMS

The CBI received the case in March 2011, and they requested the Director AIIMS to depute a doctor for forensic assistance in the case. The author was chosen for providing the expert opinion.

The CBI submitted a questionnaire along with the entire necessary documents and other relevant inquest papers, which included the FIR, photographs of the deceased, postmortem report of ESI Dispensary, Nalagarh, District Solan, subsequent opinion of the doctor who conducted the autopsy and forensic lab report.

Crime Scene Visit

On the author's insistence, the CBI arranged for a crime scene visit in June 2011; the place of occurrence was Baddi, Himachal Pradesh (Figures 4.40 and 4.41). The author also interacted with the doctor who conducted the postmortem examination, initial investigating officer/constable and the

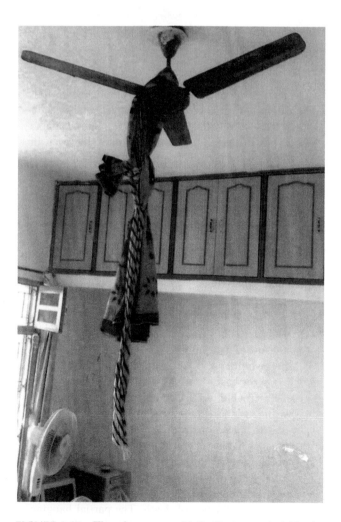

FIGURE 4.40 The crime scene with the ligature material in situ tied to the ceiling fan.

first eyewitness. Reconstruction of the original scene of occurrence was done for better understanding of the crime scene and position of the ligature. The author also interacted with the aggrieved father and uncle of the deceased, who were present for any input to shed light in the medical conclusion of the case.

The author answered the queries given in the questionnaire so that it can give more clarity to the court for judgement. Here are the following queries asked and their answers:

1. **What is the medico-legal inference of injury in neck as described ligature mark? Whether the death is due to strangulation by ligature and subsequent postmortem hanging? To mimic death due to hanging? It is the point of contention and requires the clarity.**

    The Geometry of the mark is important in interpreting fatal events. In strangulation, unlike hanging, the mark tends to encircle the neck horizontally and at a lower level. Typically it crosses immediately above or below the prominence of the larynx and passes back to the nape of neck. In homicide where a single turn is used, there is often a cross over point where the two ends of the ligature mark overlap. This may be at the front, side or back of the neck depending on the relative position of assailant and victim.

    As per medical science, the imprint of ligature material in the neck will appear in both cases of ante-mortem or postmortem hanging or strangulation which is called pressure abrasion or imprint/pattern abrasion. In case of death due to strangulation by ligature and subsequent postmortem hanging, there will be two ligature marks seen: one for the strangulation which will be more or less horizontal and another for hanging which will be more or less obliquely present in the neck. The ligature mark will be most likely separate or even if overlapping each other that will be only partial in whole circumference of neck in case of ante-mortem strangulation by ligature and subsequent postmortem suspension of the body to mimic ante-mortem hanging as cause of death it is evident that there will be two ligature marks on the neck: one mark will be of strangulation and another ligature mark will be of post mortem hanging; however, on examination of the photographs in record of CBI, Postmortem Report and after thorough discussion with the doctor who had conducted the PM examination, and initial police investigating personnel who were the eye witness of the case found nothing suggestive of the presence of double ligature mark in front of the neck of the deceased except a single faint oblique ligature mark. An oval-shaped injury seen in photograph is also simple in nature.

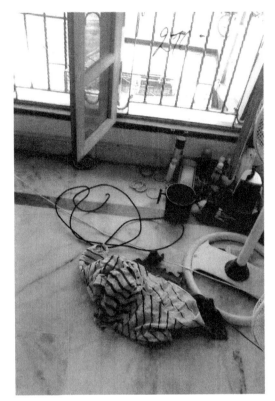 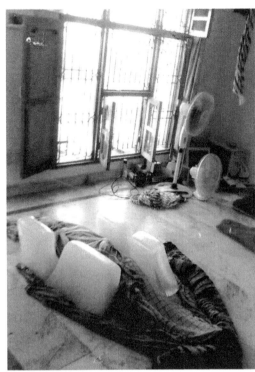

FIGURE 4.41   Photos of the crime scene taken during the recovery of the dead body.

OPINION-1

In given examined circumstances and evidences in record of CBI it may be concluded that the cause of death as a result of strangulation by ligature and subsequent postmortem hanging is ruled out.

2. **What is the medico-legal inference of injury in neck described as ligature mark? Whether it is a case of ante-mortem homicidal hanging by use of force/overpower/poisoning?**

    This is also a necessary component of medico-legal perusal. The FSL report of viscera of the deceased is negative for common poison in this case means the victim was not under influence of intoxication or poisoning prior to the sad incidence of death and suggests that she may be in normal physical condition. On further examination, neither in PM report nor in the photograph nor in the observation of eye witness, there are any findings found suggestive of signs of active struggle/resistance offered in the form of injuries on the body of deceased as well as in the clothing. Homicidal hanging is a much more violent form of asphyxial death and is not feasible without complete physical overpower/mouth is gagged/limbs are tied and struggle leaving significant injuries in the body of normal victim. Further as per medical literature, the homicidal hanging is extremely rare and generally seen in the form of lynching and judicial hanging where it is a complete hanging means foot will be above the ground and complete body weight of the victim will act as constricting force to make sure the death of victim by assailant; however, in this case the type of hanging is partial hanging—means the feet of the deceased was touching the cot at the level of knee and only partial body weight was working as constricting force on neck.

OPINION-2

It may be concluded that in the given situation of the case, the cause of death as ante-mortem homicidal hanging or homicidal hanging by use of force/overpower/poisoning is ruled out.

3. **Whether it is a case of death due to asphyxia as a result of ante-mortem hanging or not? If yes then whether it is a case of suicidal hanging?**

    On the basis of all the material evidences available in record of CBI in this case and exclusion of various probabilities I am of considered opinion that the cause of death in this case is combined effect of Asphyxia and ischemia as a result of ante-mortem partial hanging by alleged Ligature found at the scene of incidence on ceiling fan which has been examined by me on 4th June 2011 at the scene of incidence of death. The partial hanging is generally suicidal in nature and on the above exclusion in this case it is a case of suicide.

BASIS OF OPINION: Opinion is derived on of examination/perusal of the initial inquest papers, photographs of the deceased, recorded findings in postmortem report, FSL reports, and discussion on recall memory of the doctor who had conducted the PM examination and initial police investigating team who were eye witness and to the best of my knowledge the following evidences are sufficient to derive the above conclusion. The faint ligature mark as mentioned in postmortem report/seen by them could be possible by the examined dupatta in the CBI record at the scene on 4th June 2011 The body of the deceased was in compatible position with self-suspension FSL report is negative for common poison. Ligature mark encircles on the entire neck except on the left side below left ear, Ligature mark above the level of thyroid cartilage, between the larynx and the chin. Width of groove of ligature mark was one inch to 1.5" compatible with ligature. Scalp, skull and vertebrae along with thorax; thorax; pleura, larynx and trachea, right and left lung, pericardium, heart, large vessels, walls of abdomen, peritoneum, mouth, pharynx and esophagus are normal. Ligature was high up in neck and incomplete. It is a case of partial hanging no injuries on the hands and other part of the body of victim in the form resistance.

Dribbling of saliva is considered to be a sign of ante-mortem hanging but it is not necessarily seen in all the cases of hanging since the secretion of saliva in hanging is dependent upon, the stimulation of salivary glands which are situated in the neck by ligature material during the course of hanging due to its mechanical force as well as it depends upon the positioning of ligature material on neck during the ante-mortem period/exactly prior to death. It is a case of partial hanging and only partial body weight is working as constricting force on neck and this is the reason that the ligature mark is faint. Hence in this case or any other case of hanging particularly partial hanging where the salivary glands are not stimulated by the constricting force of ligature there is no dribbling of saliva seen and the same in this case cannot be ruled out.

The neck of the deceased will not be stretched and elongated in this case since as it is a case of partial hanging and complete body weight is not working as stretching force. The eyes may remain open in a case of ante-mortem hanging. As per literature only in approximately 25 percent cases suicide notes are left.

4. **What is the medico-legal inference of oval shape injury in neck and another injury in left face? Is the above two injury are ante-mortem or post-mortem in origin? Means injuries originated prior to death, during death or after death and what is the nature/is it simple/grievous or dangerous injury?**

Both the injuries are ante-mortem in nature as evident with color of injuries seen in photograph and both the injuries are simple in nature individually as well collectively. The color of the oval shape injury on neck as seen in photograph (Figure 4.42) is either due to contusion an injury appreciated by coloration or its redness is due to inflammatory changes as seen in burn injury. The injury due to knot of ligature will be an abrasion particularly in a case of partial hanging and there will be no such coloration of injury on skin because the pressure abrasion is appreciated by epidermis of skin (a blood less layer of skin) which are void of blood vessel and there will be no coloration. In view of this the oval shape injury as an imprint pattern abrasion due to knot of ligature is ruled out.

The doctor who had conducted the postmortem examination had written in PM Report that injury oval in shape in neck could have been produced by hot liquid and his appreciation as a doctor and eye

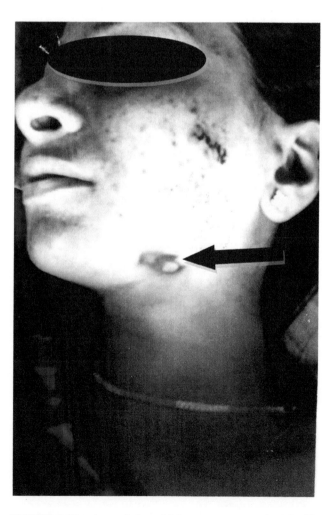

FIGURE 4.42 An oval-shaped injury present over the left side of the neck, reddish in color.

witness of injury as well my discussion with the doctor during my visit in Nalagarh PM House on 4th June 2011 the injury caused by hot liquid/tea a burn injury cannot be ruled out since the visual appreciation of a bum injury is a routine matter of any practicing doctor.

5. **What is the forensic importance/explanation of injury in left face? What is the significant and forensic importance of injury on Left face in a case of suicide of a young newlywed woman?**

The photographs are showing acne vulgaris on face with slight bleeding red in color on left side of cheek (Figure 4.43). Bleeding is an ante-mortem phenomena hence it is an ante-mortem injury means prior to death and may be of fresh in origin or of few hours prior to death. The acne doesn't bleed during the process of hanging even oozing of blood is unlikely seen. It is a laceration injury caused by blunt force. The injury as self-inflicted is also ruled out since self-inflicted injury may be multiple and in the form of scratch abrasion during the process of death due to hanging.

It is further clarified that both, injury on face and oval shape injury in neck are simple in nature

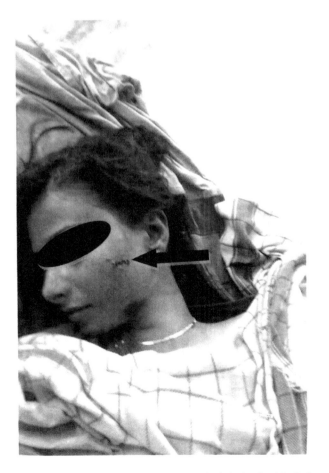

FIGURE 4.43 Acne vulgaris seen over the left cheek with slight bleeding.

have no physical bearing into the cause of death. However, the presence of injury on the face along with an ante-mortem burn injury on neck is a subject matter of investigation.

It can be seen that in the postmortem, findings remained the same. However, based on the same findings, different opinions have been given at various stages. It can surely create confusion and lack of trust in the eyes of the judiciary and the investigators. In criminal cases, medical conclusions are based on a reasonable degree of certainty, and in the court of law doctors as an expert witness is expected to provide this evidence clearly beyond any reasonable doubt.

A definitive opinion on the basis of clear facts can solve much confusion and help the court in framing a judgement. The same facts are to be explained with a reasonable degree of certainty in the medico-legal opinion so it gives assistance to court because sometimes a simple confusion leads to delay in justice.

DISCUSSION ON A CASE OF PARTIAL HANGING WITH DECEASED IN STANDING POSTURE AND ALLEGATION OF HOMICIDE

A young fashion designer had married the proprietor of a local newspaper in 2008, but the relationship soured by 2011 and the two had been living separately for some time. In August 2017, she was found dead at her in-law's house in standing posture with a chunni tied around her neck, the other end of which was attached to the ceiling fan above (Figure 4.44). A few dried drops of blood were found on the floor immediately beneath the body, and a bucket was seen nearby that had not been toppled. All this made her parents suspicious about possible foul play. They accused her husband and in-laws of murdering their daughter. After two separate investigations (first by Rajpur police and the next one by a Special Investigation Team headed by a Superintendent of Police-level officer), the death was opined as suicidal in manner. Her parents then approached the High Court for justice, and a case of murder was registered and handed over to the CBI. The room where the dead body was discovered had been found locked from inside. Postmortem examination of the deceased was conducted at a nearby government hospital by a team of two doctors, who reported a ligature mark as the only injury present over the body and described it as 'Ligature mark around the neck: below the chin & above the thyroid going backwards and interrupted oblique towards right side. Base of the groove is brownish and is hard, parchment-like, margins abraded. Subcutaneous tissue underneath the ligature mark; white, hard and glistening'. Cause of death was given as 'asphyxia due to ante-mortem hanging'. Chemical analysis of the preserved viscera did not yield any poison.

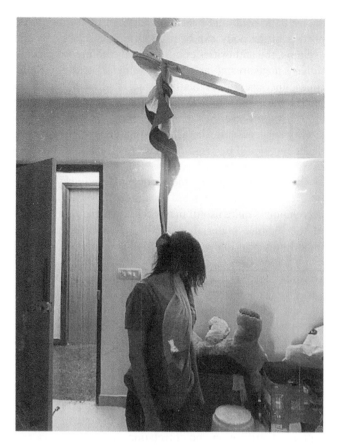

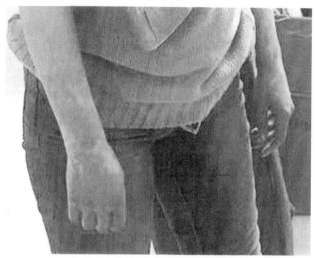

FIGURE 4.45   Glove and stocking pattern of postmortem lividity was seen in the body. This picture shows the distribution of livor mortis in the lower part of the hands, indicating that the body remained in the suspended position for a considerable duration of time.

FIGURE 4.44   The deceased was found in partial hanging position with her legs touching the ground and her knees slightly flexed. The bucket seen next to the deceased was presumably used to reach the desired height for fixing the ligature material. The ligature material was chunni suspended from the ceiling fan in the room, which was bent due to the weight of suspension.

Then the CBI requested an expert medico-legal opinion from AIIMS under the chairmanship of the author. All the related documents, including scene of occurrence photographs, postmortem report, previous expert opinion given by a board of forensic doctors from a state-run medical college and forensic science laboratory reports, were submitted for perusal. After considering all the facts and findings related to the case, the AIIMS Medical Board opined it to be a case of partial hanging, suicidal in manner. The presence of some blood-stained fluid was noted over the nostrils, which is not rare in hanging cases, and the same could have produced the blood stains seen on the floor. A glove and stocking pattern of postmortem lividity was appreciable in the photos submitted (Figure 4.45). Since there was no breach of skin anywhere over the body, the blood drops were concluded to originate from the nostrils, which is sometimes seen in cases of partial hanging as the degree of congestion in these is more than that in complete hanging. Since the knot was at the back and the neck was in flexed position, the blood drops could have hit the ground without touching the front of the chest region or the clothes.

CLASSIFICATION OF HANGING ACCORDING TO THE POSITION OF KNOT

TYPICAL HANGING

Many authors categorize hanging based on the placement of knot or the point of suspension. The term 'typical hanging' refers to cases wherein the knot or the point of suspension is positioned at posterior midline. In these cases, there is a symmetric occlusion of blood vessels of the neck bilaterally, resulting in complete cerebral anoxia.

ATYPICAL HANGING

Atypical hanging represents all other knot positions. In these, complete blockage of the vessels of one side with partial compression of arteries on the other side may happen, theoretically producing unilateral congestion and petechiae, but such a finding is rarely seen during routine case work. Atypical hanging is the commonest variety and is further divided into subclasses by some authors.

Mental Knot Position

Here the knot is placed over the mentum in the front midline. Based on the vertical placement of the knot, it is further divided into supra and sub-mental. The supra-mental knot commonly does not produce knot impression. Since the mouth is directed upwards in mental knot positions, salivary dribble marks at angles of mouth are generally not seen. Compression of blood vessels at the back and the sides results in death with manual airway compression. Vertebral fractures are possible in sudden fall as the entire body weight gets transferred to the posterior aspect of neck.

Mandibular Knot Position

The knot is placed along the mandible in between the mentum and the angles. A knot position below the level of mandible is called sub-mandibular and above it over the face is called supra-mandibular. In such types of knot placements, the head will be seen turned to the side opposite to the knot with dribbling of saliva occurring from the contra-lateral angle of the mouth. The tongue may remain inside the oral cavity, and hypostasis of face occurs on the side opposite to the knot.

Auricular or Mandibulo-Mastoid Knot Position

The knot is placed between the angle of the mandible and the mastoid process. The impression of the knot may not be present in many of these cases. Dribbling of saliva occurs from the contra-lateral side since the head gets turned towards the opposite direction.

Mastoid Knot Position

The knot is positioned over the mastoid process. A knot impression may not be seen at all in the supra-mastoid position or if seen may be very faint due to the high density of hair.

Occipitomastoid Knot Position

In this type, the knot is situated between the posterior midline and the mastoid process. The head shows a forward tilt and dribbling of saliva is commonly seen over the front of the chest or the abdomen at the side opposite to the knot.

ACCORDING TO THE MANNER OF DEATH

On the basis of manner, hanging cases can be classified into suicidal, homicidal and accidental. Determining the manner of death in hanging cases is important like it is in any other type of death. The possibility of getting variable autopsy findings in cases with similar circumstances makes this a complicated exercise in some instances. Scene of occurrence examination clears any doubt about the manner in most of the cases of hanging, and the same has to be carried out whenever the forensic surgeon is in doubt. Since hanging deaths account for a huge proportion of the total caseload in any autopsy center, all forensic surgeons should be well trained and always focused in this regard. A more detailed discussion on these medico-legal aspects is given later in the book.

LIGATURE MATERIAL

Ligature material is one of the key factors in hanging deaths, and it includes a wide variety of materials such as ropes, shawls, sarees, kurtas, towels, neck ties, belts, chains, etc (Figure 4.46 a-h). Virtually any object that can encircle the neck and bear the weight of the unsupported portion of the body can be used as a ligature. In jails and asylums, the authorities commonly take numerous precautionary measures so as to avoid suicidal attempts. Many times, unconventional ligature materials like multiple torn pieces of a cloth that have been joined together or even the elastic waist bands of underwear may be used. The possibility of accessing the alleged ligature material by the decedent should be cross-checked in all cases of hanging to rule out foul play.

Ligature material and the corresponding injury need to be examined and correlated in almost all cases, and this correlation is quite useful in concluding these cases. Fibers of the ligature material generally get transferred to the underlying skin due to friction and can be demonstrated using cellophane tape lifts from the ligature mark. It is advisable to preserve and analyze these in all suspicious cases.

Harder materials produce more prominent ligature marks due to the greater friction and pressure produced. Very hard and broad materials like leather belts can produce friction marks at both borders with an intervening pale pressure band. The specific pattern of the ligature material surface gets imprinted on the ligature mark and is more appreciable under an oblique illumination. Use of a hand magnifying lens yields better results for imprint pattern identification and correlation. In cases of very soft material, the ligature mark may be absent even after hours of suspension.

Any rimmed structure can act as a ligature material if the neck gets compressed over it in prone position and cause death by 'hanging' when the body weight in part or whole acts as the compressing force. These partial hanging cases usually show some degree of incapacitation of the individual commonly due to drugs, alcohol or some natural disease like seizure disorder/epilepsy.

Type of Knot

In the case of a loop, the mark will be deepest on the side of the neck to which the head has inclined. The knot mark is not usually seen. But in the case of a running noose, the mark more or less encircles the neck and is prominent beneath the knot.

- *Slip knot (Figure 4.46 i):* It is a simple knot through which a ligature material can slip freely. It allows the noose to tighten if the dragging force is maintained. In hanging cases, a slip knot allows the noose circumference to get smaller with time and produce a continuous ligature mark completely encircling the neck. The ligature mark caused by a running noose in such cases may mimic ligature strangulation due to its continuity.
- *Reef or granny knot (Figure 4.46 j):* It is formed when the ligature end is knotted in conventional manner to itself forming a fixed noose.

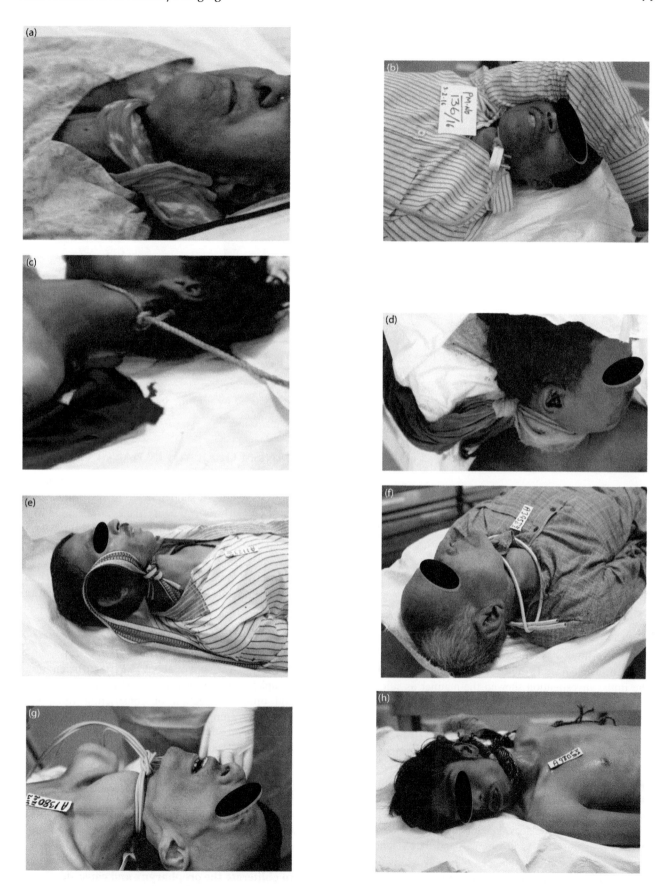

FIGURE 4.46 Examples of some of the ligature materials that have been used for hanging: (a) dupatta, (b) electric cord, (c) rope, (d) gamcha/shawl, (e) cot strap, (f) and (g) electrical wire, (h) double ligature material with rope and cloth. *(Continued)*

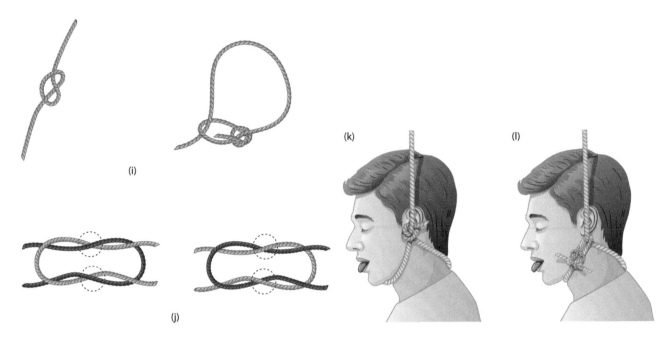

FIGURE 4.46 *(Continued)* (i) Slip knot. (j) Reef or Granny knot (k) Running noose and (l) Fixed noose.

TYPE OF NOOSE

Noose refers to the circle formed by the ligature material which causes constriction of neck during hanging. It can be of the following types:

- *Running Noose (Figure 4.46 k):* The noose formed by passing the ligature through a slip knot.
- *Fixed Noose (Figure 4.46 l):* The noose formed using a reef knot or a granny knot.

DISCUSSION ON A CASE OF SUICIDAL HANGING USING VARIOUS LIGATURE MATERIALS

A 23-year-old male had visited his female friend's house for an overnight stay. He was found hanging from the ceiling fan at his friend's place the next morning. Although the initial investigation showed the manner as suicide, the relatives of the deceased alleged murder as they were suspicious of the events and the narration of his friends.

Post-mortem examination was done at AIIMS mortuary, and the ligature material used in the case was an off-white maxi dress with a transparent plastic button and an irregular border at one end. The other end was tied to a blue *'nara'* (draw cord/draw string) having a knot and two free ends which were tied to the ceiling fan. The ligature material was loosely encircling the neck. During the postmortem examination, a ligature mark, incomplete and parchmentized at places, was present over the neck obliquely, going upwards and backwards, in both the directions (Figures 4.47a and 4.47b). The manner of death in this case was suicidal. The ligature material used had a very close correlation with the ligature mark injury present on the neck as well as the injuries produced by it in the internal neck structures seen on dissection.

MECHANISM OF DEATH IN HANGING

The neck provides a conduit to various vital structures throughout its length. A sudden insult to any of them individually or collectively can cause the death of an individual. These structures mainly include the carotid arteries, the jugular venous system, the airway, which includes pharynx, larynx and trachea, and the upper spinal cord. The constrictive force in hanging causes variable mechanical and/or functional disruption of these vital structures, resulting in death. The quantum of force needed to disrupt the vital structures is different and has been extensively studied.

- *Asphyxia:* A weight of about 15 kg is sufficient for complete tracheal obstruction. Due to the oblique and upward direction of constricting force in hanging, it commonly does not completely occlude the trachea or larynx. However, this compressive force is sufficient to cause elevation and posterior displacement of the root of the tongue and adjacent structures, resulting in their approximation with the posterior pharyngeal wall. This obstructs the airway completely and results in asphyxia. In most cases, the placement of ligature is above the level of the larynx and the hyoid, and the upward and backward force transmitted through it **is sufficient to obliterate the oropharynx and cause death**.
- *Venous occlusion:* Since the vessel walls of veins are less muscular, veins of jugular system are easily compressible. Even a compressive force

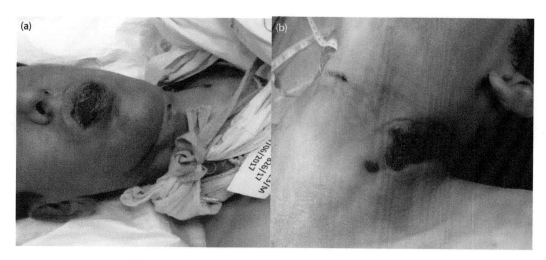

FIGURE 4.47 (a) Two ligature materials used. (b) Ligature mark on the neck.

exerted by a 2 kg weight is sufficient for complete jugular obstruction, which results in back pooling and stagnation of deoxygenated blood above the level of ligature. Venous pressure above the level of the constricting force gradually rises, resulting in rupture of smaller vessels like venules and capillaries. The hypoxic atmosphere also results in oozing out of intravascular fluids, and its sequelae include severe congestion, cyanosis and edema of the face and the upper neck with multiple petechiae. The congestion, cyanosis and edema generally fade or even disappear when the body is taken down from hanging position and the noose is loosened. Even then, visible petechial hemorrhages persist. Death occurs relatively slowly by this mechanism. Such a mechanism is common in incomplete suspensions where the compressive force is relatively less.

- *Arterial occlusion:* Internal carotid arteries and vertebral arteries are the sole arterial supply to a highly oxygen-dependent organ and hence hypoxia-prone brain. Many scientists studied the minimum force needed to compress and completely occlude these arteries and found that the force transmitted by about a 5 kg weight is sufficient for complete occlusion of common carotid arteries and about 20 kg occludes the vertebral arteries. In complete hanging, the fall produces sudden complete occlusion of all these arteries, and critical brain hypoxia supervenes within a few seconds. Abrupt stoppage of arterial supply to the brain generally results in unconsciousness in around 5–11 seconds. If all these arteries are suddenly occluded and the compression is maintained, hanging does not show any facial congestion, edema or petechiae. Rather, cases of complete suspension generally show facial pallor instead. If asymmetrical pressure dissipation happens due to the peculiarity of noose, one may see mixed findings of paleness on one side and congestion and petechiae on the other.

- *Reflex vagal stimulation:* In many cases of hanging, the noose at anterior aspect of the neck is settled at the level of the carotid bifurcation. As a result, the underlying carotid sinuses get compressed, thereby exciting pressure sensors and activating the afferent pathway of the vagal cardiac inhibition reflex. This postulated mechanism explains the pale face and 'spontaneous' motionless deaths in many cases.

- *Vertebral fractures:* Generally, cervical vertebral fractures occur only in unsupported 'long drops'. When a body falling with reasonable velocity suddenly stops due to the noose around neck, the transmitted force is generally sufficient to fracture one to two cervical vertebrae (Figures 4.48a and 4.48b). A judicial hanging, where an unsupported free fall of about six feet or more is maintained beneath the trap door, generally ensures these fractures. Fracture of the odontoid process of the axis (C2) is a common fracture of this kind, and has been termed as hangman's fracture. C3 and C4 fractures are also not uncommon. Since long drops are rare in suicidal settings, these fractures are not encountered in everyday forensic practice and are only seen when a person jumps from the branch of a tree or from higher stories of a building, resulting in a long, unsupported fall followed by sudden stoppage due to the noose around the neck. The fractured vertebrae may directly injure the enclosed spinal cord in many cases. For example, Hangman's fracture may result in the separation of the lower medulla and spinal cord. Fracture separations cause the neck to elongate with time, and in cases where the ligature material used is very thin, even decapitation may occur.

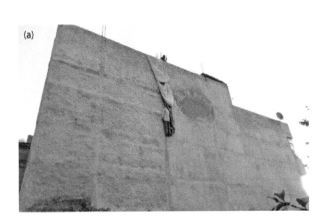

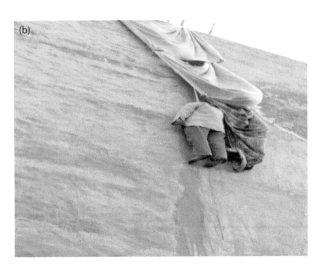

FIGURE 4.48 (a) Case of complete hanging from a building with a long drop resulting in the fracture of the cervical vertebrae. (b) Closer view of the case of complete hanging from a building.

REVIEW OF PATHOPHYSIOLOGY OF HANGING

Vertebral artery is placed relatively deep in the neck and has a protective covering provided by the cervical vertebrae, and hence, greater pressure is needed for its occlusion. Old studies conducted on cadavers at the end of the 19th and beginning of the 20th century have reported the pressures needed to occlude the neck structures as follows: jugular veins- 2 kg, carotid arteries- 5 kg, trachea- 15 kg, vertebral arteries- 30 kg. These values have doubtful credibility in cases of hanging, as during these cadaveric experiments, the pressure vectors were applied perpendicularly, but in real life ante-mortem hanging, the pressure vectors are diagonally oriented at various angles to the neck depending on the position of ligature and knot, the suspension point, etc.

Austrian author Hoffman shared his view that hanging was a form of respiratory asphyxia, but he believed that the cartilaginous structures of the larynx and trachea could not be sufficiently compressed to cause obstruction. Instead, he proposed that it was the compression of these structures against the posterior pharyngeal wall that caused the respiratory obstruction, sometimes in association with occlusion by the base of the tongue.

In 1893 in England, Dixon further emphasized the crucial role of respiratory asphyxia in death by hanging. In support of his theory he had been able to directly visualize the effects of neck compression on the laryngotracheal area and he cited the work of Langreuter, a German researcher who did experiments by tying a rope around the neck of cadavers who had died of natural cause. He demonstrated that with moderate neck compression, the epiglottis became crushed against the posterior pharyngeal wall, obstructing the upper airways. With more intense compression, not only the epiglottis but also the base of the tongue was pushed back against the posterior pharyngeal wall. Apart from this interesting autopsy study, Dixon also substantiated his point of view by reporting a case seen by his colleague, Ecker, in which the frozen body of a hanging man was found and similar anatomic evidence of compression was observed at autopsy.

Brouardel stated in his book that by applying a 15 kg of weight on the neck, the pressure exerted by the base of the tongue on the pharynx is sufficient to completely block any airflow. To further support this opinion, he described large retropharyngeal ecchymoses in victims of judicial hangings.

Balthazard, Smith and Webster continued to publish that the principal mechanism of death in hanging was respiratory asphyxia and that vascular occlusion was a minor contributor.

Studies done by Tardieu, Hofmann, Dixon, Guy and Ferrier, Brouardel, Lacassagne, Balthazard, Smith and Webster all conclude that respiratory asphyxia is the main mechanism of death in hanging, and most of them also consider vascular occlusion as a possible mechanism of death in hanging.

Compressing the bilateral carotids will produce loss of consciousness. The loss of consciousness can reduce the muscle tone, which may further lead to compression of other vital structures in the neck. There are no studies conducted wherein prolonged neck pressure has been applied only to the carotids to see if death occurs. The loss of consciousness is mainly due to transient ischemia suffered by those areas supplied by the anterior circulation of the brain. The posterior circulation, which feeds the vital center for respiration, is supplied by the vertebral system and is usually unaffected by neck compression unless there is a traumatic injury to vertebral system. Such injuries are especially seen in cases of judicial hangings where the drop heights are longer.

CONCLUSION ON CAUSE OF DEATH IN HANGING

The author, based on his experience in dealing with hanging cases and observing the autopsy findings in relation to the position of the ligature, knot, suspension point and the study of existing literature, would like to conclude that one

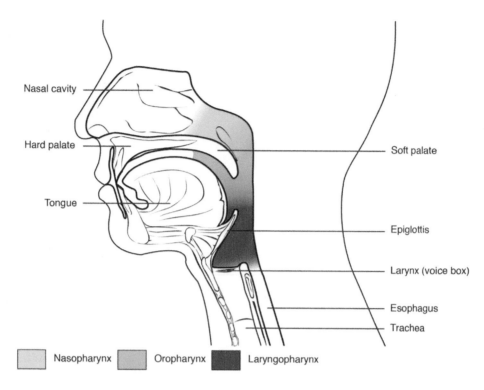

FIGURE 4.49 The various sub-divisions of pharynx, and it is seen that the oropharynx connects the oral cavity, nasopharynx and the laryngopharynx.

of the primary mechanisms of death in a case of hanging is due to posterior pharyngeal obstruction due to pressure on the soft structures of neck and floor of mouth, finally leading to respiratory asphyxia. The oropharynx is the most critical passage in the respiratory system, which joins the oral cavity and nasopharynx with the larynx and laryngopharynx. The oropharynx consists of the tongue base, tonsillar region and lateral and posterior oropharyngeal walls (Figure 4.49).

These all play the essential function in inspiration/ expiration, swallowing and speech, which involves over 30 muscles, multiple motor and sensory nerves, and coordination by the brainstem, and cortex and sub-cortical structures. Mechanical blockage and obstruction of the pharyngeal cavity by ligature pressure results in paralysis of the function of oropharynx and leads to complete deprivation of oxygen to brain. This in turn leads to necrosis and death of neurons of respiratory centers in pons and medulla, resulting in apnea, loss of spontaneous respiration and brain stem death. The intrinsic and extrinsic tongue muscles and other muscles responsible for opening/closing of jaws and the pharynx, especially those innervated by hypoglossal nerve, which prevents tongue from being bitten or falling behind to obstruct the air passage, also get paralyzed in some cases. Constriction and drawing of the posterior pharyngeal wall forward, and backward displacement of the back of the tongue due to mechanical constricting force applied by the ligature pressure on oropharynx almost immediately closes the airway, causing asphyxia and unconsciousness due to compromise and collapse of the pharynx. Author would like to present the proof of this

consideration with a comparison between postmortem CT finding of the neck in a case of hanging with the ligature material still present in situ encircling the neck, which shows that the critical passage of oropharynx is obstructed by pressure applied by the ligature (Figure 4.50) even when the vertical pull of the ligature in hanging is removed while recovering the dead body in the crime scene, and the postmortem CT finding of neck in a control case with no compressive force over the neck where the oropharynx is patent (Figure 4.51).

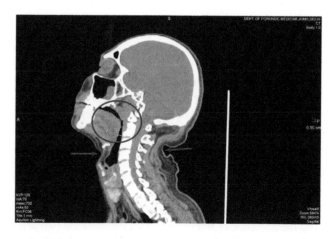

FIGURE 4.50 Postmortem CT examination of the neck in a case of hanging with ligature present in situ compressing the neck (*red arrows*) and causing narrowing and closure of the oropharynx (*red circle*) even when the vertical pull of the ligature hanging is removed while recovering the dead body in the scene of occurrence.

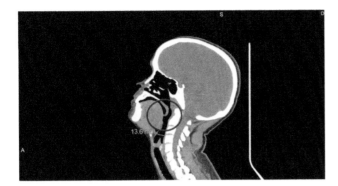

FIGURE 4.51 Postmortem CT examination of a control case without any compressive forced applied on the neck. The oropharynx remains patent with neither the base of tongue pushed back nor the posterior pharyngeal wall pushed front (*red circle*).

Obstruction of this critical passage due to this mechanical force results in loss of speech and capability to shout or make noise, and that is the reason for encountering cases where a person commits suicide by hanging and remains unnoticed/unheard by wife/husband/individual sleeping in same room. In the author's experience, the below-mentioned case is a good example for this phenomena. In this case, postmortem examination was conducted by the author in 2013 on the body of a 35-year-old male who was arrested as an accused in the Nirbhaya gang rape case (Figure 4.52). He was found hanging by a rope inside the barrack of Tihar central jail. Along with the deceased, on the night of the incident, about 40 other inmates were present, sleeping inside the barrack. None of them reported hearing any shouting or crying by the deceased. In the author's 27 years of experience, no case of hanging has been encountered by him where any shouting or crying by the deceased was reported by the relatives or police.

In most of the cases of death due to smothering by means of closure of mouth and nostrils, similar absence of hearing of crying or shouting has been observed. Though some vague moaning sounds may be heard by nearby persons.

For making an audible cry or shout, an intact communicating airway is needed for the complete resonance of the vocal cords. Whenever the free passage of air flow to the exterior is obstructed by neck compression as in hanging or by occlusion of the external respiratory orifices like mouth and nostrils as in smothering, this mechanism of sound production is compromised, hence no audible crying or shouting is present.

Vascular occlusion is also a possible mechanism, but it is less likely the primary cause in most cases of hanging deaths due to the facts explained before, which include the auto-regulatory mechanisms of increasing the cerebral blood flow, compensatory supply by collateral circulations and the presence of inter-connection between the two arterial systems through the Circle of Willis and also the fact that the vital centers of the brain are supplied by the vertebral system, which is not easily compressed by a neck ligature in the absence of some traumatic disruption to stop this blood supply as they are protected by cervical vertebrae.

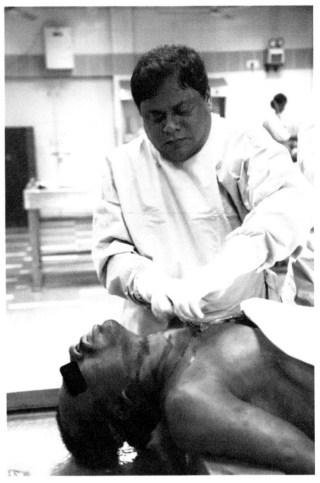

FIGURE 4.52 Author Dr. Sudhir Gupta conducting layer-wise neck dissection under bloodless field in the case of suicide of the accused in the Nirbhaya gang rape case.

Other causes like venous obstruction are also less likely to be the possible mechanisms in hanging deaths due to the interconnections between the various venous sinuses and absence of severe venous congestion or hemorrhages in the brain in hanging cases. Also, considering clinical scenarios like venous thrombosis of the brain have shown that death occurs only after a certain duration and not immediately even in the presence of venous obstruction.

Vagal inhibition is another frequently debated possible cause of death in hanging, but it is a diagnosis of exclusion, which itself is very tough in matters regarding the cause of death especially when most of the authors and forensic surgeons only consider it a rare possibility. This could be only considered for medical opinion in case of strong eyewitness and circumstantial evidence and on the basis of eliminating any other cause of death after thorough postmortem examination and viscera analysis.

FATAL PERIOD IN HANGING

Death is almost instantaneous in judicial hangings and in cases where there is injury to the spinal cord or reflex cardiac inhibition. When the occlusion of the air passage is incomplete, it takes about 3–8 minutes for death to ensue. When the body is brought down before death takes place, the person usually lingers in coma for several days and death eventually results from complications such as pneumonia.

NEAR HANGING

'Near hanging' represents a person who survives the immediate aftermath of an attempted hanging. Broken ligature materials, broken suspension supports or early rescue by witnesses can result in an unaccomplished hanging attempt. However, the external outcome of this 'survival' depends on the degree of already established cerebral anoxia. Other local injuries may also cause delayed deaths in a survivor of hanging. Generally, only few victims overcome 'near hanging'. The ligature mark may not be appreciable in these cases. After the loosening of the noose, facial congestion, edema and cyanosis disappear in a few minutes. Petechiae, if already established, stay appreciable for one to two days. In most of these cases, the victim presents in a comatose state due to the already established hypoxic, ischemic cerebral injury. Swollen root of tongue gives a typical 'hoarseness of voice' in many cases, and on palpation, fractures of the laryngo-hyoid complex present as bony crepitations. Injuries to the neck structures present as local edema and tenderness. Edema of the upper respiratory mucosa often progresses rapidly, causing airway obstruction and death if prompt interventions are not carried out. Injury to the carotid artery intima initiates thrombus formation and distal embolization, which may result in death following cerebral infarction.

The survival rate in near hanging depends on many factors, among which the duration and degree of suspension are the most important. If the victim hung for less than 5 minutes and prompt resuscitation efforts were made, the chances of survival are more. As the duration of suspension and the time delay in starting the resuscitation increase, the chances of survival decrease. In complete unsupported suspensions, where arterial occlusions occur or possible reflex cardiac inhibition occurs, the chances of survival are relatively less. Severe hypoxic ischemic encephalopathy with irreversible neuronal damage results in death in many cases of near hanging. Survivors of such pathologies generally end up in a persistent vegetative state. In global ischemia, the brain becomes edematous and the distinction between grey and white matter becomes difficult with the passage of time. Early microscopic changes like micro-vacuolization and cytoplasmic eosinophilia followed by pyknosis and karyorrhexis start to appear after 12 hours of the incident. These acute changes develop first in neurons and later in the astrocytes and the oligodendrocytes. Neutrophilic infiltration follows as a reaction of the body to tissue damage. This stage is followed by necrosis, neovascularization and scarring. The uneven scarring of regions of the neo-cortex is termed as pseudolaminar necrosis. Brains of hypoxic ischemic encephalopathy patients on ventilators show autolysis of cells followed by

evident liquefaction, i.e., the 'respirator brain'. Near hanging deaths commonly show pulmonary edema on autopsy as the efforts of forceful breathing result in alveolar epithelial injuries, causing increased permeability and also hyperemia of the lungs, which is a common finding.

DELAYED DEATH

When the body is brought down before death takes place, the person usually lingers in coma for several days and death eventually results from complications such as:

- Pneumonia
- Infections
- Pleural edema
- Laryngeal edema
- Infarction of brain
- Hypoxic ischemic encephalopathy

As in other forms of asphyxial deaths, the heart may continue beating up to a few minutes after the cessation of respiration. The brain cannot withstand the lack of oxygen for a period exceeding 5 minutes, and beyond this, permanent cerebral damage occurs. Hocking (1961) had reported a case of a man who died seven days after hanging. The death was due to complications arising from the fracture of the larynx sustained during the attempt.

TREATMENT IN CASE OF HANGING

Resuscitation should commence immediately. The constriction should be removed, the tongue pulled out, the mouth and the nostrils should be cleared, and artificial respiration started. If the body is warm, cold affusion may be applied to the head. If the body is cold, the body temperature may be restored by the application of warmth to the chest, abdomen and limbs. If the victim is able to swallow, stimulants may be given orally or otherwise injected hypodermically. Venesection may be useful to relieve the load on the right side of the heart and the congestion of the lungs and the brain.

POSTMORTEM APPEARANCE

EXTERNAL EXAMINATION

- Neck may be elongated and stretched due to prolonged suspension, especially in complete hanging. The pressure on the cervical sympathetic ganglia due to compression by the knot results in excitation and discharge, causing ipsilateral opening of eye and papillary dilation (Le facies sympathique) (Figure 4.53). This is considered as an ante-mortem phenomenon by some authors.
- Salivary trickle/dribble marks from dependent angle of the mouth are seen in many cases of hanging (Figure 4.54). This is explained by the excess salivary secretion that follows excitation

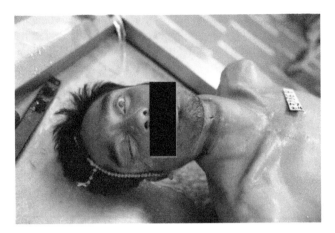

FIGURE 4.53 Le facies sympathique is present on the left side due to compression on the cervical sympathetic chain by the knot of ligature on left side.

of submandibular and submental glands due to mechanical stimulation by the compressing noose and is considered another ante-mortem phenomenon by some authors. Vertical salivary trickle marks are seen in front of the chest and the abdomen in many cases.

- In many cases, tip of tongue is seen protruded between rows of teeth due to uplifting of the root of tongue (Figure 4.55). With time, this exposed area gets dry and has a brownish to blackish color mimicking injury.
- Facial congestion, edema and cyanosis are seen in incomplete suspensions, but these may subside with time. In complete hanging, the face will be pale due to sudden onset of arterial occlusion. In incomplete suspensions, multiple petechiae are seen, mainly over the eyelids, posterior aspect of auricles and the oral mucosa. In severe congestion (Figure 4.56), engorged blood vessels may rupture and result in bleeding from nostrils or mouth.

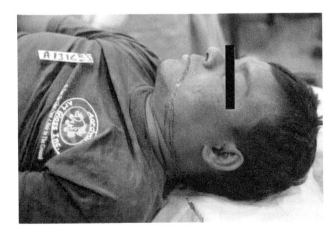

FIGURE 4.54 Dribbling of saliva from the dependent angle of the mouth in a hanging case.

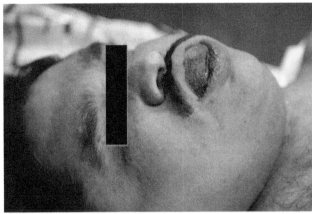

FIGURE 4.55 Protrusion of tongue with blackish discoloration in a case of hanging.

- If the body has not been removed for over a few hours after death, postmortem staining will be present over the lower dependent portions of the body, including the lower aspects of all the four limbs and the genital region. If the staining is not fixed, this 'glove and stocking' pattern fades

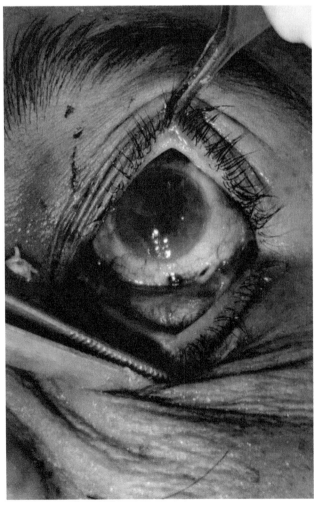

FIGURE 4.56 Congestion of the eye in a case of partial hanging.

after removal of body from hanging position and redistributes to the posterior aspect of the body. In cases where fixation has occurred either partially or completely, the same will be maintained. In rare instances, the history of suicide by hanging is hidden by the relatives due to some reasons such as to avoid social taboo or for insurance purposes. Identification of the pattern of postmortem staining is of much importance to reach a conclusion regarding the cause and manner of death in such cases. Intense postmortem staining at external genitalia may be misinterpreted as genital injuries in bodies suspended for longer duration. In prolonged suspension, postmortem hypostatic petechiae are common at dependent portions due to rupture of small blood vessels subjected to gravitational pooling causing increased pressure. In rare instances, these petechiae rupture and result in 'bleeding spots' that are often misinterpreted as ante-mortem injuries by untrained eyes.

- Swelling of the penis is a common finding in hanging. Some authors correlate it with sexual arousal due to cerebral hypoxia while others have proposed hypostatic seepage of fluid due to their dependent position. Discharge of semen is another common finding in hanging cases. Development of rigor mortis in the muscles of the seminal vesicles is a postulated reason for this occurrence, but some authors consider it to be an ante-mortem phenomenon occurring as a result of increased sexual arousal due to cerebral hypoxia. Blood or blood-stained fluid may also be seen coming out from the vagina or anal cavity in some cases.

Ligature Mark

Generally, hanging produces a pressure abrasion due to friction between the noose and the underlying skin. This is a mechanical injury and is possible in postmortem suspensions too, especially when the dead body is hung within 2–3 hours after death. As a rule, the greater the duration of suspension, the more evident is the impression. The weight of the body and the duration of suspension also show positive associations with better visibility of the ligature mark. Compression of the skin and underlying tissues by the noose displaces the fluid content of that area, making it dry. This dryness, if longstanding, gives a typical desiccated consistency commonly described as 'parchment-like' in postmortem reports. The friction by the ligature mark can even cause peeling of the skin (Figure 4.57). Initially, the ligature mark is pale, but as time passes, the area gets more dried up becoming dark brown in color. Zones of erythema may be seen immediately above or below the ligature mark, but this is not a sign of vitality. The upper erythematous zone may be caused by obstructed gravitational seepage as per some authors. Mechanical milking out of the underlying blood by the pressure transmitted by the noose is

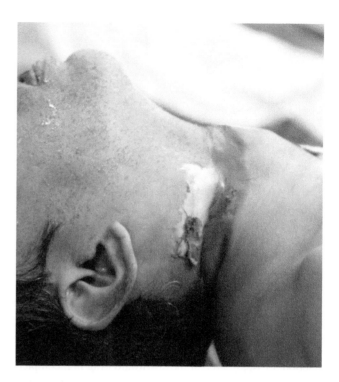

FIGURE 4.57 Ligature with skin peeling due to the friction between skin and the ligature material.

another postulate for these. These have been proven to be possible in postmortem suspensions and are no longer considered an ante-mortem phenomenon. The ligature mark rises to the point of suspension due to the tension built by the gravitational drag. This obliquity is a characteristic sign of the ligature marks seen in hanging with few exceptions. Since the entire weight of the body acts as the dragging force, commonly the nooses settle at the highest possible position, immediately below the jaw, and in the anterior midline, the ligature mark is generally at or above the level of the thyroid cartilage.

The suspension point at the knot generally forms the apex of an inverted 'V'-shaped ligature mark, and this is a sure-shot sign of suspension of body for a considerable duration of time. Generally, the ligature mark is discontinuous near the apex of the inverted 'V'. In cases of a very tight and fixed noose, this obliquity may not be appreciable since the noose is not free to move up. A horizontal ligature mark can be expected in a few cases of running noose too, such as when the ligature material is very thin like a metallic wire and gets tightened before the drop. The grooving produced by the ligature mark is generally more over the side opposite to the knot as this represents the area of maximum pressure bearing and replicates some morphological peculiarities of the contacting surface of the noose as imprints or patterned abrasions (Figure 4.58). Magnifying lenses, oblique illumination and scaled high-resolution photography with suitable post-processing technique help in identifying and interpreting these. Identification and documentation of these imprints has medico-legal significance for correlating the ligature material with the injury mark. If the ligature is wound

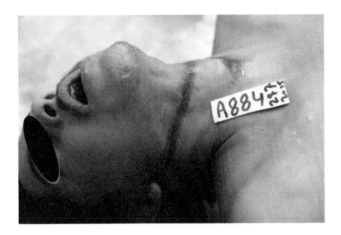

FIGURE 4.58 Patterned ligature mark replicates some morphological peculiarities of the contacting surface of the noose.

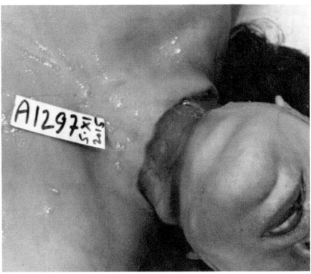

FIGURE 4.59 Broad ligature causing shallow ligature marks.

around the neck in multiple turns, the skin in between the strands may get entangled or pinched, producing hemorrhagic bands between imprints of these individual strands, but this does not suggest an ante-mortem nature of their production. Lesser degree of the downward drag in incomplete suspensions generally produces transverse ligature marks. These may be present below the level of the thyroid cartilage. A combination of congestive facial appearance and transverse ligature mark situated at a lower level, which is common in incomplete suspension, mimics ligature strangulation. In a few instances, where there are no reliable witnesses or a proper scene of crime examination, reaching a conclusive opinion regarding the manner of death is virtually impossible. The pattern of hypostasis, if established and fixed before removal of the body, generally provides some clues regarding the mechanism behind death.

- The appearance of the ligature mark around the neck depends on the type of ligature used, the duration for which the body was in suspended position and the overall postmortem interval. If the ligature material is soft and the duration of suspension is less, a visible ligature mark is commonly absent. Harder objects generally give visible pressure abrasions with some recognizable imprint pattern. Broad ligature materials leave shallow marks (Figure 4.59), while narrow ones cause deep and grooved marks, and in extreme cases cause deeper injuries by 'cheese cutter' mechanism. Friction and pressure built due to suspension may produce some fluid-filled epidermal blisters immediately above or below the level of ligature mark. These blisters are not proven to be having any significance in assessing the vitality of hanging.
- *Slippage of the ligature mark:* The noose may get tightened first at one level around the neck followed by its upwards slippage to finally settle beneath the mandible. This process produces many visible slippage abrasions below the level of the final ligature mark, and assessing the direction

of these can give a forensic surgeon the confidence to rule out any possible foul play. Similar abrasions if found above the level of ligature mark should raise some suspicion. The ligature may fix at one level first, producing a pressure abrasion. In some cases after getting fixed at one level, the body may slip down further, causing the noose to settle at a higher level, resulting in two pressure abrasions from a single noose (Figure 4.60). This scenario may mimic that of ligature strangulation followed by suspension of the body.

Discussion on a Case of Suicidal Hanging with Slippage of Ligature Material Leading to Formation of Two Ligature Marks with a Single Noose

The author has come across multiple cases where the ligature material encircles the neck in a single loop but two ligature marks are seen around the neck. This becomes more confusing when the direction of one ligature mark is

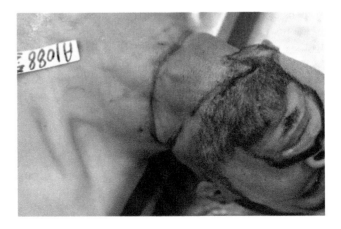

FIGURE 4.60 Slippage of the ligature causing double ligature mark from a single noose.

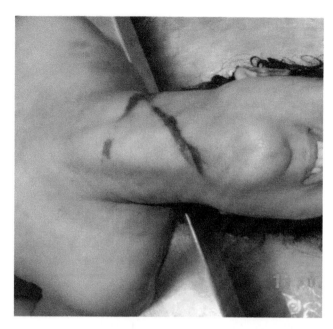

FIGURE 4.61 Two ligature marks are seen over the neck caused by a single ligature encircling the neck in a single loop. The lower horizontal ligature mark is the initial position of the ligature and the upper, oblique one is its final position after slippage.

horizontal and the other one is oblique (Figure 4.61). Such cases usually trigger the doubts regarding the possibilities of strangulation and postmortem suspension of the body. In this case, evidence showed that the deceased had spoken to her mother and told her that she was going to hang herself. All the circumstances were that of a suicidal hanging. The postmortem was conducted at AIIMS under the author's guidance, and it was observed that there was no injury in the soft tissues beneath the skin or in any other part of the neck (Figure 4.62), and nothing was found suggestive of strangulation and finally the case was concluded

as 'Ante-mortem hanging, suicidal in nature'. Internal neck structure could be clearly seen on layer-wise dissection in a bloodless field. The two ligature marks were explained as one being a horizontally placed pressure abrasion produced at the initial position of the noose and the second being an obliquely placed pressure abrasion produced by the noose as it finally settled higher up. The relocation of the noose happened due to slippage of the ligature over the neck produced by the downward pull of the weight of the body. This upward slippage of ligature mark is usually seen in cases of hanging and sometimes creates confusion with regard to the possibility of it being a combination of ligature strangulation and postmortem suspension. Careful evaluation of the external features of ligature mark, proper neck dissection and analysis of all the circumstantial evidences will be helpful in opining on similar cases.

Histopathology and Immunohistochemistry of Ligature Mark

The macroscopic appearance of the ligature mark mainly depends on the duration and the amount of the pressure applied to the region. If the intra-vital period is shorter, the chances of getting histological signs of vitality are less. Histopathology is an ancillary investigation in forensic practice and is not routinely used for cases of hanging. Universally acclaimed forensic histopathology atlases and textbooks mostly do not describe any histopathological findings in the neck in hanging cases. We have attempted an extensive review of the available literature and found that only a handful of authors have attempted to explore the medico-legal importance of histopathology of neck tissues in hanging cases.

The histopathological findings that can be seen in the skin of the ligature mark are compression of the epidermis with flattening of the cells (Figures 4.63 and 4.64), abraded epidermis, collagen condensation, breaking, wrinkling,

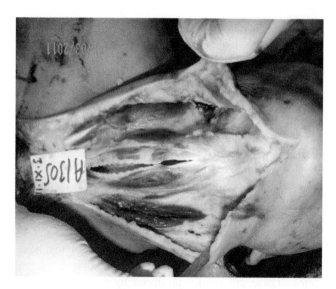

FIGURE 4.62 Bloodless neck dissection of the case shows absence of any other injury in the neck, ruling out other possible causes of fatal neck violence.

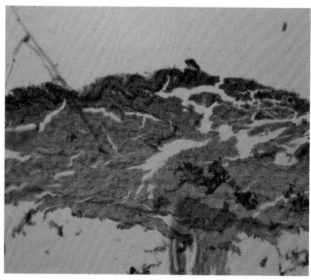

FIGURE 4.63 Compression of epidermis and dermis.

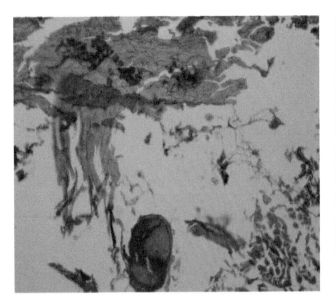

FIGURE 4.64   Compressed and edematous hair follicle.

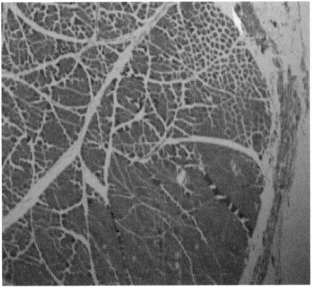

FIGURE 4.66   Coagulative necrosis of muscle.

dermal congestion and hemorrhagic infiltration. The dermal hemorrhage was more pronounced in ligature strangulation than in hanging. The subcutaneous tissue under the ligature mark can show congestion, hemorrhage and cellular infiltration. The histopathology of the skin and the subcutaneous tissue has been studied by multiple authors, and their unanimous suggestion was to implement the practice in differentiating ante-mortem suicidal hanging from postmortem suspension and other manners of death. They also suggested that immunohistochemical studies were better for assessing the vitality of the ligature mark. The literature on this concept is insufficient to reach conclusions for formulating any general recommendations.

Histopathology of blood vessels, lymph nodes, muscles and any osseo-cartilaginous fracture sites has also been attempted by a few authors. The findings that have been noted regarding the carotid artery are intimal, medial and adventitial tears, disruption of the intimal layer (Figure 4.65), subintimal hemorrhages and perivascular

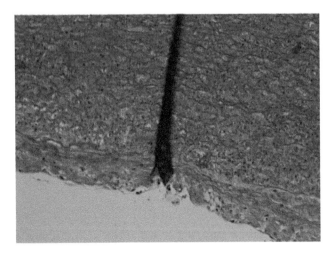

FIGURE 4.65   Disruption of intimal layer from the medial layer.

congestion. The most common finding was that of disruption of the intimal layer from the medial layer, and it was commonly seen in cases of complete hanging. Congestion and infiltration were the prominent findings seen in the lymph nodes. Muscles in some cases showed features of coagulative necrosis (Figure 4.66). Congestion alone was commonly seen in hanging, and congestion associated with infiltration was seen more in cases of strangulation. Despite these, the unanimous conclusion of all these studies was that more research is required in this regard before commenting on the medico-legal value of these findings in the differentiation of antemortem hanging vs postmortem suspension and hanging vs strangulation.

Histopathology and immunohistochemistry studies of the lung tissue show promising results in evaluating the vitality of the hanging incident. The commonest histological findings in hanging deaths include emphysema, alveolar septal oedema, hyperemia and micro-hemorrhages. Some of the markers used for immunohistochemical evaluation of lung tissues in asphyxial deaths include CD68, LN-4, 27E10, AMH152 and Ki-67.

Other Injuries

Many cases of hanging show injuries of recent or old failed suicidal attempts. Atypical recent injuries create doubts about involvement of foul play and the accessibility of the injured areas; the possibility of these injuries being self-inflicted need to be analyzed with the utmost care before reaching a conclusion. Identification of presence of non-fatal injuries of assault in a suicidal hanging case takes a pivotal role in the trial of abetment charges. Suicidal hanging cases show many superficial injuries over trunk and limbs. These are mostly produced by rough surfaces of nearby objects that come in contact with the body during hanging especially in the convulsive phase. These aberrant injuries need detailed scrutiny keeping in mind assault and homicidal hanging being the possible causes. Scene of occurrence examination is useful whenever there is even a trace of doubt regarding the manner of causation.

Fingernail Marks and Other Injuries in Neck in Hanging Cases

In hanging death, the ligature mark on the neck is the main finding, and its characteristics are well described in literature. Sometimes, peri-ligature injuries, which are caused by rope burns or nail marks, are found around the ligature mark. A few authors have discussed medico-legal significance of peri-ligature or non-ligature injuries in suicidal hanging.

The author studied a total of 2,409 cases (1,556 males and 853 females) of suicidal hanging from the autopsy cases conducted during a 9-year period from 2006 to 2014. Peri-ligature injuries were present in only 119 (67 males and 52 females) cases, which comprised 4.93% (4.3% among males and 6.1% among females) of all suicidal hanging cases, with non-ligature injuries in hanging cases showing that the most common body region involved was upper limb (45.4%) followed by lower limb (35.3%), head and face (31.9%). Injuries over upper limb and head and face were more common in females than in males; the difference was statistically significant (p = 0.011). In 11 males and 28 females, multiple injuries were found over more than one region of the body; the difference between the two groups was statistically significant (p = 0.002). The most common mechanism for production injury was during the process of bringing down the victim for rescue and due to breakage of ligature (29.4%) followed by self-infliction of injury (28.6%). Self-inflicted injuries were in the form of incised wounds over the wrist, lower part of the forearm of upper limbs and chest and abdomen. In one case, self-inflicted nail mark was present on the neck and lower part of the face. In 11 cases (9.2%), the injuries were inflicted by others before suicide (2 males and 9 females). These injuries were in the form of abrasion, nail marks, bite marks and railroad contusions.

The victims of suicidal hanging may attempt to pull away the ligature as a reflex action to preserve life, thus inflicting nail marks on the neck around the ligature. Rarely such injuries can also be seen over the chin (Figures 4.67

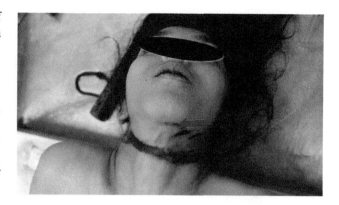

FIGURE 4.68 An abrasion seen below the chin and above the ligature mark in a case of suicidal hanging possibly due to victim's reflex action to preserve her life and resulting nail abrasions.

and 4.68). In attempted resuscitation or rescue, nail marks can also be produced by the rescuer while trying to remove the ligature. In certain cases, suicide can be initially attempted by cutting the throat, but on failing, hanging can be performed by the deceased (Figure 4.69).

Artifacts

Hanging deaths present with many 'injuries' that are unrelated to hanging and are produced as postmortem artifacts. In many cases, the body may fall down on the ground while removing it from the noose. This fall may result in injuries like abrasions, contusions, lacerations and fractures. The postmortem nature of these injuries makes the interpretation easy in most of the instances, but these can create suspicion of foul play in some cases. Thus, a thorough evaluation will be useful to rule out other possibilities. Fracture of lower cervical level (C6–C7) is a common postmortem artifact due to rough handling of the dead body and has been termed as 'undertakers fracture'. This postmortem fracture may be mistaken as a fracture due to hanging. Hangings that happen in outdoor or non-secured areas show many postmortem artifacts following ant, maggot and other

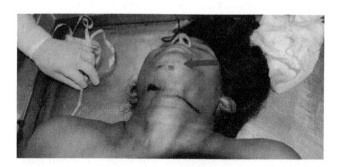

FIGURE 4.67 Multiple abrasions are seen in the neck below the chin and above the ligature mark in a case of suicidal hanging possibly due to victim's reflex action to preserve her life and resulting nail abrasions.

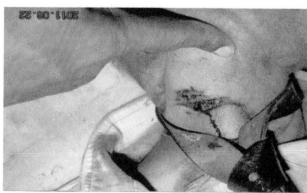

FIGURE 4.69 Superficial incised wounds (hesitation cuts) seen over the neck in a case of suicidal hanging where the person had multiple hesitation cuts over the neck, wrist, thigh and after that committed suicide by hanging using a leather belt as the ligature material.

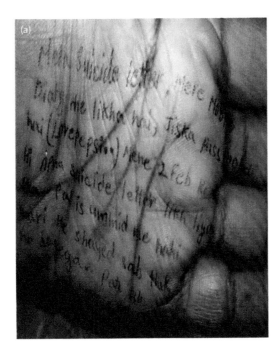 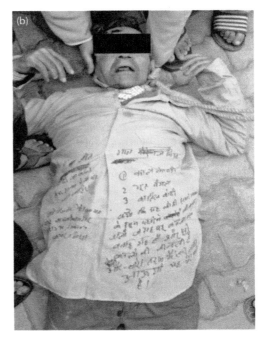

FIGURE 4.70   (a) Suicide note written over the palm. (b) Suicide note written over the shirt.

predator activity. Decomposition changes generally do not affect the appreciation of ligature mark. The relative dryness under the mark due to the persistent pressure through the noose is the postulated reason for this preservation of findings. Discoloration due to skin folds or prolonged refrigeration may produce external neck images similar to that of a ligature mark in some cases.

RADIOLOGICAL EXAMINATION (VIRTUAL AUTOPSY)

Combination of postmortem computed tomography (PMCT) and postmortem magnetic resonance imaging (PM-MRI) examination has proven useful in detecting most of the structural injuries found in hanging. Cervical vertebral injury is one important finding identifiable with PMCT. Detection of these fractures is difficult with traditional dissection techniques especially when the fracture is at the upper level or if without separation between segments. Most of the hyoid and laryngeal fractures are also detectable in PMCT. Directions of displacement of the fractured segments are demonstrable with virtual autopsy, which helps in identifying the direction of force applied. Muscular injuries and subcutaneous tissue hemorrhages are better seen with PM-MRI. Carotid artery injuries are demonstrable with PM angiography, which demonstrates the leaking of the contrast medium from the rupture site.

Medico-legal Importance

Suicidal Hanging

Hanging is the commonest modality adopted for ending one's own life. As a norm, all deaths due to hanging are considered suicide until the contrary is proven. All the types described above, i.e., complete or incomplete suspension

and typical or atypical knot positions, are possible in suicides. Circumstantial evidences like the room being latched from inside, the presence of a suicide note (Figures 4.70a and 4.70b), accessibility of the ligature material, use of supporting devices like stools, etc. to help achieve the desired height, etc. should be considered before commenting about the manner if in doubt.

Absence of any other injuries on the body, a negative toxicological report and lack of any infirmity or weakness together support a suicidal manner.

Sometimes, multiple methods are used for committing suicide, which might complicate the process of determining the cause of death. In a few cases, the deceased strapped himself to ensure complete hanging, leaving no chance of survival. However, on first look, these cases may appear to have a homicidal component, but on systemic examination of the other aspects, a proper conclusion can be reached.

DISCUSSION OF A CASE WITH MULTIPLE HESITATION CUTS ALONG WITH HANGING IN A DEATH IN JAIL

Inadequate knowledge and lack of expertise in the forensic field sometimes mislead a case, which leads to unnecessary confusion and delay in justice. The author encountered such a case of a Senior Medical Officer of Lucknow. The arrest of this Senior Medical Officer was due to his alleged link with killing of his previous Chief Medical Officers by a motorcycle-borne assailants. The local police had found his connection with the murder cases and had called him for interrogation. An FIR was later registered against him in case of embezzlement of National Rural Health Mission (NRHM) funds for which he was arrested and sent to prison.

In June 2011, after some days after the arrest, the dead body of this Senior Medical Officer was found in an unused toilet of the minor operation theater located on the first floor of the jail hospital. His body was found in sitting position on the commode of a western style toilet with him facing the reverse side and a belt was seen encircling his neck and the other end was tied with the grill of the window. Postmortem was conducted by a panel of five doctors at Lucknow and the report was as follows.

POSTMORTEM EXAMINATION REPORT

External Examination

Height 158 cm, Weight 75 kgs. Clothes worn-Shirt-l, Underwear-I, White Metallic Finger Ring-I with red stone. Clothes were blood stained. Rigor mortis passing off from upper extremity, present in lower extremity. Average built body and eyes closed, mouth closed.

Injuries

1. Incised wound 6 cm × 2 cm × muscle deep present on lateral aspect of right side of neck, 1 cm below right angle of mandible. Tailing present towards mid line of neck. Margins are clean cut, wound is spindle shaped, red clotted blood present in and around the wound (Figure 4.71).
2. Incised wound 3 cm × 0.5 cm × muscle deep present on front of neck, 6 cm below chin, starting from midline going towards left. Margins are clean cut, spindle shaped (Figure 4.72).
3. Incised wound 4 cm × 1.5 cm × muscle deep, present on frontal aspect of right elbow joint. Margins are clean cut, spindle shaped, red clotted blood present in and around the wound (Figure 4.73).
4. Incised wound 3 cm × 1 cm × muscle deep, present on anterior medial aspect of right elbow, 2 cm medial to injury no. 3. Margins are clean cut, spindle shaped, red clotted blood present in and around the wound (Figure 4.73).

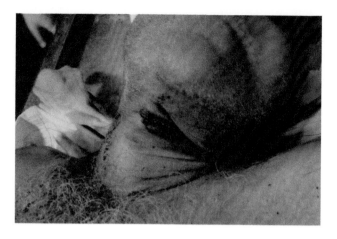

FIGURE 4.72 Muscle-deep incised wound present on front of neck, 6 cm below chin, starting from midline going towards left.

5. Incised wound 3 cm × 1 cm × muscle deep present in anterior medial part of left elbow joint. Tailing present towards medially. Margins are clean cut, spindle shaped, red clotted blood present in wound (Figure 4.74).
6. Incised wound 6 cm × 1.5 cm × muscle deep present on anterior lateral aspect of left elbow joint. Margins are clean cut, spindle shaped, red clotted blood present in wound.
7. Incised wound 4 cm × 1 cm over lateral aspect of left wrist joint, 13 cm from the tip of left thumb. Margins are clean cut, spindle shaped, red clotted blood present in wound.
8. Incised wound 9 cm × 1 cm × muscle deep present on front of right thigh extending medially, 3 cm below right inguinal fold. Margins are clean cut and sharp, red clotted blood present in wound (Figure 4.75).
9. An Obliquely placed ligature mark 37 cm × 3 cm present on all around the neck above thyroid cartilage in front of neck passing obliquely upwards in front of right ear along the line of mandible ligature mark is interrupted by 4 cm area in front

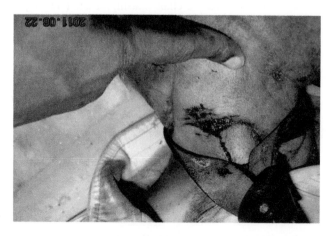

FIGURE 4.71 Muscle-deep incised wound present on lateral aspect of right side of neck below the belt, which was the ligature material.

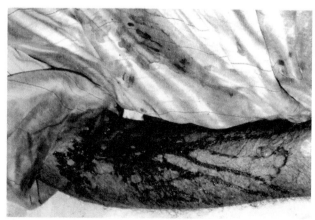

FIGURE 4.73 Two muscle-deep incised wounds, present on anterior and anterior medial aspect of the right elbow.

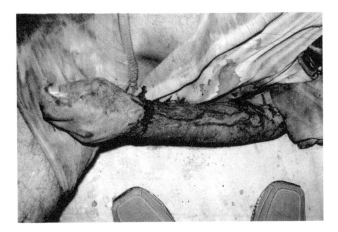

FIGURE 4.74 Muscle-deep incised wounds present over the left elbow joint and lateral aspect of left wrist joint.

of mastoid process & involving right ear lobule. Ligature mark is situated 1 cm below right ear lobule (posteriorly) and 6 cm below left ear lobule.

Internal Examination
No abnormality was found in internal organs.

Opinion
Probable time since death: About one day

Cause and manner of death: The cause of death to the best of my knowledge and belief is:

    a. Immediate cause — Shock and haemorrhage
    b. Due to — Ante-mortem injuries

Injuries no. 1,2,3,4,5,6,7,8 are ante-mortem and fresh in duration. Injury No. 9 is post-mortem.

Manner of causation of injuries- Injury No. 1,2,3,4,5,6,7,8 caused by sharp edged weapon. Injury No. 9 caused by the ligature (Figure 4.76).

The Senior Medical Officer found dead under mysterious circumstances in the district jail was initially investigated

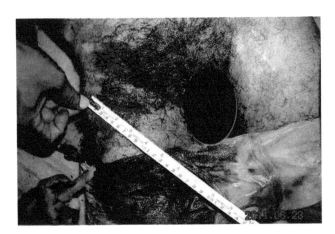

FIGURE 4.75 Muscle-deep incised wound present on front of right thigh extending medially, 3 cm below right inguinal fold.

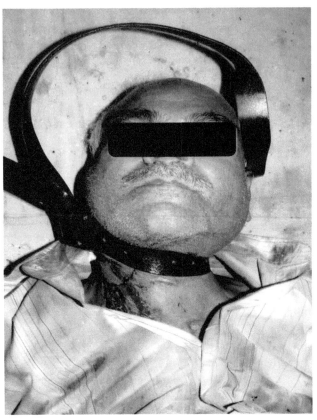

FIGURE 4.76 Ligature material, i.e., belt present around the neck.

by the local police, but later, a public interest litigation (PIL) filed in the High Court caused the transfer of the case to the CBI.

First Opinion of CBI from AIIMS Medical Board
On 17.10.11, the HOD of Department of Forensic Medicine, AIIMS, New Delhi was requested by the CBI to constitute a board of doctors for furnishing opinion on the cause of death/nature of injuries, weapons of offence, etc. The board was constituted under the chairmanship of Dr. T D Dogra, to give their relevant opinion regarding the enquiries sent. All the relevant records and reports were submitted.

As Per Central Forensic Science Laboratory (CFSL) Report (Fingerprint Division)
No identifiable finger/palm/footprint could be detected/developed from the scene of crime.

As Per CFSL Report (Chemistry Division)
- The exhibit 1 (Dirty pant), 2 (Dirty shirt), 3 (Dirty underwear) and 8 (four polythene packets) gave negative test for the presence of common poisons/drugs including sedatives/tranquilizers.

As Per CFSL Report (Physical Division)
- The belt examined as ligature material was not a new one.

- Laboratory examination revealed that the belt is long and strong enough for hanging/committing suicide of a normal human being.
- The slippers examination revealed no signs of wiping out of the blood could be detected to the backside of the slippers.

In consideration of above reports and along with the findings mentioned in postmortem report, video recording of postmortem examination and photographs were also examined; the following were the medical board observations.

Observations of the Medical Board

- Injury No. 2- Incised wound 3 cms × 0.5 cm × muscle deep present on front of neck, 6 cms below chin, starting from midline going towards left. Margins are clean cut, spindle shaped. This injury was completely within the boundaries of ligature mark. There was not much bleeding from the wound.
- All the injuries were on approachable body parts and were superficial in nature. Further, there was no involvement of underneath major vessels (artery or vein) in the vicinity of any injury mentioned in post-mortem report.
- All the injuries are ante-mortem in nature and fresh before death and are produced by sharp edged weapon like shaving blade.
- All the injuries are present on the suicide sites because they are accessible and having underneath vein and arteries, if these arteries are cut, the bleeding is faster and produces haemorrhagic shock due to loss of blood, therefore, such sites are selected for committing suicide. Once artery is cut, there may be not much pain but bleeding may be profuse with each heart beat often associated with spurt.
- The blood clot on the body of the deceased at the site of injuries indicates the bleeding for some time after infliction of injuries. No cut was seen in any of the clothing corresponding to the injuries.
- The pant/trousers were not worn by the deceased, the trouser was found lying close to the door of the toilet.
- The amount of blood on the clothing and on the tiled floor does not seems to be sufficient to cause acute haemorrhagic shock in a healthy person like the deceased (Figures 4.77 and 4.78). Because, about minimum 1.5 l of blood is required to cause death due to haemorrhagic shock in case of such acute bleeding. The visual impression of total amount of blood seems to be much lesser than the aforesaid amount.
- On removal of skin and dissection of underneath structure. There was no extravasation of blood underneath the ligature mark. The thyroid complex was intact.

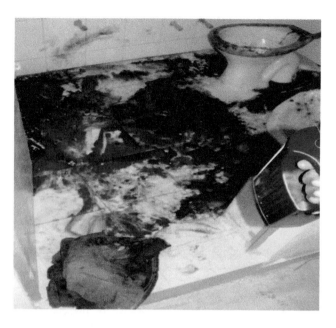

FIGURE 4.77 The trouser was found lying close to the door of the toilet. Blood over the tiles does not seems to be sufficient to cause acute hemorrhagic shock in a healthy person.

- The pattern of injuries is suggestive of being possible by a right handed person as the tailing of wounds is as under:
  - Injury on Right side neck (tailing Right to Left)
  - Injury on Left Cubital Fossa (tailing Left to Right)
  - Injury on Right Thigh (tailing left to right)
- Trickling marks of blood stains were in vertical directions. No spurt was observed at the scene of occurrence.
- The deceased was found to be in sitting position on the commode of toilet (Figure 4.78) hanging with a belt around his neck and tied to the window bar (Figure 4.79).

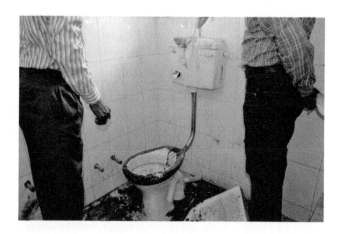

FIGURE 4.78 Crime scene photos of the commode of the toilet on which the deceased allegedly sat while hanging himself from the nearby window bar.

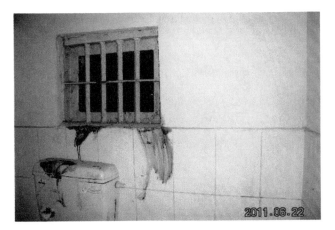

FIGURE 4.79 Crime scene photos of the window panel, the bar of which was used to tie the end of the belt used as ligature material.

- There is no evidence suggestive of presence of second person at the time of bleeding or applying ligature.
- The place of incidence is quite secluded and not in use.
- Prof TD Dogra informed the board that it was verified at the site by him using a belt of the same size and dimension as worn by the deceased, and it was observed that the deceased could have hanged himself by tying the ligature at the point it was found at the scene of occurrence as described by the persons who first saw the deceased.
- The description of ligature mark in the region of neck is consistent with that of ante-mortem hanging.
- On examination of the video clips, it is observed that there is a streak coming from close to the left angle of mouth and running downwards to the mandible, faint yellowish in colour suggesting the salivary secretion from the mouth which is seen in case of ante-mortem hanging. Some of the authors consider it as a sure sign of ante-mortem hanging.
- In one of the photographs, taken after removal of the dead body from the toilet shows a posture of the body with flexed limbs suggesting the onset of rigor mortis, indicating that the deceased was in sitting posture on the commode for at least a period of 1-2 hrs after death (Figure 4.80).
- The pattern/impression of the ligature mark as visible in photographs and video is consistent with that of the ligature material (belt).

The board is of the considered opinion that the deceased could have first attempted to kill himself by inflicting incised wounds on the suicidal sites where arteries and veins are situated, i.e., wrist, elbow, and inguinal region, but (he wounds produced did not cut any major artery or vein instead only superficial veins were cut from which there bleeding but it was very slow, hence, after sometime when (the deceased

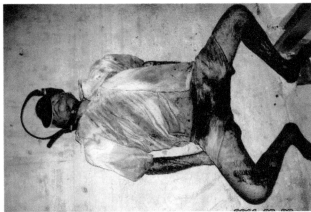

FIGURE 4.80 Posture of the body with the flexed limbs suggesting the onset of rigor mortis, indicating that the deceased was in sitting posture on commode at least for a period of 1–2 hrs after death.

could have realised that these are not killing him fast, he could have attempted to hang himself with the help of belt which he has succeeded. Therefore, the immediate cause of death in this case is asphyxia as a result of hanging associated with bleeding from the injuries inflicted.

Questions Submitted Subsequently

Q.1. Whether the death of the deceased is a case of suicide or homicide?

Ans. In view of the above mentioned observations, the board is of the considered opinion that the findings mentioned in post-mortem report in this case are consistent with that of a suicide. However, it is the prerogative of the investigating agencies to decide the issue of suicidal or homicidal death.

Q.2. Whether injuries mentioned in the post-mortem report and shown in photographs/videos are self-inflicted or otherwise?

Ans. The injuries mentioned in the post-mortem report and shown in photographs/videos could be self-inflicted in nature.

Q.3. Whether the half blade contained in sealed packet can inflict the injuries as mentioned in post- mortem report and shown in photographs/videos or otherwise?

Ans. The half blade (Figure 4.81) as provided in sealed packet could have caused the injuries as mentioned in the post mortem report or as seen in photograph and video.

Q.4. What was the sequence of injuries?

Ans. The board is of the considered opinion that the deceased could have first attempted to kill himself by inflicting incised wounds on the known suicidal sites where arteries and veins are situated, i.e., wrist, elbow, neck and inguinal region, but the wounds produced did not cut any major artery or vein instead only superficial veins were cut from which there was bleeding but it was very slow, hence, after sometime when the deceased could have realised that

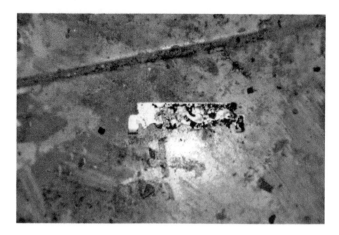

FIGURE 4.81 Half blade recovered from the scene of occurrence which had blood stains.

these are not killing him fast, he could have attempted to hang himself with the help of belt which he has succeeded. Therefore, the immediate cause of death in this case is asphyxia as a result of hanging associated with bleeding from the injuries inflicted. It is difficult to give the correct sequence of these injuries sustained.

Q.5. Whether a right handed person can inflict the injuries on his person as mentioned in postmortem report and shown in photographs/video?

Ans. It could be possible for a right handed person to inflict the injuries on his person as mentioned in post-mortem report and shown in photographs/video.

Q.6. What was the approximate time taken for death to occur after inflicting the injuries in instant case?

Ans. The approximate time taken for death to occur after inflicting the injuries in instant case could be within half an hour of the infliction of injuries.

Q.7. How did post-mortem staining on the back of the deceased has appeared as visible in photographs, while his body was found in sitting position?

Ans. The post mortem staining takes about 6–12 hrs to get fixed. Within this period if the dead body is removed and kept in another position, the Post-mortem staining may appear on new dependent part. It indicates that the dead body could have been removed before the fixation of PM staining.

Q.8. Whether the ligature mark on the neck of the deceased is post-mortem or antemortem and how it had appeared?

Ans. The ligature mark on the neck in hanging is usually partly ante-mortem and partly post-mortem in nature. In the first part till the death has occurred, the ligature produces ante-mortem ligature mark after 3–7 minutes when the person is dead but remains suspended depending upon the duration of suspension, the ligature mark changes are post mortem in nature. Thus, the ligature mark in hanging is likely to have both ante-mortem and post mortem changes.

Q.9. What was the time gap between death and ligature mark present on the neck of the deceased?

Ans. On an average it takes 3–7 minutes to cause death in case of hanging.

Q.10. Whether the discharge of yellow fluid from mouth of deceased as seen in the photographs, is indicative of something which had bearing on the cause of the death of the deceased?

Ans. This was examined in detail and it was observed that it could be salivary secretion coming out close to the left angle of mouth running downwards as a salivary streak to the mandible. This is considered to be a sure sign of ante-mortem hanging by many of the authors. Hence, it is a significant evidence of hanging being ante-mortem in nature.

Q.11. What was the cause of death?

Ans. Asphyxia as a result of ante-mortem hanging could be produced by a ligature material like belt associated with multiple suicidal wounds.

Q.12. Any other point of relevance.

Ans. NIL

On 9.3.12, it was again asked if the skin peeling of neck could be seen in a hanging case and also if asphyxia could occur if hips of deceased were partially resting on commode of toilet. A reply was sent on 15.03.12, stating that the skin peeling could be due to friction of ligature material and skin and could be seen in case of partial hanging; also, it was opined that asphyxia could occur in the specified position of the deceased, and the position could only be attained when the person was alive. Thus, the case was opined to be of antemortem partial hanging by a ligature.

On 27.7.12, it was requested to clarify if the pattern of flow of blood from the injuries on the body and clothes of deceased were possible, if the injuries are self-inflicted. On 30.7.12, it was opined by the board of doctors that the injuries as mentioned in the PM report and as seen in photographs and video recording are self-inflicted, and can produce the pattern of flow of blood as specified.

As no foul play was found in the death of the deceased, the closure report was filed in the court of special judicial magistrate for CBI cases at Lucknow.

COURT REJECTION OF CBI CLOSURE REPORT

The honorable court rejected the Closure Report in early 2013 citing differences between the opinion provided by the board of doctors from AIIMS, who gave their opinion after scanning the videography of the post-mortem examination, photographs of the body and visiting the spot. The postmortem report submitted by a panel of doctors from Lucknow claimed that some of the injuries were caused by a sharp-edged weapon and there were no signs of asphyxia on the body; also, the ligature mark was postmortem in nature.

The court referred to a Supreme Court judgment that if there was a difference of opinion between two doctors, then priority will be given to one who had examined the injured or the body of a deceased. The honorable court directed the CBI to carry out further investigation mainly on two queries:

Query 1. Can a person cause so many self-inflicted injuries without being incapacitated and without any injury to his hands?

Query 2. Even if the injuries were muscle deep only, whether a person committing suicide would be able to inflict upon himself so many injuries especially when the injuries let out blood and then go on to hang himself in order to commit suicide?

Third Medical Opinion in 2017 from AIIMS, New Delhi

A request was sent to Department of Forensic Medicine, AIIMS, New Delhi in 2017 by the CBI to form a board and provide second considered opinion on the above-mentioned queries. A Medical Board was formed under the chairmanship of Dr. Sudhir Kumar Gupta (author) to provide opinion regarding the same. The Medical Board perused the postmortem report, photographs, opinion given by the previous medical board and other submitted documents related to the case. The six photographs of the deceased taken at the scene of death were studied in detail for injuries, their location on the body, pattern and dimension of these injuries with reference of injuries as per standard established forensic literature.

QUERIES

Query 1. Can a person cause so many self-inflicted injuries without being incapacitated and without any injury to his hands? The nature of injuries appears to be such that both hands have to be used to cause the injuries.

Opinion: As per the PM report multiple incised injuries are located in the wrist, elbow, groin and neck, which has affected the superficial veins and not the major vessels (arteries and veins). It also shows that there was clot formation in the injury which is a natural body mechanism to control bleeding. The amount of bleeding was not sufficient to incapacitate him from inflicting multiple injuries to his body. The location of injuries suggests that the person could have used either hand to inflict the injuries on his body. It is also observed that it is possible to cause self-inflicted injuries as mentioned in the PM report by the weapon of offence, i.e., half blade, without causing injury to his hands.

Query 2. Even if the injuries were muscle deep only, whether a person committing suicide would be able to inflict upon himself so many injuries especially when the injuries let out blood and then go on to hang himself in order to commit suicide?

Opinion: As per literature and our experience it is well known that a person determined to commit suicide can inflict multiple injuries to his body till he is incapacitated and also he can use more than one means to complete the suicide as in this case.

Final Opinion: After detailed perusal of the available materials and deliberation of the case, the Medical Board is of the considered unanimous opinion that the eight antemortem incised injuries on the body of deceased are self-inflicted and suicidal in nature. The Cause of Death in this case is Asphyxia due to Antemortem Partial Hanging. The Medical Board observed that the deceased was found sitting on commode in rigor mortis suggesting antemortem phenomena as a sequence of hanging. The type of hanging in this case is partial (semi suspension) which are invariably suicidal in nature.

CONCLUSION

Insufficient knowledge and experience sometime lead to ignoring the findings. Interpretation of self-inflicted injuries is the need of the hour, so as to avoid the deviation of justice. As in this case, misinterpretation of self-inflicted injuries as fatal one leads to confusion. So this case summarizes the great importance of the forensic specialist in delivering justice.

DISCUSSION OF A CASE OF SUICIDAL HANGING WITH HANDS AND FEET STRAPPED TOGETHER CAUSING SUSPICION OF HOMICIDE

The body of an adult man was brought to AIIMS Forensic Medicine Department with an undisputed history of hanging. Both hands (Figure 4.82) were seen tied together by a cable wire and a similar tie was noted between the ankles. A cloth was seen tied around the mouth (Figure 4.82) to avoid any sound. There were no other injuries suggestive of homicidal hanging or postmortem or peri-mortem suspension, and the viscera analysis of the deceased did not yield any poison or incapacitating drug. The case was concluded as 'asphyxia due to ante-mortem hanging'.

In such situations, the pattern of the ties has to be analyzed for the involvement of a second person. For further evaluation, the removed ties should be sent to the Forensic Science Laboratory. This phenomenon of strapping of body parts is seen in a small proportion of suicidal hangings. The victims are trying to ensure their death by removing the possibility of backing out due to a possible change of mind during the agonal period.

DISCUSSION ON A CASE OF SUICIDAL HANGING IN JAIL

In 2013, a 35-year-old male arrested as an accused in a gang rape case was found hanging using a rope inside Tihar Central Jail. The family of the deceased alleged foul play in his death due to the presence of multiple ligature marks over his neck. The postmortem examination conducted at Department of

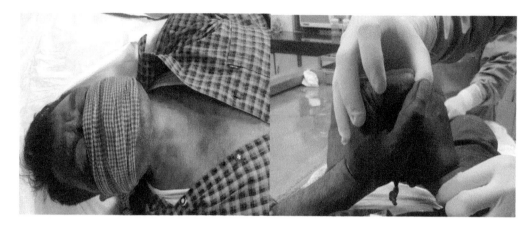

FIGURE 4.82   The picture shows that the deceased had tied a cloth around his mouth to avoid sound being heard by any possible rescuers, and also tied his hands together to ensure death by hanging and to avoid change of mind during the act.

Forensic Medicine, AIIMS found four ligature marks over the neck (Figure 4.83), none of which were situated over the upper part of the neck nor were they oblique, and all the ligature marks were completely encircling the neck. On dissection, the underlying structures were pale, white and glistening, and no extravasation of blood was seen in the region, but there were muscular contusions underneath all ligature marks (Figure 4.84). The multiple turns of ligature around the neck, which were actually caused by the slippage of ligature material around the neck as the deceased was under heavy influence of alcohol, had raised suspicion about a homicidal manner among the peers of the deceased. On autopsy, no evidence of any mechanical violence was found on the body of the deceased, and AIIMS Medical Board opined the cause of death as suicidal hanging, and the same was corroborated by the investigating agency.

HOMICIDAL HANGING

If judicial hanging is excluded, homicidal hangings are extremely rare. Homicidal hangings are commonly seen only if the victim is a child or an adult is incapacitated

due to drug, injury, old age or infirmity. In case of a conscious adult person, homicidal hanging is accompanied by multiple injuries of resistance, which usually do not miss the notice of an autopsy surgeon. These cases generally show finger grip contusions over the inner aspect of arms and many other injuries suggestive of physical restrain. Injuries of other attempted modalities for homicide like those of smothering and ligature strangulation should also be expected and screened for. Most assailants do not prefer this method mainly due to the difficulty in accomplishing the desirable outcome in everyday settings and due to the availability of easier modalities. Scene of crime examination and analysis of visceral organs for detecting the presence of any intoxicant has to be done in all suspected homicidal hanging cases. In homicidal hanging, gags may be present inside the mouth to silence the victim.

Assailants may tie the limbs together to avoid resistance. Though rare, ties at wrists and ankles may be present in suicidal hanging cases also as have been discussed previously. Generally in homicides, these ties are accompanied by underlying skin and soft tissue injuries in the form of

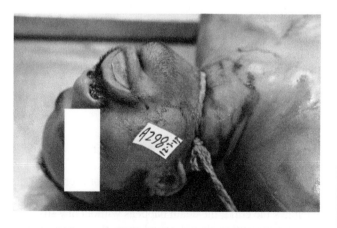

FIGURE 4.83   Neck shows three ligature marks present below the level of the final settled ligature mark, without any overlapping. This was due to the slippage of the ligature before it reached its final position and caused death.

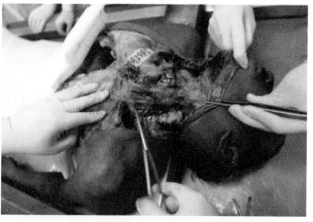

FIGURE 4.84   Muscular contusions underlying the ligature marks on neck dissection under a bloodless field; layers did not show any other internal injuries in neck structures.

abrasions, contusions or lacerations. A detailed examination of the knot pattern also helps in clarifying doubts in these situations.

LYNCHING

Lynching is a form of homicidal hanging wherein there is extrajudicial killing of a person by a mob motivated to do so due to severe personal differences and enmity. Cases of lynching have been reported all over the world, including India, and it was commonly practiced during the late 18th century in North America.

JUDICIAL HANGING

Judicial hanging has long been used in our country for capital punishment. Other countries where judicial hanging is practiced include Afghanistan, Bangladesh, Botswana, Iraq, Japan, Kuwait, Malaysia, Nigeria, the Palestinian Authority in Gaza and Sudan. In judicial hanging, ligature is applied to the neck with a submental knot (knot under the chin) and the person is dropped from a height according to his weight. During the fall, the ligature gives a forceful jerk to the neck, leading to fracture and dislocation of cervical vertebrae especially C2–C3, and less commonly C3–C4. This is also called as 'hangman's fracture'. The cervical vertebrae fractures are also associated with lacerations and contusions of the spinal cord.

The execution of death penalty in India, under the Code of Criminal Procedure, is being carried out using 'hanging by the neck till death' since more than a 100 years. The execution of the death penalty is carried out in accordance with section 354(5) of the Code of the Criminal Procedure, 1973, and the Jail Manuals of the respective states.

The actual execution process has to be carried out in accordance with paragraphs 868 to 873 of CrPC, briefly stated as follows:

1. The officers required to be present at the execution are—Superintendent and Medical Officer of the jail and Magistrate of the district.
2. The execution is to be carried out by the public executioner, or some other trustworthy individual who has been locally trained to be assigned to this job. The duty is entrusted to the Superintendent to satisfy himself or herself that the person thus assigned is competent to fulfill the job.
3. *Regulation of the drop:* It is the most important factor in deciding the death in a judicial execution by hanging. The slightest error in deciding the length of the drop may lead to a lingering death for the condemned man. The drop is regulated according to the height, weight and physique of the prisoner. The following scale suggesting the recommended drop in proportion to the weight of the prisoner is included for general guidance:

- A prisoner under 100 lbs weight is dropped 7 feet.
- A prisoner 100–120 lbs weight is dropped 6 feet.
- A prisoner 120–140 lbs weight is dropped 5½ feet.
- A prisoner 140–160 lbs weight is dropped 5 feet.

4. The Superintendent and the Deputy Superintendent reach the cell of the condemned prisoner and identify him or her. The warrant of death should be read over to the prisoner, and various legal documents such as a will, etc. may be signed by the prisoner in the presence of the Superintendent.
5. *Marching towards death:* The condemned prisoner shall be marched to the scaffold under the charge of the Deputy Superintendent.
6. The wardens holding the arm of the convict also mount the convict to the scaffold and place him under the direct beam to which the rope is attached.
7. The executioner straps his or her legs tightly together, places the cap over his or her head and face and adjusts the rope around his or her neck. The noose should be placed one and half inches to the right or left of the middle line and remain free from the flap of the cap.
8. The wardens holding the condemned prisoner's hand will withdraw the same on receiving the signal from the Superintendent, the executioner shall draw the bolt.
9. The body of such condemned prisoners remains suspended for half an hour and is not taken down till the medical officer declares the life extinct. The Superintendent is required to return the warrant with the endorsement to the effect that the sentence has been carried out.

There are many types of ligature materials used for hanging like ropes, dupattas, sarees, wires, scarves, strings, pajama cords, bed sheets, belts, nighties and numerous other objects, depending on their availability. In prison or police custody, considerable ingenuity may be employed to overcome the efforts of the custodians to remove anything from reach that may be used to cause self-harm. Shoelaces, stockings and torn bed-sheets have been used for hanging in prison cells.

ACCIDENTAL HANGING

Accidental hanging rarely occurs, and if it does, it mostly involves children. Here, the neck gets entangled in any ligature or other structure like side rails of a crib and the body gets suspended. Since sudden cerebral hypoxia incapacitates the child, the death happens without any struggle. Scene examination should complement the theory of accidental death, and all other possible circumstances should be analyzed before ruling out a homicide angle. Accidental hanging is very rare among adults. It can happen following sudden unexpected malfunctioning of some machinery or sudden collapse of an individual when a potential noose or any other object like scarf, chain, etc. is present around neck. These incidents generally happen with people incapacitated due to drugs, injury, infirmity, senility or any other serious natural disease. All these circumstances need to be considered and worked up meticulously by the forensic surgeon before the conclusion of the case. Another group of accidental hanging is death following autoerotic practices. These mishaps are discussed in a separate chapter.

POSTMORTEM SUSPENSION

A dead body may be suspended for many reasons; the commonest of which is to conceal some crime related to that death. Postmortem examinations show signs of violence and struggle in most of these cases in the form of other injuries in addition to the ligature mark. Dribbling of saliva through angles of mouth does not happen in most of the cases, but some studies have shown it to be possible, so this is not a definitive sign of postmortem suspension. If death happened within 2–3 hours before suspension, a ligature mark indistinguishable from that of an ante-mortem hanging may be seen. Commonly, ligature marks of hanging show erythematous lines near their upper and lower margins, and these are considered to be a sign of vitality by some authors. But the same is proven to be possible with postmortem suspension also and hence is not a sign of vitality during the hanging process. Properties of ligature marks of hanging such as their higher placement, obliquity, imprinted pattern of the

ligature material and parchment-like consistency are present in cases of suspensions during the early postmortem period. If suspension occurred after few hours have passed since the death, the ligature mark commonly looks pale and lacks any vital reaction, just like a pressure imprint. In cases where the body is hanged within a few hours of death, postmortem staining reestablishes to give the typical 'glove and stocking' pattern depending on the duration of suspension. If the pre-suspension duration is more, the body shows postmortem staining pattern fixed in its previous posture. Homicide cases like smothering or strangulation consistently present with injuries and associated signs. Ligature strangulation cases generally show two ligature marks, i.e., a transverse ligature mark of strangulation and an oblique mark of postmortem suspension. Postmortem suspension generally does not produce injuries at carotid arteries due to the lack of tensed blood column at the time of suspension. Facial signs do not correlate with the anticipated mechanism of death in hanging and commonly suggest more violent mechanisms. Point of suspension and the use of a support should be analyzed in relation with their accessibility, possible height of the drop and the degree of suspension. Generally, while suspending a body after death, the perpetrator fixes the noose first and then pulls the body up. The direction of pinning of the fibers of the ligature material reveals the direction of pull and gives a vital clue towards it being a case of postmortem suspension. Viscera analysis for presence of incapacitating drugs helps in differentiating cases of homicidal hanging and postmortem suspension (Table 4.1). There is no

TABLE 4.1
Difference between Hanging and Strangulation

S. No.	Hanging	Strangulation
1.	Face is pale	Face is congested and livid with petechial hemorrhages
2.	Tongue protrusion and swelling less marked	Tongue protrusion and swelling are well marked
3.	Dribbling of saliva is present	Dribbling of saliva is absent
4.	Blood-stained fluid from nose, mouth and ears are less frequent	Blood-stained fluid from nose, mouth and ears are more frequent
5.	Generally, the neck is stretched and elongated	Neck is neither stretched nor elongated
6.	Ligature mark is oblique, incomplete and placed high up over the neck	Ligature mark is transverse, complete and placed low down over the neck
7.	Base of the ligature mark is pale and parchmentized	Base of ligature is soft and reddish
8.	Knot is simple, single and on one side of the neck	Knots are multiple, granny type and tied tightly
9.	Abrasion and ecchymosis along the ligature mark are not common	Abrasion and ecchymosis are commonly seen along the ligature mark
10.	Involuntary discharge of urine and feces is less common.	Involuntary discharge of urine and feces is more common
11.	Involuntary discharge of semen is more common	Involuntary discharge of semen is less common
12.	Contusion of neck muscles is generally absent	Contusion of neck muscles is always present
13.	Subcutaneous tissue under the ligature mark is white, hard and glistening	Subcutaneous tissue under the ligature mark is contused and lacerated
14.	Thyroid cartilage fracture is generally absent	Thyroid cartilage fracture is generally present
15.	Larynx and trachea fracture are rare	Larynx and trachea fracture may be present
16.	Injury to the intima of the carotid arteries may be present	Injury to the intima of the carotid arteries is less likely
17.	Emphysematous bullae may or may not be present on lungs	Emphysematous bullae are mostly present on lungs
18.	Signs of struggle are absent	Signs of struggle are often present
19.	Intoxication and drugging are generally absent	Intoxication and drugging may be present

rise in serotonin and histamine around the ligature mark on histochemical examination, and emphysematous bullae are mostly present over the lungs.

DISCUSSION ON A CASE OF ANTE-MORTEM HANGING WRONGLY JUDGED AS POSTMORTEM SUSPENSION WITH SMOTHERING AS CAUSE OF DEATH

In 2010, the body of a 23-year-old unmarried female journalist was found at her residence hanging from the ceiling fan in her bedroom with a suicide note recovered from the scene of crime. Postmortem examination done by a team of three doctors revealed a ligature mark around the neck, 1–3 cm wide (Figure 4.85). The underlying skin was pale and the subcutaneous tissues didn't reveal any ecchymoses either. The autopsy surgeons opined that the ligature mark should be regarded as postmortem in nature based on its appearance, and the initial postmortem report stated the cause of death as asphyxia due to smothering; a 12-week fetus was found in utero during the autopsy.

The woman's boyfriend accused her family of killing their daughter as they were continuously opposing her marriage with him. Based on the allegations and the opinion given by the autopsy surgeons, a murder case was registered, and the main suspect, the mother of the deceased, was arrested by the police. The Government of Jharkhand requested AIIMS to peruse the postmortem report, photographs, Forensic Science Laboratory reports and other relevant documents and give an opinion as to whether the hanging was ante-mortem suicidal in nature or she was murdered first and then her body suspended to mimic hanging. After perusing all documents, the Medical Board opined that 'Cause of death in this case is antemortem hanging by ligature which could be suicidal in nature'. After the police investigation, the boyfriend was finally arrested for abetment of suicide of the deceased. The alleged suicide note

found at the scene of occurrence was analyzed by handwriting experts in Forensic Science Laboratory and was found to have been written by the deceased herself.

DISCUSSION ON A CASE WHERE A CLOTH PIECE IN THE MOUTH CONFUSED A PARTIAL HANGING WITH POSTMORTEM SUSPENSION

The body of a boy was found hanging inside a school room that was allegedly locked from inside. He was wearing a school uniform. The room was allegedly broken into, and the corpse was shifted to a nearby mortuary. Postmortem examination was carried out, and a piece of cloth was found inside the mouth extending into upper airway up till the voice box (Figure 4.86). Postmortem staining was noted over both the lower limbs and over the back. The conjunctivae showed congestion. The tip of tongue was seen protruded out from between the rows of teeth. The lip was contused. The ligature mark was present higher up, obliquely and discontinuously over the front and sides of neck. It was dry and parchment like. Neck dissection did not reveal any internal injuries. The doctor gave his opinion as to the cause of death as: 'Asphyxia as a result of choking of airways, i.e, trachea due to a piece of towel, i.e, thick cloth present in mouth and voice box. Hanging is post-mortem in nature'. Accordingly, a case under murder charges was registered, and the crime branch division took over the investigation. Forensic scientists confirmed that the door was locked from the inside at the time of incident and was broken open to recover the hanging body. They also confirmed that no one from outside could lock the door from inside by any mechanism. An alleged suicide note was also recovered from the scene of crime. Forensic calligraphic analysis proved that the suicide note was written in the victim's handwriting.

An expert medico-legal opinion was sought from AIIMS to get more clarity regarding the cause and manner of death.

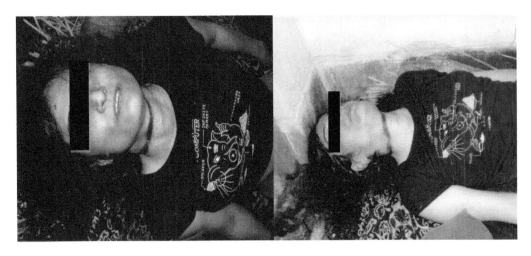

FIGURE 4.85 Picture shows the ligature mark of ante-mortem hanging, which was erroneously labeled as an injury of postmortem suspension by doctors conducting the postmortem examination. No other injuries were appreciated in this case, which had been suspected to be present initially.

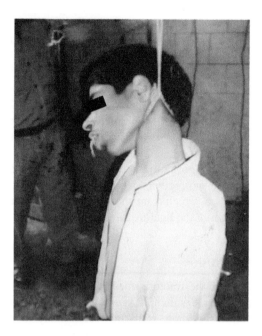 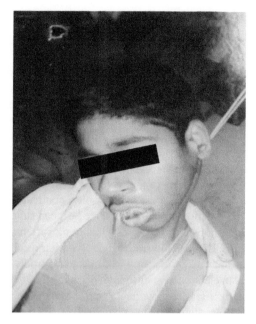

FIGURE 4.86   Pictures show a portion of the piece of cloth that was present in the mouth of the deceased, which created the confusion and suspicion of postmortem suspension.

Photographs and all relevant documents were submitted for perusal by the AIIMS Medical Board. The AIIMS Medical Board concluded it as a case of suicidal partial hanging. The 'lip contusion' was identified as a misinterpretation of an inexperienced autopsy surgeon. The cloth in the upper airway was a part of the victims attempt to conceal any possible sounds or gesture for seeking help during the attempt.

The autopsy surgeon should reserve his opinion till consultation with seniors or more experienced forensic experts whenever he or she is in doubt. Otherwise, as was seen in this case, misinterpretations can become a cumbersome task for the law enforcement agencies to solve.

HOLISTIC APPROACH TO AVOID MISINTERPRETATION OF FINDINGS

Asphyxial deaths due to hanging are the most common kinds of death to be misinterpreted. Proper evaluation and following a holistic approach, including giving due consideration to all circumstantial evidences, before formulating the postmortem report will decrease the chances of error.

SIMON'S HEMORRHAGE

Hemorrhage that is appreciated in the ventral aspect of intervertebral disc beneath the anterior longitudinal ligament is termed as Simon's hemorrhage (Figure 4.87). This was first described by German Forensic Pathologist Axel Simon in cases of hanging where he observed this pattern of hemorrhage. This is also termed as Simon's sign and is seen usually in the lower thoracic and lumbar vertebral region. The hemorrhage is restricted to the region below anterior longitudinal ligament and does not extend into the vertebral body. It is seen more common among young people than in

elders with degenerative changes of the vertebral column. The hemorrhage is seen more commonly in hanging cases with complete suspension than the ones that have incomplete hanging.

Simon's hemorrhage is observed to occur in the following cases:

- Hanging
- Other asphyxial deaths
- Electrocution, lightning strike
- Hypothermia
- Road Traffic Accidents (RTA)
- Fall from height

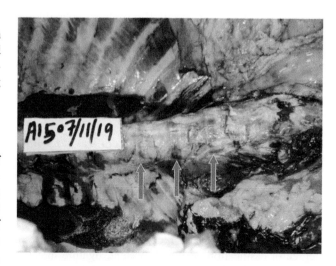

FIGURE 4.87   Simon's hemorrhage: Hemorrhage in the intervertebral disc near anterior longitudinal ligament in the lumbar vertebral region in a case of complete hanging.

MECHANISM OF SIMON'S HEMORRHAGE

Simon's hemorrhage occurs in hanging and other asphyxial deaths due to the forceful or violent movement of the person usually during the convulsive stage of asphyxia and the following decorticate rigidity causing extension of the vertebral column and sudden contractions of the muscles leading to rupture of vessels originating from the arteries in the lumbar or lower thoracic region. In addition to this, in hanging, the traction of the body due to gravity can also cause some bleeding in the intervertebral region due to the caudo-rostral hyperextension of the vertebral column.

In hypothermia, intense shivering and violent contraction of muscles in a protective attempt to produce heat can cause bleeding into the iliopsoas muscles and adjoining vertebral region. In cases of RTA and fall from height, a similar mechanism of violent contraction of muscles or injury can produce such bleedings. In electrocution or lightning strike cases too, the violent contraction of para-vertebral muscles can cause such a pattern of bleeding in the intervertebral discs.

INTERPRETATION OF SIMON'S HEMORRHAGE

Simon's sign is an important finding strongly indicating ante-mortem hanging. It is also a vital sign which is not specific and whose absence does not rule out a hanging death. However, the presence of Simon's sign in hanging strongly predicts its ante-mortem nature of occurrence.

FRACTURE OF NECK STRUCTURES AND RELATION TO KNOT POSITION

The fracture of hyoid and thyroid can be seen in asphyxial deaths due to pressure over the neck or local violence. The factors deciding the vulnerability of these structures are complex and are less understood due to the multiple factors at play here. A few studies done by Khokhlov determined a so-called vulnerability coefficient of hyoid bone/thyroid cartilage, which showed that the highest susceptibility to these injuries was in complete hanging of the body with the co-efficient being 1.75, whereas in cases of partial hanging, the susceptibility was found to be less with the vulnerability co-efficient from highest to least being in the following order of positions, that is, standing 0.88, kneeling 0.63, sitting 0.33 and prone 0.25.

A few studies also showed that there was no significant difference in the frequency of fractures between the left and right greater horns of the hyoid bone in relation to eight different positions of the ligature knot, which were anterior, posterior, right, left, right anterior, right posterior, left anterior and left posterior. All these findings were in persons older than 30 years recognizing the importance of degree of ossification, age, body weight, ligature material and various other factors playing a role in determining the outcome. It was also concluded that the absence of any form of hyoid-laryngeal fractures in cases of hanging in persons older than 30 years usually indicated that the knot position was anterior, but the presence of either hyoid bone or thyroid cartilage fracture indicates that the knot position could be posterior.

MECHANISM OF NECK INJURY

The mechanism of inner neck structure injuries is considered to occur in two ways: either directly at the location of highest compression by the ligature, which occurs on the side opposite to the position of the knot (Figures 4.88–4.90), or indirectly because of the neck structures being too stretched, which is mostly seen in the area surrounding the position of the ligature knot.

CONCLUSION

Hyoid bone fracture doesn't indicate the knot position in persons older than 30 years, which could imply that direct pressure is more important for fracture development and that it could also depend on the contact area between the ligature and the neck skin – the thinner the ligature, the higher the applied pressure per square unit of skin area (Figures 4.88 and 4.89).

It could also be said that the superior horns of thyroid cartilage get fractured usually due to stretching on the same side as the ligature knot, and it does not depend on ligature thickness but instead on the weight of the body or body part suspended by it. The force can propagate across the anatomic neck structures, including the throat skeleton, as these form a physiological unit, and get transmitted indirectly to the side opposite to the knot.

According to studies, the absence of hyoid and laryngeal fractures could indicate an anterior position of the ligature knot. An anterior subluxation of the cervical vertebrae could indicate the same as well.

The author would like to illustrate a case of complete hanging with thin ligature material. In this case, injuries to the neck muscles and cartilage show a similar mechanism as described above. The deceased in this case used the kitchen slab to reach the desired height for tying the ligature (Figure 4.88). The complete suspension of the body with a thin ligature caused the entire force of the weight of the body to be transmitted to the neck, causing transmission at a narrow point leading to contusion of the neck muscles (Figure 4.89) and also left ala of thyroid fracture at the point of contact (Figure 4.90).

TWIN SUICIDAL PACT BY HANGING

A suicide pact is an agreement between two or more people to kill themselves. Hanging is a common method of suicide reported in case of suicidal pact. Usually one or more than one member may choose hanging as a method of suicide in suicidal pact. The author has conducted many such cases of suicide. An elderly couple committed suicide by hanging from an iron bar in their bedroom. They were depressed due to physical illness (Figures 4.91a, 4.91b).

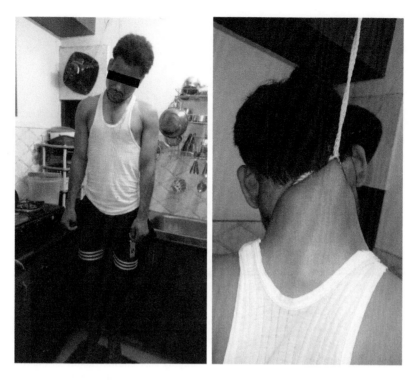

FIGURE 4.88 Shows a case of complete hanging using a nylon rope as the ligature material with a running knot present over right posterior aspect of the neck. The deceased used the kitchen's slab to reach the desired height for tying the ligature above and then jumped from it to hang himself.

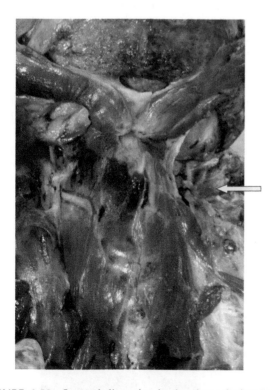

FIGURE 4.89 Internal dissection in the above-depicted complete hanging case shows that contusion of the neck muscles is present corresponding to the ligature mark position over the neck and is seen over the right side, middle and a little to the left of the midline of the neck. This shows the mechanism where the pressure is applied directly by the ligature on neck structures and the ligature material being thinner resulted in more force being applied per square inch of the skin.

DOUBLE SUICIDAL HANGING WITH A SINGLE LIGATURE: A CASE REPORT

The author conducted postmortem examination of a case at AIIMS, New Delhi along with Dr. C. Behera, Additional Professor, in which a single ligature was used by a couple to commit a suicide pact by hanging. A 30-year-old male and a 26-year-old female who were working as casual labor had committed the suicide pact in their bedroom by using a single chunni. They had used the ends of a single chunni as a ligature around the neck and the middle part was crossing an iron bar and there was no fixation of the ligature material. As the ligature was not fixed at any point, the male being comparatively heavier than the female, the male was found in kneeling position and the female was in standing position, possibly due to the free movement of the ligature material over the iron bar (Figure 4.92).

The male victim who was moderately built had the ligature mark which was reddish-brown in color and obliquely placed. The knot was located on the right side of his neck just behind the ear near the mastoid tip (Figure 4.93a).

The female victim had reddish-brown, incomplete ligature mark over the front of the neck above thyroid cartilage; the knot was positioned near the left angle of the mandible (Figure 4.93b).

Suicide pacts are rarely encountered in forensic practice. This case is very unique for the reason that it's a suicide pact where two deceased who are a couple have used only a single ligature for completing the process of double hanging, which has not been cited earlier in the literature. A single ligature may have been used by the couple to ensure

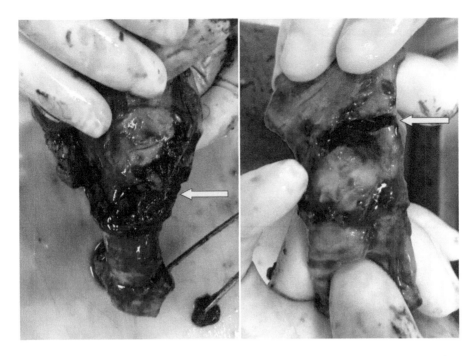

FIGURE 4.90   Internal dissection in the above-depicted complete hanging case shows fracture of the thyroid cartilage over left ala and near the left side inferior horn. This position corresponds to the place where ligature's highest compression force is experienced, and it is opposite to the position of the knot. The jump from the kitchen slab in this case and the nature of the ligature material, a nylon rope, could have caused a great amount of local sudden compressive force causing these features.

both die together. They were depressed due to severe finan-cial constraint. Emotional stresses due to the death of a close relative coupled with financial constraint might have triggered them to take such an extreme step.

POSTMORTEM ARTIFACTS IN HANGING LEADS TO SUSPICION OF A MURDER CASE

The author has seen many instances of misinterpretation of the postmortem artifacts by relatives, police and even a few inexperienced autopsy surgeons, resulting in confusions

during the investigation. This is more frequently seen when the circumstances were suspicious. Careful evaluation of the entire case as a whole, including the timeline and chro-nology of events, position and state of the deceased body at the scene of crime, internal and external postmortem exam-ination findings and other forensic evidences, including the viscera analysis report, is needed to rule out criminality in such cases. Knowledge and awareness regarding all pos-sible peri-mortem and postmortem artifacts is needed while giving expert medico-legal opinions in similar cases. The below-mentioned case is an interesting example of misin-terpretation of postmortem artifacts. This case was referred

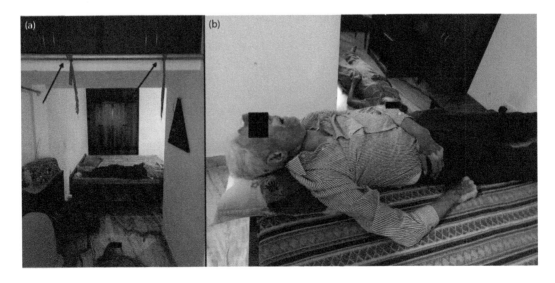

FIGURE 4.91   (a) Arrows showing hanging points. (b) The bodies of the elderly couple.

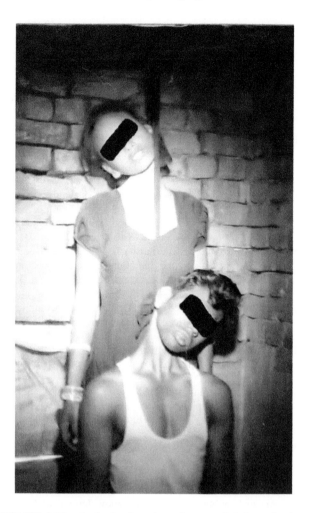

FIGURE 4.92 A single chunni used suspended from the iron bar and both ends of the chunni acting as ligature around the neck of the male and female. The position of the male is seen to be kneeling and that of female being standing.

to the author to obtain expert medico-legal opinion regarding the cause and manner of death of an adult male who was first found in partial hanging position in a bamboo tree plantation. After postmortem examination, the doctor opined the case as death due to hanging. The allegation from the part of relatives was homicide committed during the post-poll violence in the state of West Bengal. The case was referred to CBI by the honorable High Court, and an expert medico-legal opinion was requested from the author. One of the main doubts regarding this case was the presence of 'blood stains' over dhoti (cloth worn on lower half) of the deceased. The image captured when the deceased body was still at the alleged scene of occurrence (Figure 4.94) showed the lower limbs of the deceased in flexed position with an angulation of about 90 indicating that rigor mortis is well developed in the body of the deceased. This limb position in rigor mortis is consistent with partial hanging as in kneeling or sitting posture.

Purging fluid dribbling marks were noted around the nostrils and the right cheek of the deceased (Figure 4.95). There was no open injury present over the body of the deceased, which could result in bleeding in this case. The color of the fluid stain is exaggerated by the orange color of the dhoti, resulting in the false interpretation of 'blood stain'. The dark fluid stains present over the dhoti were due to postmortem artifact of staining by fluids from natural orifices/handling. Frothing, vomitus or blood can be seen in similar cases over mouth and nostrils in various stages of changes of decomposition. Feces and urine stains can also be seen. A medico-legal expert should consider these possible postmortem purging artifacts potentially misinterpreted as fatal 'hemorrhages' and should correlate the same with other circumstantial and scientific evidences to reach a logical conclusion of the case.

In the absence of any relevant injuries other than the oblique, noncontinuous ligature mark and absence of any

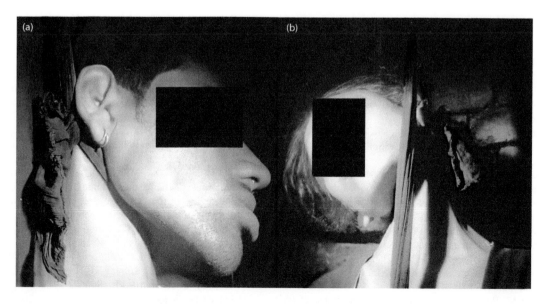

FIGURE 4.93 (a) The knot in case of the male victim was present over the right side of neck near the mastoid tip. (b) In case of female victim, the knot was present over the left angle of the mandible.

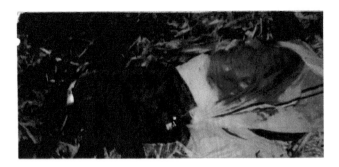

FIGURE 4.94 Lower limbs seen flexed at knees and dark purging fluid stain found over dhoti, which was perceived as blood due to grave injuries.

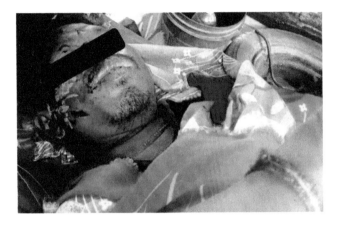

FIGURE 4.95 Purging fluid dribbling marks around nostrils and right cheek.

intoxicating drugs in the viscera analysis report, considering the details of postmortem report and other circumstantial and forensic evidences, the author concluded the case as a suicidal partial hanging.

BIBLIOGRAPHY

1. Kanchan T, Menon A, Menezes RG. Methods of choice in completed suicides: gender differences and review of literature. Journal of Forensic Sciences. 2009;54(4):938–42.
2. Rao D. An autopsy study of death due to suicidal hanging—264 cases. Egyptian Journal of Forensic Sciences. 2016;6:248–54.
3. Simonsen J. Patho-anatomic findings in neck structures in asphyxiation due to hanging. Forensic Science International. 1988;38:83–91.
4. Talukder MA, Mansur MA, Kadir MM. Incidence of typical and atypical hanging among 66 hanging cases. Mymensingh Medical Journal. 2008 Jul;17(2):149–51.
5. Badkur DS, Yadav J, Arora A, Bajpayee R, Dubey BP. Nomenclature for knot position in hanging: a study of 200 cases. Journal of Indian Academy of Forensic Medicine. 2012 Jan–Mar;34(1):34–6. ISSN 0971-0973 36.
6. Bowen D. Hanging—a review. Forensic Science International. 1982;20:247–9.
7. Bohnert M, Pollak S. Complex suicides—a review of the literature. Archiv fur Kriminologie. 2004;213(5–6):138–53.

8. Sauvageau A, Godin A, Desnoyers S, Kremer C. Six-year retrospective study of suicidal hangings: determination of the pattern of limb lesions induced by body responses to asphyxia by hanging. Journal of Forensic Sciences. 2009;54(5):1089–92.
9. Marcus P, Alcabes P. Characteristics of suicides by inmates in an urban jail. Hospital and Community Psychiatry. 1993;44(3):256–61.
10. Tumram NK, Ambade VN, Bardale RV, Dixit PG. Injuries over neck in hanging death and its relation with ligature material: is it vital? Journal of Forensic and Legal Medicine. 2014;22:80–3.
11. Clément R, Redpath M, Sauvageau A. Mechanism of death in hanging: a historical review of the evolution of pathophysiological hypotheses: mechanism of death in hanging. Journal of Forensic Sciences. 2010 Sep;55(5):1268–71.
12. Russo MC, Antonietti A, Farina D, Verzeletti A. Complete decapitation in suicidal hanging—a case report and a review of the literature. Forensic Science, Medicine and Pathology. 2020;16:325–9.
13. Kodikara S. Attempted suicidal hanging: an uncomplicated recovery. The American Journal of Forensic Medicine and Pathology. 2012 Dec;33(4):317–8.
14. Rao VJ, Wetli CV. The forensic significance of conjunctival petechiae. The American Journal of Forensic Medicine and Pathology. 1988 Mar;9(1):32–4.
15. Ambade VN, Tumram N, Meshram S, Borkar J. Ligature material in hanging deaths: the neglected area in forensic examination. Egyptian Journal of Forensic Sciences. 2015;5(3):109–13.
16. Leth P, Vesterby A. Homicidal hanging masquerading as suicide. Forensic Science International. 1997 Feb 7;85(1):68–70.
17. Bhosle SH, Batra AK, Kuchewar SV. Violent asphyxial death due to hanging: a prospective study. Journal of Forensic Medicine, Science and Law. 2014 Jan–Jun;23(1):1–8.
18. Howard RS, Holmes PA. Koutroumanidis M. Hypoxic-ischaemic brain injury. Practical Neurology. 2011;11:4–18.
19. Clement R, Guay J-P, Redpath M, Sauvageau A. Petechiae in hanging: a retrospective study of contributing variables. American Journal of Forensic Medicine and Pathology. 2011;32:378–82.
20. Bohnert M, Faller-Marquardt M, Lutz S, Amberg R, Weisser H-J, Pollak S. Transfer of biological traces in cases of hanging and ligature strangulation. Forensic Science International. 2001;116:107–15.
21. Suárez-Peñaranda JM, Alvarez T, Miguéns X, Rodríguez-Calvo MS, De Abajo BL, Cortesão M, Cordeiro C, Vieira DN, Munoz JI. Characterization of lesions in hanging deaths. Journal of Forensic Sciences. 2008 May;53(3):720–3.
22. Tumram NK, et al. Injuries over neck in hanging deaths and its relation with ligature material: is it vital? Journal of Forensic and Legal Medicine. 2014;22:80–3.
23. Ben Dhiab M, Jdidi M, Nouma Y, Ben Mansour N, Belhadj M, Souguir MK. Accidental hanging: a report of four cases and review of the literature. Journal of Clinical Pathology and Forensic Medicine. 2014 Feb;5(1):1–5.
24. Ahmad M, Hossain MZ. Hanging as a method of suicide: retrospective analysis of postmortem cases. Journal of Armed Forces Medical College Bangladesh. 2010 Dec;6(2).
25. Ali E, Maksud M, Zubyra SJ, Hossain MS, Debnath PR, Alam A, Chakrabarty PK. Suicide by hanging: a study of 334 cases. Bangladesh Medical Journal. 2014 May;43(2):90–3.

26. Krywanczyk A, Shapiro S. A retrospective study of blade wound characteristics in suicide and homicide. American Journal of Forensic Medicine and Pathology. 2015 Dec;36(4):305–10.

27. Nouma Y, Ben Ammar W, Bardaa S, Hammami Z, Maatoug S. Accidental hanging among children and adults: a report of two cases and review of the literature. Egyptian Journal of Forensic Sciences. 2016;6:310–4.

28. Khan MK, Hanif SA. Accidental hanging on loaded sugarcane trolley—a case report. Egyptian Journal of Forensic Sciences. 2012;2:139–41.

29. Kodikara S, Alagiyawanna R. Accidental hanging by a T shirt collar in a man with morphine intoxication: an unusual case. American Journal of Forensic Medicine and Pathology. 2011 Sep;32(3):260–2.

30. Sauvageau A, LaHarpe R, King D, Dowling G, Andrews S, Kelly S, Ambrosi C, Guay JP, Geberth VJ. Agonal sequences in 14 filmed hangings with comments on the role of the type of suspension, ischemic habituation, and ethanol intoxication on the timing of agonal responses. American Journal of Forensic Medicine and Pathology. 2011 Jun;32(2):104–7.

31. Matsumoto S, Iwadate K, Aoyagi M, Ochiai E, Ozawa M, Asakura K. An experimental study on the macroscopic findings of ligature marks using a murine model. American Journal of Forensic Medicine and Pathology. 2013 Mar;34(1):72–4.

32. Dayapala A, Samarasekera A, Jayasena A. An uncommon delayed sequela after pressure on the neck: an autopsy case report. American Journal of Forensic Medicine and Pathology. 2012 Mar;33(1):80–2.

33. Patel JB, Bambhaniya AB, Chaudhari KR, Upadhyay MC. Study of death due to compression of neck by ligature. International Journal of Health Sciences and Research. 2015 Aug;5(8).

34. Bamousa MS, AL-Madani OM, Alsoway KS, Madadin MS, Mashhour MM, Aldossary M, Kharoshah M. Importance of tissue biopsy in suicidal hanging deaths. Egyptian Journal of Forensic Sciences. 2015;5:140–3.

35. Behera C, Chauhan M, Sikary AK. Body coloration artifacts encountered at medicolegal autopsy in India. American Journal of Forensic Medicine and Pathology. 2019 Jun;40(2):129–35.

36. Boghossian E, Clement R, Redpath M, Sauvageau A. Respiratory, circulatory, and neurological responses to hanging: a review of animal models. Journal of Forensic Sciences. 2010 Sep;55(5):1272–7.

37. Doberentz E, Schyma C, Madea B. Histological examination of the carotid bifurcation in case of violence against the neck. Forensic Science International. 2012;216:135–40.

38. Bhausaheb NA, Baburao CS, Banerjee KK, Kohli A. Pattern of external and internal findings in deaths owing to hanging: a study in northeast Delhi. International Journal of Medical Science and Public Health. 2015;4(11):1536–9.

39. Ozer E, Yildirim A, Kırcı GS, Ilhan R, İşcanlı MD, Tetikçok R. Deaths as a result of hanging. Biomedical Research. 2017;28(2):556–61.

40. Sharma N, Shrivastava A, Vyas PC. A Study of Morphology and Histopathology of Ligature Marks in Asphyxial Deaths by Compression of Neck in Jodhpur Region, Rajasthan. JMSCR. June 2018;06(06):923–929.

41. Polacco M, D'Alessio P, Ausania F, Zobel B, Pascali VL, d'Aloja E, Miscusi M, De-Giorgio F. Virtual autopsy in hanging. American Journal of Forensic Medicine and Pathology. 2013 Jun;34(2):107–9.

42. Kokatanur CM, Havanur B. Histopathological study of skin and subcutaneous tissues at ligature mark in cases of hanging and strangulation. Medico-Legal Update. 2014 Jul 1;14(2).

43. Yadav A, Gupta BM. Histopathological changes in skin and subcutaneous tissues at ligature site-in-cases of hanging and strangulation. Journal of Indian Academy of Forensic Medicine. 2018 Dec;31(3):200–4.

44. Perju-Dumbravă D, Rebeleanu C, Ureche D, Pop O, Bulgaru-Iliescu D, Radu CC. The medico-legal value of histopathological examination in hanging. Romanian Journal of Legal Medicine. 2018;26:349–53.

45. Singh D, Vohra V. Histopathological study of blood vessels in hanging and strangulation deaths. Journal of Punjab Academy of Forensic Medicine and Toxicology. 2013;13(1):17–9.

46. Ghodake D, Mohite S, Desai H. Histopathological study of carotid arteries in deaths due to hanging. Medico-Legal Update. 2014;14(1):82.

47. Singh D, Vohra V. Histopathological study of lymph nodes in hanging and strangulation deaths. Journal of Indian Academy of Forensic Medicine. 2013;35(2):137–9.

5 Fatal Pressure Over Neck by Strangulation

MANUAL STRANGULATION

Manual strangulation, or throttling, is the constriction of the neck by hands. It's a common method of homicide as no weapon or tool or instrument is required, i.e., bare hands of the perpetrator are sufficient. The frequency of deaths following throttling is higher in comparison with deaths following ligature strangulation. Commonly, homicidal throttling happens between two individuals with a reasonable disparity in the physical attributes. Females are the victims in most cases and perpetrators are generally males. If a female is the perpetrator, victim is usually a child. High variability in the inflicted injuries makes diagnosis of throttling deaths difficult, especially when findings are not of a typical nature.

Manual strangulation can be one of the multiple modalities attempted in a homicidal case. Though injuries consistent with manual strangulation are present, in cases of a suspected violent homicide, the examination for other causes of death should be carried out thoroughly.

Mechanism of Injury

All combinations of mechanisms of death that have been described for hanging are possible in manual strangulation also. The compression of larynx and windpipe results in complete occlusion of the lumen. Jugular veins are compressed in most of the cases. Carotid artery compression is also common, but the waxing and waning grip may allow some arterial blood flow in between. Complete occlusion of vertebral artery is generally not possible in adult victims if there is only one perpetrator. Hence, most of the cases of manual strangulation show signs of congestion above the level of neck constriction. Many cases of manual strangulations present with minimal or no evident external injuries and facial congestion. The possibility of carotid sinus stimulation followed by reflex cardiac arrest due to stimulation of the 10th cranial nerve center at brain stem is the most acceptable reason for these cases.

Autopsy Findings

External Examination

Typical Fingernail Abrasion

The 'typical' external injuries are crescent-shaped abrasions and oval or circular dermal contusions on the neck.

Abrasions on the neck in cases of manual strangulation can be broadly classified into two categories. One is the abrasions produced by static pressure of the fingernail tips when it indents into the soft tissues of the neck. Crescent-shaped abrasions (Figure 5.1) generally depict injury caused by the tip of fingernails of the perpetrator during the act. Attempts have been made to correlate the placement of these curvilinear abrasions and the handedness of the perpetrator, but have not yielded any conclusive results. Generally, the concavity of the fingernail abrasion is directed towards the pulp of that finger, but it can also be crescent shaped in the reverse direction, linear or even 'S' shaped (Figure 5.2). Generally, in manual strangulation, fingernail abrasions are situated more towards the sides of the neck at and above the level of thyroid cartilage. They are seen at the front and back aspects of the neck, but are less frequent.

The second category of abrasions is due to the dragging effect of nail tips over the skin of the neck, which may be those of the assailant or the victim. Abrasions caused by the fingernail tips of the victim generally follow a linear and vertical course, and are parallel if multiple fingertips are involved. These dragging abrasions are struggle marks and can show different orientations as well. Differentiation between the nail tip abrasions due to the struggle of victim from those of the nails of the perpetrator by merely analyzing the objective findings during autopsy is considered unrealistic by many authors. Moist skin may not reveal all these abrasions during a naked eye examination. So it is advisable that in those cases, the neck examination should be done only after the body surface has become dry. Unique peculiarities of the nail tips of the assailant may be reproduced as imprints. Analysis of shapes of fingernail tips and scientific comparison with the abrasions may be helpful in the course of investigation and trial if the identity of the assailant is in question. Examination of the perpetrator within a few days of the incident shows similar nail tip abrasions, commonly on the upper limbs. Any case of suspected manual strangulation requires preservation of the fingernail clippings or nail scrapings for further comparative analysis of physical or biological trace evidences. These comparative forensic analyses are proven to be useful in fixing the identity of assailants and in identifying the exact scene of crime. The shape of the tips of nails and any breakage if present should be noted in detail during the postmortem examination. Ornaments like rings produce abrasions of

DOI: 10.1201/9780429026317-5

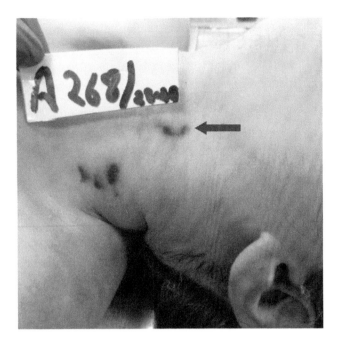

FIGURE 5.1 Fingernail abrasions seen over the neck. 'Crescent'-shaped fingernail abrasions (red arrow) along with other fingernail abrasions seen over the neck.

peculiar shapes and sizes, and the same should be noted in detail during the postmortem examination for possible future comparisons.

Harm and Rajs studied fingernail injuries and classified them into three:

1. *Impression marks:* Where the nails dig into the skin perpendicular to the surface and penetrate the epidermis and dermis. The marks are usually curved, comma-shaped, exclamation-shaped, oval or triangular with length of about 1–1.5 cm.
2. *Claw marks:* Where the nails dig into the skin at an angle and undermine the skin, usually penetrating up to the dermis. They are usually smaller than impression marks.

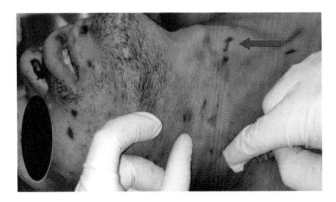

FIGURE 5.2 Fingernail abrasions seen over the neck and around the mouth and nostrils. 'S'-shaped fingernail abrasions (red arrow) along with others fingernail abrasions seen over the neck.

3. *Scratch marks:* Where the nails are drawn over the skin parallel to the surface. These usually involve only the epidermis and appear as multiple, parallel scratch abrasions.

These injuries may be evident in cases of strangulation where the body is disposed in a way to simulate suicides. Meticulous external examination will help the autopsy surgeons to conclude these cases.

Nail Mark and Injuries in the Neck in Case of Manual Strangulation

Fingernail abrasions are one of the characteristic features of manual strangulation and are usually appreciated as curvilinear abrasions produced by nails. In manual strangulation, abrasions and bruises caused by the pressure of the fingers and thumb are usually seen on either side of the neck (Figures 5.3a and 5.3b). The mark by the thumb is usually situated at a higher level than other fingers. Crescentic abrasions are found if the fingernails are pressed into the skin. In rare cases, bruising may be absent on the skin but may be present in deeper tissues. There are multiple factors that take a dynamic part in the production of a fingernail mark, which include the force applied for compression, the shape of the nails, the elasticity of the skin, pigmentation of skin of victim, the duration of compression, direction of compression of neck, presence of any intervening cloth or soft material and also the struggle by the victim to free from the compressive force.

Sometimes, abrasion can be caused by the victim themselves when trying to remove the grasping force of the assailant, or other injuries due to the presence of intervening clothes or chain can cause friction rub with the skin, producing abrasion. Rarely, bite marks or other injuries can also be produced especially when there was involvement of sexual assault or consental sex on the female prior to

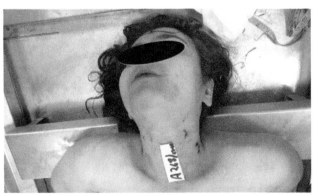

FIGURE 5.3a Anterior view of the neck shows multiple crescentic abrasions and bruises in a case of manual strangulation. Abrasions are seen on both sides of the neck, but more abrasions are seen on the left side, which could be due to compression of the neck by assailant's right hand where the four fingers lie on one side causing multiple injuries and only thumb on the other side causing only a few injuries.

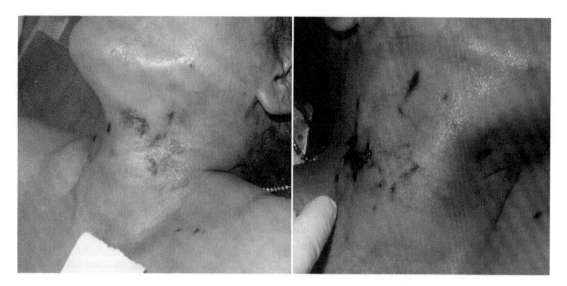

FIGURE 5.3b Anterior view of the neck shows multiple abrasions and bruises in a case of manual strangulation. Injuries are seen on both sides of the neck.

or during strangulation. In Figure 5.4, the deceased female was involved in a consensual sex with her friend; during the act, the friend accidentally compressed the neck, causing the death of the victim.

- *Superficial contusion:* The second set of external injuries is superficial contusions (Figure 5.4). A typical case where a single firm grip was used shows one circular or oval dermal contusion on one side of the neck, and a few over the other side represent pressure from fat pad of thumb and other fingers respectively. The grip of the palm of the perpetrator also produces contusions of skin, which involves a larger area. The contusions are often asymmetrically distributed over either side of the neck, with a larger affected area on one side and just a few small contusions on the other.

Although contusions over the neck in a case of manual strangulation are suggestive of the site of contact of the assailant's finger pads, such a pattern of asymmetric distribution must not be used to determine the handedness of the assailant as these can lead to inaccurate conclusions.

However, in real-life scenarios, the victims defend themselves during the entire struggle till they become unconscious, hence the grip tends to run over the front and sides of the neck. In practice, most of the finger poke contusions of manual strangulation represent irregular dermal contusions that are a confluence of multiple circular or oval contusions. These contusions may also show corresponding nail tip abrasions. Dermal contusions at the front of the neck at midline are common in manual strangulation cases (Figure 5.5). Cases of manual strangulation rarely produce

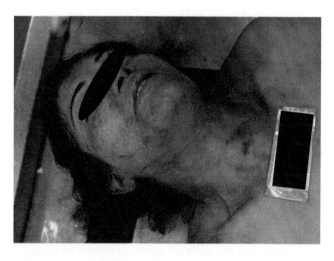

FIGURE 5.4 Multiple abrasions and contusions are found over the anterior aspect of the neck with a few petechial hemorrhages also appreciable over the neck and face.

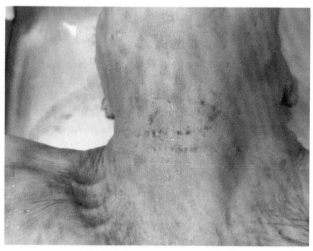

FIGURE 5.5 Superficial contusion present over the anterior midline of the neck seen commonly in manual strangulation.

contusions at the posterior aspect of the neck. Contusions are generally positioned higher up on the neck, just under the chin region. Superficial contusion at the under-chin area reflects friction with dorsum of hand of the assailant while the victim tries to flex the neck during his struggle to survive. These contusions are generally superficial, and if deeper extension is noted, the possibility of any blunt impact injury should be considered. Adjacent areas like the front of upper chest and lower aspect of face also show dermal contusions and abrasions. In many instances, dermal contusions may be minimal or even absent, creating difficulty in interpretation of objective observations. Darker shades of skin preclude identification of small dermal abrasions in many cases. Careful examination of the reflected skin has to be done mandatorily in all these cases to identify the real extent of dermal injuries. Since death follows shortly after the fatal incident, contusions of manual strangulation during postmortem examination show bluish red or purplish color suggestive of a recent contusion. Since slippage of palms is common in throttling due to the resistance from the victims, cheek and lip contusions mimicking injury pattern of smothering are seen in many cases.

- **Associated external injury**: There can be associated external injuries of assault or sexual violence that throw light on the circumstances and motive of the crime. Counter pressure injuries in the form of abrasions and contusions are common at the posterior aspect of the body over occiput, back of shoulder blades, sacrum, buttocks and dorsal projections of all joints of limbs. Forced restrain of the victim causes multiple abrasions and contusions around wrists and forearms. These injuries may show some pattern of the restraint used or circular or oval contusions of finger pads along with larger contusions produced by the palm of the assailant. Failed attempt of manual strangulation followed by homicide by some other mechanism can be identified in many violent homicidal deaths. Identifying injuries of manual strangulation along with evidence of cause of death of homicidal manner is also not rare. These cases represent deaths following combined effects of multiple modalities of homicide.
- **General findings**: Manual strangulation produces facial congestion, petechiae, cyanosis and edema. Subconjunctival hemorrhages are common. Deaths following manual strangulation show less congestive findings in comparison with those of ligature strangulation. Though common in ligature strangulation, throttling deaths generally do not show nasal and oral bleeding. Otoscope examination of tympanic membrane shows hemorrhages in some cases. A thorough external examination should be carried out under proper lighting. The visible external injuries may look trivial for many inexperienced eyes. Many cases show discharged urine and fecal matter like in many other asphyxial deaths.

Internal Examination

- *Hemorrhages:* Minimal or even absent external neck injuries can show extensive hemorrhage in the underlying tissues. Hemorrhages are common in subcutaneous fat, platysma and strap muscles. The carotid sheet structures, lymph nodes, salivary glands of the under-chin area and outer aspect of the larynx also show contusions in many cases. The parenchyma and sub-capsular regions of the thyroid gland show areas of hemorrhages in certain cases. The base of tongue also shows multiple superficial hemorrhagic areas.
- *Fractures of thyro-hyoid complex:* Virtually all cases of manual strangulation involve direct pressure over the larynx. Since a larger area at the front of the neck is involved, manual strangulation shows more fractures of the thyro-hyoid complex than seen in hanging and ligature strangulation. Mechanisms of causation of the fractures are the same as those in hanging or ligature strangulation, i.e., direct pressure or the transmitted pressure through the thyro-hyoid membrane. These fractures do not directly cause death of the individual but are suggestive of force applied over the voice box. Unilateral isolated fracture of the superior horn of thyroid is the commonest fracture. The second most common fracture in manual strangulation is that of greater cornua of the hyoid bone (Figure 5.6).
- Scientific literature regarding the absolute frequency of these fractures shows great variability. Usually these fractured segments show an inward displacement in most cases. However, both inward and outward fractures are seen in combination in many cases. The side where the thrust from pulp of thumb is applied shows fractures more frequently. Considering the variability of these fractures, opining on the cause or manner of death and the handedness of the assailant solely based on the fracture pattern should not be attempted. These fractures are generally ante-mortem and show hemorrhagic infiltration in the surrounding soft tissues. Vitality of these fractures should be confirmed grossly and microscopically, if in doubt. The autopsy surgeon should be aware of the fact that postmortem fractures may show some artefact hemorrhage around the fracture site. A fracture site has to be dissected for minute details, including position of tear in the periosteum and subperiosteal hemorrhage. Laminar fractures of thyroid cartilage and fractures of cricoid cartilage are rare in manual strangulation, but if present, they indicate severe antero-posterior compression of the neck structures between the external force and the anterior aspect of bodies of cervical vertebrae. Since ossification of hyoid bone and laryngeal cartilages starts late, these structures are elastic in early decades of life and fractures are

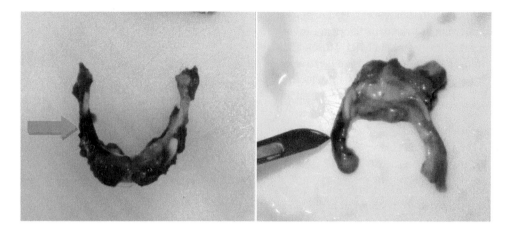

FIGURE 5.6   Fracture of greater cornua of hyoid bone with surrounding infiltration.

less frequent in the younger age group. Hyoid bone fractures are more commonly seen in victims of throttling and hanging above 40 years of age due to the calcification of bone.

Hyoid bone fractures are classified into three types:

i. **Inward Compression Fracture:** This type is commonly seen in the cases of throttling; the main force causing the fracture is inward compression of the hyoid bone. The greater horns of hyoid are compressed inwards, which causes fracture and tear of the periosteum on the outer surface of the bone, displacing the fractured ends inwards. It can be demonstrated by holding the body of the hyoid in one hand and its distal portion in between the fingers of the other hand, which could be bent inwards, but not outwards due to the intact periosteum on the medial surface.

ii. **Antero-Posterior Compression Fracture:** The hyoid bone gets compressed backwards and the greater cornu gets impacted over the cervical vertebra, causing fracture with displacement of fractured ends outwards. Here the periosteum gets torn on the inner side, making the fragment to move outwards. It can be seen in cases of hanging, ligature strangulation, etc.

iii. **Avulsion Fracture:** It occurs as a result of traction on thyrohyoid ligament caused by hyperextension of the neck, or violent movement either by lateral or downward compression. Here the hyoid bone is drawn upwards.

The joints in between greater/lesser cornu and the body should not be mistaken as fractures. Also, the ante-mortem nature of hyoid bone fracture should be confirmed by the presence of hemorrhage at the affected area.

- *Froth in trachea:* Tracheo-bronchial tree may contain white foam with streaky hemorrhages, resembling that of drowning.

- Scalp and brain show intense congestion and petechiae. Some cases of manual strangulation show patches of subarachnoid hemorrhage.
- Lungs show edema, hemorrhage, acute emphysema and areas of atelectasis.
- Many cases show internal injuries due to other modalities such as assault and sexual violence.

Samples for Collection

In all cases of manual strangulation, the possibility of incapacitation following intoxication has to be assessed by chemical analysis of visceral organs.

Radiological Examination

- **Postmortem Multislice CT (PMCT)** provides us with many details in asphyxia cases. This technique is very helpful in finding out injuries over tiny structures in neck, which is surrounded by many small soft tissues and thus difficult to be appreciated in traditional autopsy. Findings that are seen in PMCT are ligature mark by 3D reconstruction, fracture of greater horns of hyoid bone and superior horn of thyroid cartilage. MSCT is an important tool in detecting injuries due to laryngeal trauma such as fractures. 3D reconstruction shows us ossification of triticeous cartilages, fractures of horns of thyroid cartilage as displaced fragments or discontinuity. Many forensic surgeons suggest performing PMCT before the traditional autopsy and with special concern for strangulation cases because it gives us an idea for choosing the right dissecting technique. Reformatted MSCT shows fracture of greater horns of hyoid bone and lamiae of the thyroid cartilage.
- **Magnetic resonance imaging (MRI)** is an important tool in detecting soft tissue hemorrhage in strangulation cases. In MRI, muscular hemorrhage in the retropharyngeal areas and within the posterior crico-arytenoid muscles can be appreciated. Lymph node hemorrhage is seen in both manual

and ligature strangulation cases. Hemorrhages appear as hyper-intense areas in Short tau inversion recovery (STIR) - weighted MRI. Muscle that appears tumid and hyper-intense is suggestive of hemorrhage and swelling. MRI aids in detecting lymph node hemorrhage, soft tissue and muscular hemorrhage.

DELAYED DEATH IN MANUAL STRANGULATION

Asphyxia is the commonest cause of death in manual strangulation. Delayed deaths due to mechanical asphyxia may occur due to anoxic cerebral damage occurring as a complication following prolonged cerebral hypoxia. There are cases where other mechanisms like injuries sustained over the neck may cause death. This could be due to hypoxia occurring as a result of massive subcutaneous or mediastinal emphysema following tracheal or laryngeal laceration. In such cases, airway occlusion occurs as a result of edematous or hemorrhagic swelling of the pharyngeal tissues or aryepiglottic folds. In certain other cases, complications like acute respiratory distress syndrome (ARDS), aspiration pneumonia, pneumonitis or carotid artery dissection causing vascular compromise can cause death.

A review of a few of the case reports of delayed deaths due to manual strangulation that have been published shows that in some cases, the mechanism of death is not well established.

In 1996, Anscombe and Knight published a case of attempted strangulation with a survival time of seven days. The authors were convinced that the cause of death was hypoxic brain damage, although they have not mentioned any gross pathological lesion or any specific histopathological finding.

In 2005, Badkur D et al reported a case of attempted manual strangulation who survived for 19 days and then died due to cerebral infarction from occlusion of cerebral vessels.

CASE REPORT 1: DELAYED DEATH IN ATTEMPTED CASE OF STRANGULATION

A 27-year-old man from Uttar Pradesh was brought to AIIMS with complaints of breathing difficulty and stridor. History was that a few people tried to strangle him manually during an assault. A portion of the ligature mark was identified at the emergency department and documented. Airway was secured initially by endotracheal intubation and later by tracheostomy. The condition of the victim deteriorated during treatment, and he succumbed to death on the seventh day after admission. During autopsy, ligature mark was not distinctly appreciable since the scab had started to fall off and an iatrogenic artefact was also present over the front of the neck, the tracheostome. Apart from these multiple contusions and lacerations over the inner aspect of the lower lip (Figure 5.7), scabbed abrasions over the neck were present

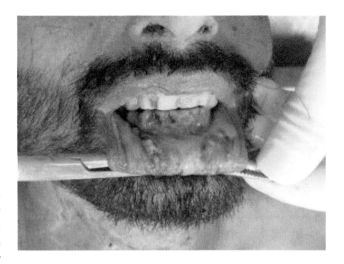

FIGURE 5.7 Multiple contusions and lacerations present on the inner aspect of the lower lip.

(Figure 5.8). On dissection of the neck, around 5 mL collection of yellowish pus was present over the left side of the neck at the level of thyroid cartilage beneath the sternohyoid muscle. Another collection of around 5 mL of yellowish pus was present between the inner aspect of thyroid cartilage and the laryngeal mucosa on the left side (Figure 5.9), with a connection with the above-mentioned pus collection and the lumen of the larynx via a laceration over the left side of laryngeal mucosa, which was stained with yellowish pus along the margins. There was also fracture of thyroid cartilage at the midline with separation of the alae (Figures 5.10 and 5.11) and fracture of superior horns of thyroid cartilage on both sides with infiltration along the fractured ends. Vertical fracture of the cricoid cartilage, 0.5 cm left lateral to the anterior midline was also present. Hyoid bone was intact. Lungs showed changes of pneumonia and pleural effusion. These fractures are consistent with the history of manual strangulation, and the opinion was given as death due to respiratory insufficiency consequent

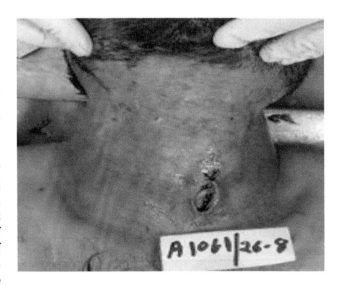

FIGURE 5.8 Multiple scabbed abrasions present over the neck.

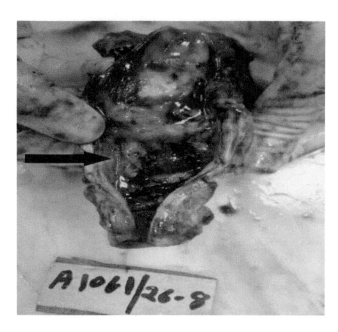

FIGURE 5.9 Yellowish pus seen in the laryngo-tracheal complex.

to manual strangulation. Laminar fractures of thyroid cartilage and cricoid cartilage usually do not happen with hanging and ligature strangulation. These injuries are seen in some cases of manual strangulation or in cases of direct blow to the neck.

MEDICOLEGAL ASPECT OF MANUAL STRANGULATION

Suicide by throttling is not possible in normal circumstances since the persistent compression of neck cannot be maintained beyond the level of cerebral hypoxia, which causes the individual to become unconscious and loosen the grip over the neck.

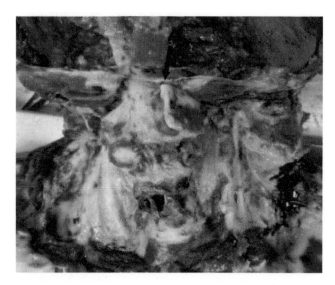

FIGURE 5.10 Fracture of thyroid cartilage at the midline with separation of the alae.

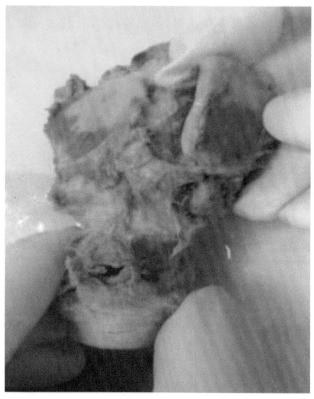

FIGURE 5.11 Fracture of thyroid cartilage at the midline with separation of the alae seen after fixation in formalin.

Homicidal throttling is the commonest manner of homicide. Women, children and those under the influence of alcohol or drugs are likely victims of throttling. Struggle injuries are often associated with homicidal throttling.

Accidental throttling can occur due to the sudden compression of neck, which may occur during an act of affection or when done just for fun.

In some cases, the line between accidental and homicidal throttling is narrow and difficult to prove on the mere basis of the objective findings of a routine autopsy, especially when the injuries in the body are less. If the victim is female, it is imperative that an examination for sexual assault be carried out prior to autopsy. This includes a thorough examination of the genitalia, breasts, thighs, lips, oral cavity, etc. for injuries as well as the collection of necessary samples such as swabs from the genitalia, oral cavity, bite mark site if any and pubic hair samples both combed and plucked.

A variation of manual strangulation is palmar strangulation, in which force is applied over the neck using the open palm, without any of the fingers, fingertips or nails coming in contact with the skin of the neck. In most such cases observed by forensic pathologists, the victims were children and the assailants were adults who were intoxicated. In such cases, there are no external injuries that can be attributed to the application of the hand, nor is there any evidence of injuries on internal dissection. Also, the classical signs of asphyxia such as congestion and petechiae in conjunctiva and peri-orbital skin may be observed only in some cases.

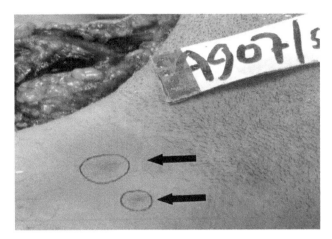

FIGURE 5.12   Two small contusions found on the left side of the neck.

CASE 2: TRIVIAL INJURY OVER THE NECK CAN BE FATAL

In 2017, the dead body of a 45-year-old male was recovered under mysterious circumstances from his friend's house, where he was last seen with three of his friends. As per friends' statements recorded by the police, all of them were drinking alcohol, eating and dancing together till around 11.30 pm, after which two of the friends left. One of the friends went to sleep in a different room, while the deceased lay down on a bedding present in the room in which they were partying. Next day, at around 5 am, the friend came to wake up the deceased, and found him dead. Post-mortem examination was conducted in AIIMS and revealed two small contusions present over the left side of the neck (Figure 5.12). On dissection of the neck, extravasation of blood was present within the muscle layers of the neck underlying the external contusions and extravasation of blood was present within the layers of the left side of thyro-hyoid muscles (Figure 5.13). All other possible causes of death were examined, investigated and finally ruled out. The opinion on the cause of death was given as asphyxia as a result of manual strangulation.

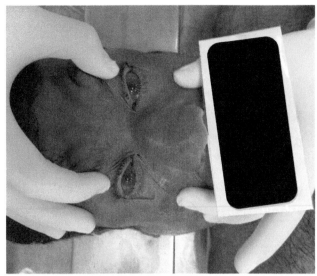

FIGURE 5.14   Congestion of bilateral conjunctivae along with congestion of face and upper chest is seen.

CASE 3: CASE OF COMBINED STRANGULATION AND SMOTHERING

In 2019, a dead body of a 40-year-old male was found on his bed in his residence with blood oozing out from his nose, at about 4:15 pm. He was last seen alive at about 11 pm the previous night when he had dinner and went to bed. Postmortem examination was conducted at AIIMS, New Delhi by a board of five doctors. On external examination, rigor mortis was present and postmortem lividity was present and fixed. Bilateral conjunctivae were congested. Congestion was also seen over the face, neck and upper chest (Figure 5.14) with blood oozing out from his nostrils. Bluish discoloration of palms, soles, lips and fingernail beds (Figure 5.15) was present. Erosion of mucosa of both sides of the nasal septum was present. Two injuries were present

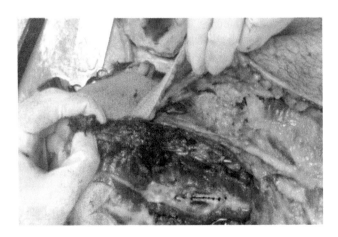

FIGURE 5.13   Extravasation of blood in internal neck muscle layers underlying contusions over the left side of the neck.

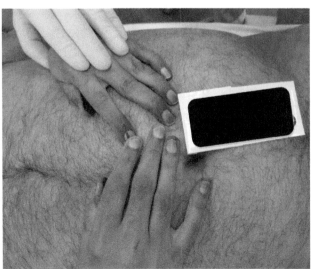

FIGURE 5.15   Bluish discoloration of the nail beds seen in both hands.

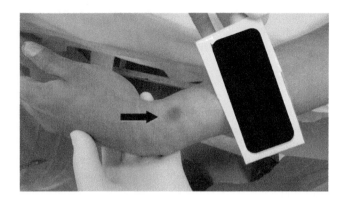

FIGURE 5.16 A contusion present over the outer aspect of the left wrist.

over the body – a contusion over the left wrist (Figure 5.16) and an abrasion over the lower abdomen (Figure 5.17).

On external examination of the neck, no obvious injuries could be appreciated (Figure 5.18). On internal examination, all organs were congested. On layer-by-layer dissection of neck structures, multiple contusions of neck muscles (Figure 5.19) and peri-laryngeal neck tissues were present. The inner surface of the epiglottis showed hemorrhages. Tracheal mucosa was congested and showed multiple petechiae.

Opinion as to the cause of death was given as 'Asphyxia due to smothering and strangulation'. The investigating officer identified the possible smothering object, a pillow from his room, and the suspects were the wife of the deceased and the servants. This is a case that was brought for postmortem examination with a history of natural death, but later the PME findings revealed a different story. Here the external injuries were not very evident, but the internal injury pattern was consistent with that of strangulation and smothering. In similar cases, meticulous layer-by-layer dissection of the neck structures under a bloodless field is highly warranted. PMCT of the neck is useful in identifying fractures of the thyrohyoid complex. In this

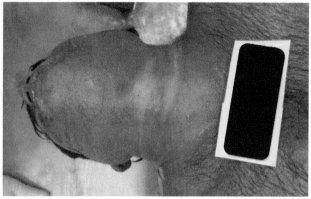

FIGURE 5.18 External examination of the neck did not reveal any obvious injuries.

case, there was no fracture of the bony or cartilaginous structures of the neck.

CASE 4: CASE OF MANUAL STRANGULATION AND SEXUAL ASSAULT

In early 2019, a 25-year-old female from Delhi went missing. She had informed her father that she was going to attend an interview for a job. When she did not return and her phone was not reachable, her father filed a missing complaint. Two days later, her dead body was found dumped in a sac at a nearby place (Figure 5.20). The female was lured with a 'Respectable job' and was invited for an interview at an apartment; when she went there for the interview, she was attacked by four accused who sexually assaulted and throttled her. They had a motive of framing three other people whom the accused were not in good terms with. They forced the victim to pen down a note mentioning the names of the three enemies of the accused as the reason if she dies

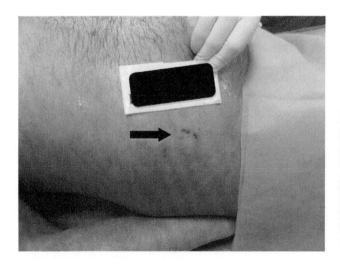

FIGURE 5.17 An abrasion present over the outer aspect of right side of the lower abdomen.

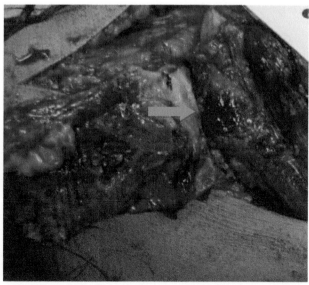

FIGURE 5.19 Contusion seen at the base of the sternocleido-mastoid muscle.

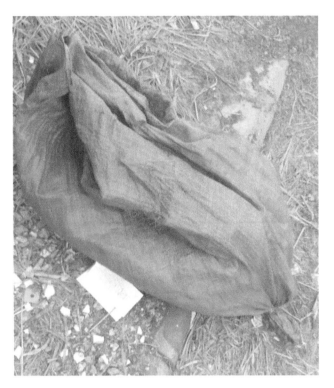

FIGURE 5.20 Dead body of the female in a sac dumped at a nearby place after sexual assault and murdering by manual strangulation (throttling).

and that she was going to meet them (Figure 5.21). After killing her, they packed her dead body in a sac along with the letter written by her placed in her pocket to misguide the police.

The dead body of the deceased was brought to AIIMS for postmortem examination, which showed there were signs of manual strangulation with multiple abrasions and contusion present over the neck (Figures 5.22 and 5.23). The autopsy examination in this case showed typical features of manual strangulation (throttling) with curvilinear fingernail abrasions and other abrasions seen more on the left side of the neck and a few seen on the right side, indicating the assailant used his right hand for throttling.

The case was solved by the police based on tracing the phone signals of the alleged accused, and when there was discrepancy, they searched for possible accused and nabbed the actual murderers.

CASE 5: ACCIDENTAL STRANGULATION DURING CONSENSUAL SEXUAL INTERCOURSE INSIDE A CAR

In August 2017, a dead body of a 38-year-old female was brought to the mortuary of Department of Forensic Medicine & Toxicology, AIIMS, for autopsy. On the night before, she was at her farmhouse in a party and left with her male friend. Her friend brought her naked body to her parents and informed them she died after being accidentally

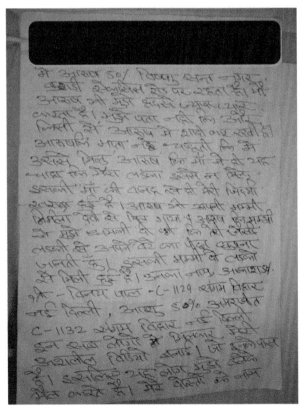

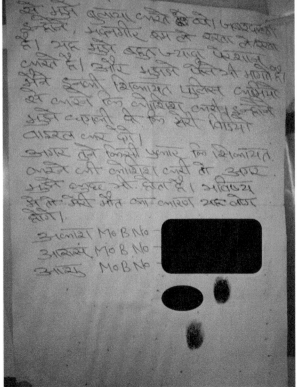

FIGURE 5.21 The letter victim was forced to pen down in her own handwriting with mentioning of the names of three persons whom the accused wanted to frame for the murder.

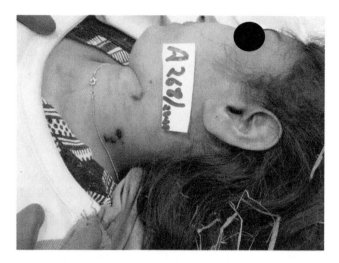

FIGURE 5.22 Shows multiple abrasions and contusions over the neck.

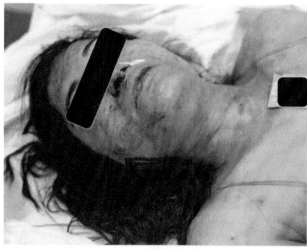

FIGURE 5.24 Congestion of the face and neck can be distinctly appreciated above.

strangled during consensual sexual act with him in his car at a parking spot. The victim's father filed an FIR that his daughter has been murdered. During autopsy, the face and neck were congested (Figure 5.24) and also both her eyes were congested (Figure 5.25). There was presence of reddish color scratch abrasions over the left cheek and contusions over thigh and back. Apart from this, multiple abrasions and contusions were present over the anterior aspect of the neck and around the mouth (Figure 5.26); on dissection of the neck, hemorrhages were present below these abrasions along with multiple patchy hemorrhagic spots within strap muscles bilaterally (Figure 5.27) and on the posterior wall of the pharynx and larynx (Figure 5.28). There was also a fracture of the left superior horn of thyroid along with hematoma (Figure 5.29). The cause of death was declared as 'fatal pressure on the anterior aspect of neck, sufficient to cause death in ordinary course of nature'. After receiving final investigation reports and analysis of the trace evidences, the Medical Board gave a subsequent opinion regarding the manner, which stated that in the absence

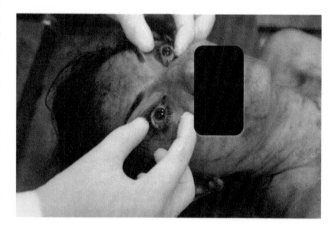

FIGURE 5.25 Congestion of both eyes along with congestion of the face could be seen.

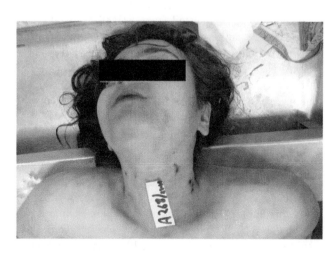

FIGURE 5.23 Shows multiple abrasions and contusions over the neck.

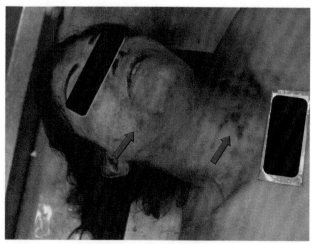

FIGURE 5.26 Multiple abrasions and contusions were seen over the neck and around the mouth.

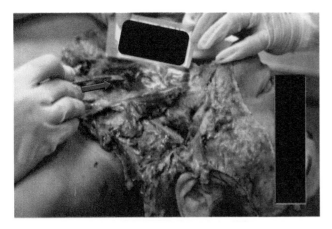

FIGURE 5.27 Dissection shows patchy hemorrhage present over the strap muscles of the neck.

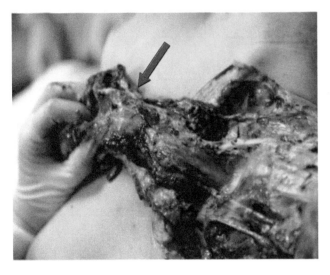

FIGURE 5.28 Congestion and hemorrhage present over the posterior wall of pharynx and larynx.

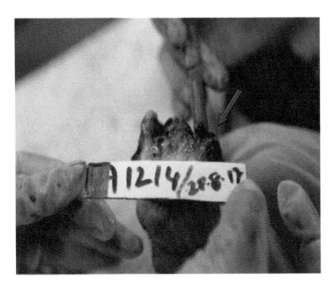

FIGURE 5.29 Fracture of the left superior horn of the thyroid cartilage with surrounding hematoma.

of defense injuries over the body, 'the manner and cause of death in the case as accidental strangulation during an intimate active sexual act in a restrained space like car seat, under influence of alcohol cannot be ruled out'.

CASE REPORT 6: STRANGLED AND BURNED, BODY RECOVERED AFTER YEARS AS SKELETON (SHEENA BORA CASE)

On 24 April 2012, Sheena took a leave of absence and she sent in her written resignation. On the same day, Rahul Mukerjea (Sheena's stepbrother who she was dating) received a breakup SMS from Sheena's phone. On questioning her whereabouts, her mother, Indrani, said that Sheena had gone to the United States for higher studies and hence a missing FIR was never filed. Sheena was never seen after 24 April 2012.

In August 2015, a partly charred and decomposed dead body of an unknown female was recovered from a forest area. Autopsy was conducted and samples were collected; the body was buried after autopsy. Due to charring and decomposition, cause of death could not be ascertained. After 3 years, Indrani Mukerjea and her aides were arrested for her daughter's murder. Indrani Mukerjea is an Indian-born British former HR consultant and media executive. She was the wife of Peter Mukerjea, a retired Indian television executive. In 2007, she co-founded INX Media with her ex-husband where she took on the role of CEO. As per the statements of the lady's aides, they drugged Sheena, strangled her and tried to destroy the body of the victim by burning it with inflammable material and later disposed it in the same forest area where the unknown female dead body was found. Assuming that the unknown dead body was of her daughter, previously buried remains of the body were exhumed for re-evaluation and identification.

CBI INVESTIGATION

The case was transferred to the CBI, and the expert medico-legal opinion was requested from AIIMS Medical Board headed by the author. The recovered skeletal remains of the victim along with all relevant documents were sent to AIIMS, New Delhi for detailed examination. On perusal of the previous reports in relation to the identity of skeletal remains, the AIIMS medical board found it consistent with standards of current medical science knowledge.

IDENTITY CONFIRMED

Identity of the victim was the next big question in relation to the case, and it was confirmed by DNA cross matching between samples collected from the skeletal remains and that of the alleged biological mother, which gave positive results of matching. Ancillary tests like cranio-facial superimposition were done, and they also gave positive results (Figures 5.30 and 5.31).

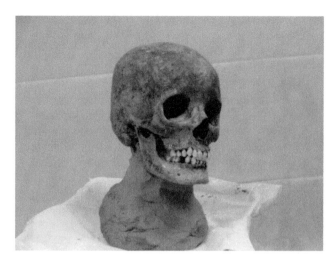

FIGURE 5.30 Articulated skull of the victim during cranio-facial superimposition.

AIIMS MEDICAL BOARD EXPERT OPINION

The Medical Board was of the opinion that the skeletal remains belonged to a female aged around 23 years with some possible variability. Calculated stature was matching with that of the victim. No ante-mortem fractures were identified, but some postmortem loss of skeletal tissue was noted. Thyro-hyoid complex was not present in the submitted skeletal remains. The Medical Board ruled out death due to sharp or blunt force injury and gunshot injury. Since there was a definite attempt to conceal the corpus delicti, the prime evidence of homicide, the Medical Board was sure about the manner of death as homicide.

The cause and manner of death in this case were opined as: The manner of death in this case is criminal homicide.

After elimination of the various causes of death as discussed above, the death in this case due to asphyxia as a result of strangulation by way of ligature or manual can't be ruled out. However, the same may be corroborated with findings of investigation.

BASIS OF OPINION

The dead body was recovered from a remote place, and it was suggestive of a discrete disposal of corpse and concealment of prime evidence i.e corpse of the deceased. The deceased had skeletal burns. It was strongly suggestive of use of inflammable material to destroy the corpse. There were pan-body burns over skeleton, which suggested that the extent of burns were massive and intention was to destroy the whole body to conceal the prime evidence of death investigation. In forensic practice this is seen in cases of criminal destruction of human corpse which is a prime evidence of corpus delecti and is seen mostly in cases of homicide. The medical board is of the considered opinion that it is case of homicide.

In deliberations regarding cause of death, the medical board took into consideration the findings of examined mortal remains and the common methods of criminal homicide which are:

- Sharp force injuries (by stabbing/knife and other sharp weapon)
- Blunt force injuries
- Gunshot injuries (firearm missile injuries)
- Head injuries

In all four above common and invariably used methods of causing fatal injuries in cases of homicide the death is

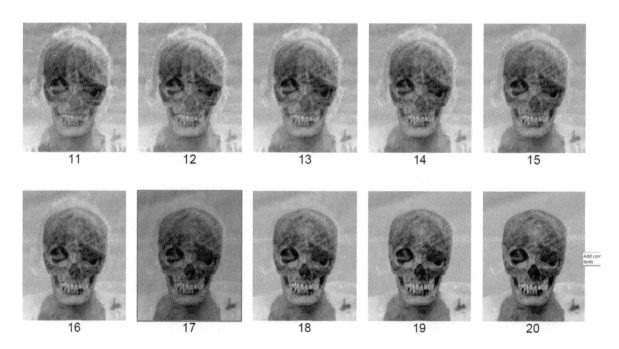

FIGURE 5.31 Cranio-facial superimposition done, which gave a positive match for deceased Sheena Bora.

due to hemorrhagic shock means person bleeds to death. The examination of the skeletal remains does not reveal any ante-mortem sharp cut/fracture. No bleeding or hemorrhagic blood spots were present on the skeleton. This observation was present in primary autopsy as well as after exhumation of the bones by TNMC.

The medical board in view of the above is of the opinion that cause of death being due to any kind of blunt force/weapon (like Iron rod/stone/brick etc) as well as by sharp cutting or pointed weapon/object (like Stab by knife etc) is ruled out. The gunshot injury is also ruled out due to above mentioned facts.

Can the death be due to head injury?

On the examination of the skull, there was no ante-mortem sharp cut or blunt force fracture of outer/inner table of frontal, parietal, temporal or occipital regions of skull bone. In cases of homicide involving head injuries, the cranium is mostly damaged due to use of excessive force or minimum there will be bleeding inside skull. In this case there was no fracture or blood stains found.

The death being caused by head injury was also ruled out.

The medical board concluded that in the absence of injuries, the above circumstances which are invariably seen in cases of homicide are being eliminated on medical examination of bony remains.

The cause of death due to strangulation either manual or by ligature in absence of any tissue including laryngeal cartilage, muscles and Hyoid bone which are completely burned and even the skeletonised remains were unavailable, the signs of strangulation are lost and could not be appreciated.

The manner of death in this case is homicide.

After elimination of the various causes of death as discussed above, the death in this case due to asphyxia as a result of strangulation by way of ligature or manual can't be ruled out. However, the same may be corroborated with findings of investigation.

OTHER VARIANT OF STRANGULATION

- **Bansdola** is a method of strangulation where a pair of hard, blunt object, for example, bamboo sticks, lathi, wooden pole or rods are placed across the front and back of the neck of victim. Pressure can be applied by various methods; one by tying a thick rope at both the ends of hard, blunt object and tightening it; second is tying thick rope at one end of the hard, blunt object and giving manual pressure at the other end; another method is by applying manual pressure at both ends of the hard, blunt object. This method of applying pressure over the neck with the help of hard, blunt object is known as Bansdola.
- **Mugging** is a variant of strangulation caused by holding the neck of the victim in the crook of the elbow or elbow bend or knee of the assailant. It

is also known as arm lock or chokehold. Here the pressure is exerted over larynx or side of neck by forearm and arm.

- **Garroting** is a variant of strangulation commonly used by robbers to kill travelers in lonely places and rob them. This method is also used for judicial execution in some countries. There are many methods of garroting; for example, in one method, the neck is grasped by a ligature or thin wire loop thrown from behind the victim and tightened, which causes loss of consciousness of the person. It is also known as **Spanish windlass** and was practiced in Spain and Turkey as a method of execution.

BIBLIOGRAPHY

1. Ubelaker DH, Cordero QR, Wu Y, Linton NF. Anthropological analysis of trauma in throat bone and cartilage: a review. Forensic Science International: Synergy. 2020;2:224–9.
2. Harm T, Rajs J. Types of injuries and interrelated conditions of victims and assailants in attempted and homicidal strangulation. Forensic Science International. 1981;18:101–23.
3. Harm T, Rajs J. Face and neck injuries due to resuscitation versus throttling. Forensic Science International. 1983;23:109–16.
4. Pydiraju Y, Sreedevi BR, Bendi N. Homicide by a road traffic accident: a case report. Journal of Evidence based Medicine and Healthcare. 2015 Apr 13;2(15):2367–70.
5. Maiese A, Gitto L, dell'Aquila M, Bolino G. When the hidden features become evident: the usefulness of PMCT in a strangulation-related death. Legal Medicine. 2014 Nov;16(6):364–6.
6. Fais P, Giraudo C, Viero A, Miotto D, Bortolotti F, Tagliaro F, Montisci M, Cecchetto G. Micro computed tomography features of laryngeal fractures in a case of fatal manual strangulation. Legal Medicine. 2016 Jan;18:85–9.
7. Aghayev E, Jackowski C, Sonnenschein M, Thali M, Yen K, Dirnhofer R. Virtopsy hemorrhage of the posterior cricoarytenoid muscle by blunt force to the neck in postmortem multislice computed tomography and magnetic resonance imaging. American Journal of Forensic Medicine and Pathology. 2006 Mar;27(1):25–9.
8. Yen K, Vock P, Christe A, Scheurer E, Plattner T, Schön C, et al. Clinical forensic radiology in strangulation victims: forensic expertise based on magnetic resonance imaging (MRI) findings. International Journal of Legal Medicine [online]. 2007 Jan 6;121(2):115–23. Available from: http://dx.doi.org/10.1007/s00414-006-0121-y.
9. Anscombh AM, Knight BH. Case report. Delayed death after pressure on the neck, possible causal mechanisms and implications for mode of death in manual strangulation discussed. Forensic Science International. 1996 Apr 23;78(3):193–7.
10. Badkur DS, Arorae A, Jain CS. Delayed death in a case of attempted strangulation; mechanism of cerebral thrombosis and infarction. A case report. Journal of Indian Academy of Forensic Medicine. 2005;27(4):263–5.
11. Rogde S, Hougen HP, Poulsen K. Asphyxial homicide in two Scandinavian capitals. American Journal of Forensic Medicine and Pathology. 2001;22(2):128–33.

12. Clarota F, Vaza E, Papinb F, Proust B. Fatal and non-fatal bilateral delayed carotid artery dissection after manual strangulation. Forensic Science International. 2005;149:143–50.

13. Di Paolo M, Guidi B, Bruschini L, Vessio G, Domenici R, Ambrosino N. Unexpected delayed death after manual strangulation: need for careful examination in the emergency room. Monaldi Archives for Chest Disease. 2009;71(3):132–4.

14. Geisenberger D, Pollak S, Thierauf-Emberger A. Homicidal strangulation and subsequent hanging of the victim to simulate suicide: delayed elucidation based on reassessment of the autopsy findings. Forensic Science International. 2019;298:419–23.

15. Green MA. Morbid anatomical findings in strangulation. Forensic Science. 1973;2:317–23.

16. Warren S. Strangulation: a full spectrum of blunt neck trauma. Annals of Otology, Rhinology and Laryngology. 1985;94:542–6.

17. Lupascu C. Letter to the editor/legal. Medicine. 2003; 5:110–11.

18. McClane GE, et al. A review of 300 attempted strangulation cases part II: clinical evaluation of the surviving victim. The Journal of Emergency Medicine. 2001;21(3):311–5.

19. Pinto DC. The laryngohyoid complex in medicolegal death investigations. Academic Forensic Pathology. 2016; 6(3):486–98.

20. Pathak AK, Sinha US. A study of findings in asphyxial deaths due to external compression of neck. Scholars Journal of Applied Medical Sciences. 2020 Feb;8(2):481–5.

LIGATURE STRANGULATION

Ligature strangulation refers to the fatal compression of the neck by a ligature, where the constricting force is applied externally and is not the weight of the body. Majority of these cases belong to the homicide category. However, very few suicidal and accidental cases have been reported from time to time. Ligature strangulation differs from hanging mainly in the source, amount and direction of the constricting force. Generally in hanging, gravitational drag of the body constricts the vital neck structures, causing the death by different mechanisms as discussed previously. In case of ligature strangulation, the constricting force is generally lesser and insufficient to cause compression of all neck arteries, especially the well protected vertebral arteries. Ligature strangulation always produces some degree of evident congestion above the level of ligature mark unless when reflux cardiac inhibition is the mechanism of death.

Mechanism of Death

All combinations of mechanisms of death that can occur in hanging are possible in ligature strangulation also. Generally, the force of constriction is transmitted from upper limbs of the assailants through the ligature used. Easy compressibility of neck veins generally results in venous flow obstruction and subsequent upstream congestion. Compression and complete occlusion of carotid arteries generally does not happen in most of the cases. Tracheal or laryngeal compression may result in airway obstruction with the normal forces of ligature strangulation. Compressive force of ligature strangulation generally does not occlude vertebral arteries, hence the 'pale face' picture of hanging is seen only in cases with reflex cardiac inhibition. All these mechanisms contribute to death in ligature strangulation with variable degree, either alone or in combination.

Ligature Materials

As in hanging, a wide variety of materials can be used as a ligature for neck compression. They include ropes, bed sheets, blankets, wires, scarves, shawls, stockings, collar of the shirt or T-shirt the victim is wearing, chains and necklaces. The presence of a specific ligature material explains the manner of death in many instances. Generally in homicides, the assailant applies the ligature in single loop, while in suicidal strangulation, multiple loops of ligature material are present. In unfortunate incidents of accidental ligature strangulations, belts or connecting parts of machines or even clothes of the deceased getting trapped in machines act as ligature and result in fatal compression of the neck. Ligature material remains around the neck in a tightly applied state until the recovery of the body in almost all cases of suicides. Cases of homicide often present with undisturbed in-situ ligature materials (Figure 5.32). In some homicidal cases, the assailant removes the ligature material after the death of the victim during his effort to conceal or destroy the evidence. Mechanisms used for tightening the ligature vary with the manner of death. Suicide cases generally show multiple turns of ligature around the neck with a rod-like material twisted to achieve a tourniquet-like effect. Multiple turns or even a single turn around neck with a simple half knot suffices in many suicide cases. Turn around neck with a heavy weight attached to the other end of the ligature causes death and can be seen in some suicidal cases, but rare (Figure 5.33). If the ligature material is present in situ, the forensic surgeon should be careful while removing the same. An advisable method is cutting the loop at a point opposite to the knot. Both cut ends should

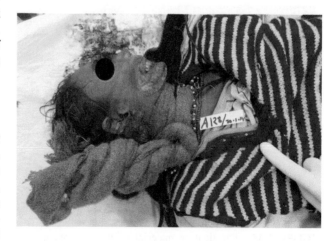

FIGURE 5.32 A case of ligature strangulation with the ligature material present in situ.

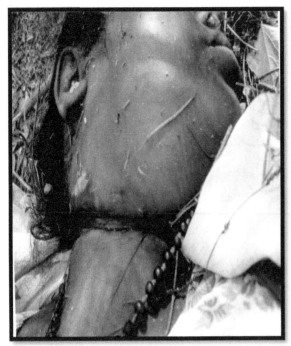
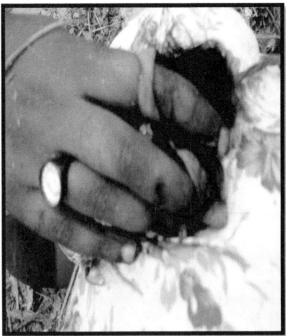

FIGURE 5.33 A case of suicidal ligature strangulation where the material used was 'naara' of pajama and the loop around the neck is seen tightly present around the neck and the ends of the ligature were tied to both her hands.

be secured by a thread. If needed, the knot may be secured by another thread. In virtual autopsy examination of the ligature material, its position (including distance from anatomical landmarks and the position of the knot) is well appreciated especially when the material used is thick and dense (Figures 5.34 and 5.35).

Postmortem Examination

External Examination

The ligature mark: A depressed mark (pressure abrasion) and a well-defined groove are seen on the neck due to the transmitted force during neck compression. A transverse,

higher up, complete ligature mark is the classical description of a mark of ligature strangulation, but the majority of cases do not show this typical finding. Many cases present with a pale compressed area with some erythematous margins. Some cases show reddish dermal contusions. If the friction is more as in cases of rough material like a rope, there may be pressure abrasions. These pressure abrasions are pale and yellowish initially and as time passes, attain a brownish color due to drying. Postmortem drying gives these abrasions a parchment-like texture. Since the pressure is not maintained continuously like in hanging, in most cases, the underlying subcutaneous tissues do not show 'dried, whitish or glistening appearance'. On the contrary,

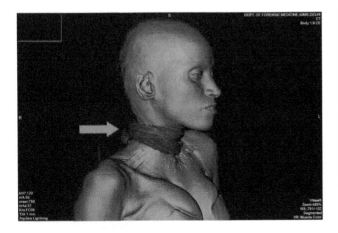

FIGURE 5.34 The ligature material position appreciated on virtual autopsy external examination of the dead body especially when the ligature is thick and dense.

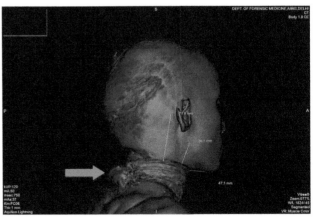

FIGURE 5.35 The position of the knot shown by the blue arrow and the distance of the ligature material from various anatomical landmarks.

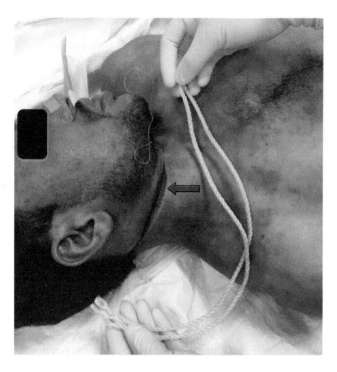

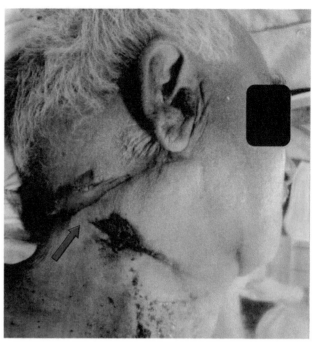

FIGURE 5.36 Very thin ligature material (rope here) resulting in a deep grooved ligature mark, also called cheese-cutter method.

FIGURE 5.37 Crossover point of the ligature mark in a case characteristic of ligature strangulation.

hemorrhages are common under the marks of ligature strangulation. The presence and appearance of the mark mainly depend upon the type of ligature material used and the manner of death. Hard materials easily produce dermal injuries in the form of abrasions due to friction. Materials like soft clothes do not produce any visible mark in many instances.

Detailed examination with the help of hand lens, oblique illumination, infra-red photography and UV lamps helps in identifying ligature impression in many cases. Imprint pattern of the ligature can be appreciated with naked eyes or with the help of these additional tools and if established, can be used as evidence in the court of law. Ligature material and mark should correspond and correlate in depth and width. Very thin ligature materials like chains or strings or narrow electric wire or cord result in a deep grooved ligature mark, also called **cheese-cutter method** (Figure 5.36). These thin materials commonly produce lacerations of the skin and other underlying structures. Broader materials produce shallow impressions, and if the pressure is released immediately after death, the mark may not be visible in many instances. Both upper and lower margins of the ligature mark in many cases show visible erythematous lines. These reddish areas are possible in ligature compression of the neck even after death and are explained as the result of mechanical displacement of blood due to the compressive force transmitted through the noose. Hence, it is not considered a sign of vitality. Contrary to hanging, the ligature mark is transverse in most of the cases of ligature strangulation, if there is no great disparity between the heights of the

victim and the assailant. Lack of vertical pull due to gravity as in case of hanging explains this transverse placement of ligature mark. If the victim is a child or when the assailant is at a relatively higher level as in the case of a lying down victim, the mark is oblique as in hanging. In these cases, the weight of a portion of the body of the victim also acts as the constricting force so an element of 'homicidal hanging' is present in many of these cases. Many homicide cases show continuous ligature mark with identifiable crossover point (Figure 5.37), a sure sign of ligature strangulation. Due to physical struggle and pull from the victim, in many cases, slippage of ligature material happens commonly upwards, which results in multiple slippage abrasions. Due to the lack of a vertical dragging force, unlike in hanging, the mark is generally situated at a lower portion of the neck, commonly at the level of the larynx. If the ligature is in situ and the pressure is maintained, tissues under the ligature mark remain as a relatively bloodless field. This is why ligature marks with in situ material show a great degree of preservation in many decomposed cases.

- **Linear abrasions:** The victim, usually with violent attempts, tries to grab the ligature and release the constriction. These attempts generally produce multiple vertical linear abrasions on the neck due to fingernail tips, above the level of the ligature mark. These abrasions may show underlying dermal abrasions/contusions. The ligature usually slips upwards, producing abrasions of the skin and settles at a higher level, and produces slippage abrasions. Though fingernail marks and

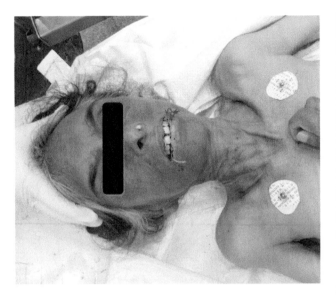

FIGURE 5.38   A case of ligature strangulation showing intense congestion of the face and portion of the neck above the ligature.

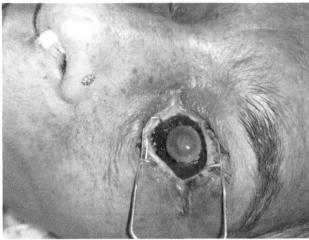

FIGURE 5.40   Ecchymosis seen in the conjunctiva in a case of ligature strangulation.

finger poke contusions of the assailants are not as common as those seen in manual strangulation, the same can be seen in some cases. If injuries suggestive of nail marks and fingertip contusions are present, the possibility of a combination of throttling and ligature strangulation should be considered.

- **Asphyxial stigmata**: The entire face and the portion of neck above the level of compression generally show intense congestion (Figures 5.38 and 5.39), cyanosis, edema and multiple petechiae. If the ligature compression is not relieved till

postmortem examination, these findings persist. Releasing the constriction results in the disappearance of congestion, edema and cyanosis in many cases, while the petechiae tend to persist. Tissue edema develops due to the oozing of fluids as a result of tissue hypoxia and subsequent membrane dysfunction. Some amount of edema develops even after death if the constriction is maintained. Severe edema of the peri-orbital region results in bulging out of eyeballs, commonly seen in ligature strangulation. Common sites of petechiae or ecchymosis are bulbar and palpebral conjunctivae (Figure 5.40), outer aspect of eyelids, upper cheeks and oral or gingival mucosa (Figure 5.41).

- **Bleeding from nostril and mouth**: Rupture of smaller blood vessels due to intense congestion and increased pressure lead to bleeding from nostrils, mouth and ears.

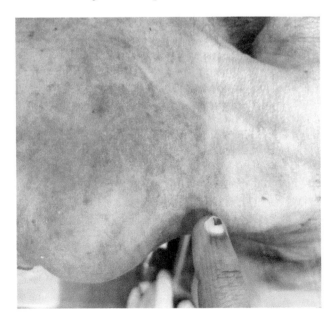

FIGURE 5.39   A case of ligature strangulation showing a definitive line of demarcation at the level of compression of the neck by a ligature, above which severe congestion with petechial hemorrhages is seen.

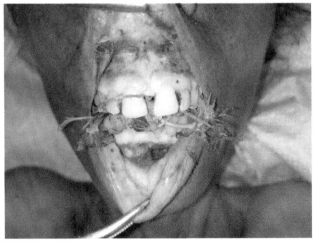

FIGURE 5.41   Petechial hemorrhages seen over the gingival mucosa in a case of ligature strangulation.

- **Other injuries**: Homicidal ligature strangulation of a normal adult shows multiple injuries of physical struggle and defense. Attempt to silence or smother the victim are not rare in ligature strangulation, and corresponding contusions and lacerations can be seen inside the lips. Involvement of multiple assailants results in different restrain attempts and corresponding abrasions and contusions commonly over the limbs.
- **Other non-specific findings**: Genital organs are congested. There may be involuntary discharge of urine, feces and semen. Cadaveric spasm of the hands may be seen since the death of the victim may be in action of defense.

Some cases of ligature strangulation do not show any of the above-mentioned signs of asphyxia like congestion, cyanosis, edema or petechiae. Cardiac inhibition due to vagal reflex mechanism can explain these cases. The ligature mark, if present, is commonly located over the anatomical position of the carotid bifurcation, at C3 vertebral level. Suicidal cases generally show less muscle and dermal contusions due to a continuous localized constricting force. Commonly, suicide cases show intense facial congestion and edema, which suggest a slower onset of death by complete venous obstruction and partial arterial patency. Asphyxia due to complete occlusion of the airway may be present in some cases.

Muscular belly of tongue along with its surfaces may show some injuries in ligature strangulation in the form of contusions and abrasions since the same is firmly in contact with the hard palate and other bony structures like teeth.

Internal Examination

Identification and interpretation of internal neck injuries is important from a medico-legal point of view. Layer-wise dissection of the neck in a bloodless field gives the best results for correlation. Ligature mark may have a dried, parchment-like appearance on dissection. Apart from this, the following are the important internal findings:

- **Hemorrhage**: The ligature mark may appear as a reddish dermal contusion without the dried, parchment-like appearance on dissection. Subcutaneous tissues immediately under the ligature mark generally show multiple streaks of hemorrhage, commonly accepted as a sign of vitality. The platysma shows layers of hemorrhages in many cases (Figure 5.42). The muscles of the neck also show hemorrhages between the broken fibers. Posterior aspect of the neck usually shows minimal dermal and muscular injuries, explained by the relatively thicker fascia and absence of abundant loose tissue.
- **Fracture of larynx and thyroid-hyoid complex**: Laryngeal cartilages generally show fractures, most commonly at the superior horn of thyroid. Though the hyoid bone enjoys a relatively safer

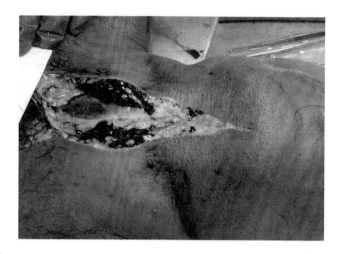

FIGURE 5.42 Hemorrhage appreciated in the subcutaneous tissue and the platysma layer corresponding to the ligature mark in a strangulation case.

and higher-up position, the greater cornua of hyoid bone gets fractured in many cases of ligature strangulation. Forces transmitted through the thyro-hyoid ligament causes fractures in most of these cases. The thyroid lamina fractures rarely, especially when the antero-posterior compression happens directly over the larynx. Cricoid fractures are the least common in this category. During neck compression, the larynx directly compresses against the anterior aspect of cervical vertebrae. If the thyroid laminae or cricoid gets fractured, the possibility of manual strangulation has to be considered. Sometimes due to lack of experience, the autopsy surgeon may misinterpret the sub-luxation of the joint between the body and the greater horn of the hyoid bone as a fracture. Sub-luxation of the joint in postmortem is commonly encountered due the decomposition changes. Uncommonly, the injury on the neck may be unilateral. Multiple peri-cartilaginous and sub-mucosal hemorrhages are possible in cases of ligature strangulation.
- **Petechiae**: Sub-pleural petechiae over the surfaces of lungs and sub-pericardial petechiae on cardiac surfaces can occur, but are not specific for ligature strangulation.
- **Froth in tracheo-bronchial tree**: Tracheo-bronchial tree contains blood-stained froth in many cases, which can be explained by the fluid leak from the alveolar capillaries and epithelial cells resulting in pulmonary edema, as a result of parenchymal hypoxia and increased respiratory struggle.

All other internal organs do not show any specific finding in ligature strangulation.

In most cases of ligature strangulation, the victims are female and the intention for committing the crime has some sexual element. Injuries suggestive of sexual assault, including bite marks, fingernail abrasions, genital and perineal injuries, are seen in many cases. Injuries of failed attempts like that of attempted smothering, throttling, stabbing, etc. may be seen.

Radiological Examination

Computed tomography scan or X-ray can be used to detect fractures and dislocations of the larynx in cases of strangulation or hanging. It has the special advantage of being able to record even minute fractures, differentiate ante-mortem fractures from dissection artefacts and also provide a permanent document for future reference in the court. Soft tissues around the fracture site will also show bruising in most cases, which could be interpreted during virtual autopsy practice and also would be a sign of ante-mortem fracture.

Artifacts

In rare instances, some postmortem findings may mimic ligature strangulation. Creases of skin folds over the anterior aspect of the neck along with superimposed patches of postmortem staining can resemble a ligature mark. Sharp margins of these purplish lesions create doubts of the application of a ligature material. This artefact is common in refrigerated bodies, especially in children or in obese individuals with a short neck. Bloating up of decomposition results in compression of soft tissues of the neck against tight neck clothing. These cases generally show a pressure band immediately after removal of the tight cloth. This artefact is often erroneously interpreted as a ligature mark, especially by inexperienced eyes. In decomposition, internal neck structures, especially those with immediate vicinity to veins, show reddish discoloration due to pigments of hemolysis. These pigmentations that mimic hemorrhages of muscles and other soft tissues of neck need cautious evaluation before interpretation. If the head is in the dependent position after death for a longer period especially while it's in a prone position, the face shows features of congestion and edema due to postmortem phenomenon of gravitational pooling of blood and fluids. If intense, these cases also show multiple petechiae over the face, but as a postmortem phenomenon. These postmortem artefacts should not be confused with congestion, edema and petechiae of strangulation.

Substantive medico-legal difficulties can arise if such hemorrhagic lividity develops in the necks of bodies that have ventral lividity due to prone position during and after death. This phenomenon can mimic soft tissue injury ('pseudo-bruising') and the internal injuries related to strangulation. Caution must be exercised when diagnosing strangulation and differentiating between hanging and ligature strangulation in bodies with anterior neck lividity.

SAMPLE COLLECTION FROM THE SITE OF LIGATURE MARK

Cellophane tape lifts from the mark become useful in all cases of suspected ligature strangulation deaths for

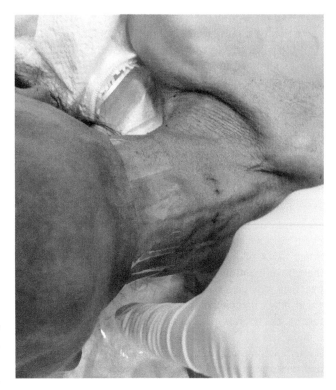

FIGURE 5.43   Cellophane tape lifting from the ligature mark in a case of ligature strangulation.

comparative analysis with the alleged ligature (Figure 5.43). Pressure and friction during strangulation generally result in transfer of dermal tissues to the ligature material used. In cases of homicidal ligature strangulation, these tissues can be used for biological testing like DNA fingerprinting.

MEDICO-LEGAL IMPORTANCE OF LIGATURE STRANGULATION

- **Homicidal:** It is a general presumption in the legal system that strangulation is homicidal in nature unless and until the contrary is proved on the basis of postmortem findings and circumstantial evidences of legal investigation. During postmortem examination, most victims have marks of injuries like scratch abrasion along the ligature mark, since it is possible that the assailants' fingers could have come in contact with the neck of the victim while applying the ligature, producing such injuries. These crescentic nail marks or abrasions are features suggestive of a homicidal strangulation. In some of the cases, the victim also tries to defend against the tightening of the ligature on the neck by the assailant and some nail marks of the victim may also be seen on their own neck, and it is a very important medico-legal finding along with other struggle injuries over the body in deciding a case of homicidal strangulation.

CASE 1: A CASE OF ALLEGED ROAD TRAFFIC ACCIDENT TURNED TO BE THAT OF LIGATURE STRANGULATION

In 2015, the mother of a young lady was informed by her son-in-law that the car in which they were travelling lost control and toppled multiple times due to which his wife died on the spot. As per the version narrated by the husband, his wife was sitting by the open window and was not wearing the seat belt. The car was moving at a speed of about 140 km/h, and suddenly, a pedestrian girl crossed the road, and in an attempt to avoid collision, he steered the car away. Since it was drizzling, the road was slippery and the car lost balance and toppled multiple times, during which she got ejected through the open window and sustained injuries and died on the spot itself (Figure 5.44). Postmortem examination was conducted at the nearby district hospital, and the postmortem report showed external injuries, including a 4 × 3 cm abraded contusion over right zygomatic arch and a 3 × 1 cm abraded contusion over the left forearm just above the wrist joint. There was fracture of five to six ribs on the left side. Left pleura showed laceration. Right lung weighed 350 g and was pale. Left lung weighted 100 g, was lacerated, and 200 mL of free and clotted blood was present in the chest cavity. As per postmortem report, the final cause of death in this case was shock and hemorrhage due to ante-mortem injury and left lung injury. It was also mentioned that injuries were sufficient to cause death. Clothes were handed over to the police officials;

no viscera for histopathology or chemical analysis were preserved.

The mother of the deceased alleged that her son-in-law showed cruelty towards her daughter, and she strongly suspected that her daughter was killed by her husband. The mother-in-law complained regarding the same and eventually the case was transferred to the CBI.

During the investigation, the Board of Forensic Experts from Forensic Science Laboratory concluded that the involvement of the car at the site of the alleged accident is found to be suspicious and they recommended investigation. Another subject expert, a Professor of Mechanical Engineering, IIT Delhi, opined the following: (1) The exterior damage on the vehicle does not indicate that the vehicle was subjected to (multiple) rollover in the crash (Figures 5.45 and 5.46). (2) Preliminary computer simulations of the crash in PC Crash ™ indicate that multiple rollovers are not possible under the circumstances. (3) Preliminary computer analysis of the boot lid indicates that its deformation could have been caused from a sequence of loads rather than that which occurs when a vehicle goes off the road or is subject to rollover.

The Medical Board of AIIMS New Delhi perused the postmortem report, photograph of the deceased, expert opinions, Central Forensic Science Laboratory reports

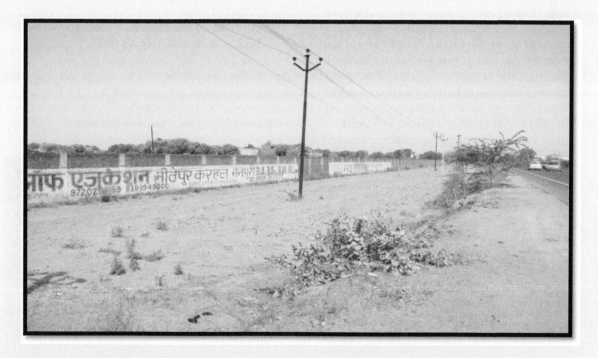

FIGURE 5.44 The alleged scene of occurrence of the incident where the deceased lady's husband told he lost control of the car and the car rolled over multiple times.

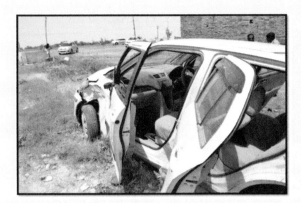

FIGURE 5.45 Dents on the side of the car not consistent with the given history of car rollover.

and other documents submitted by the investigating officer. The CBI requested to provide a holistic opinion into the cause of death. After perusal of all the reports and photographs, the Medical Board put forward a questionnaire to the CBI seeking the information on a few points from the doctor who had conducted the postmortem of the deceased.

The photograph of the victim showed a clear, transverse ligature mark on the neck. The AIIMS Medical Board opined in the case as:

1. Quantum of injuries over the body of the deceased is not compatible with the manner and severity of car accident as narrated by her husband. Inquest report shows that the deceased got ejected through the car during roll over at a speed of about 100-120 km/h and she was not wearing seat belt. If that would have been the case then due to high momentum of the body, the deceased would have suffered several and serious injuries including brush burns, multiple laceration and fracture injuries. The death of deceased due to this narrated rollover accident of car is ruled out.

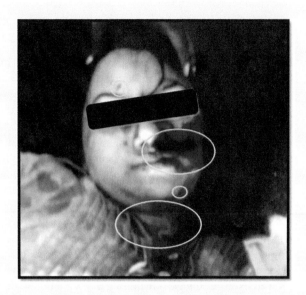

FIGURE 5.47 Injuries seen over the face along with the ligature mark over the neck.

2. Injuries over the right zygomatic arch, left forearm, left chin, left forehead and left side rib fractures without any external injury over chest are antemortem injuries inflicted upon the body of the deceased by blunt force/object during scuffle and assault (Figure 5.47).
3. On the basis of overall evaluation of the case, the ligature mark over neck and the injury over right mastoid region behind right ear are seen in case of pressure of the knuckles of an assailant in the course of ligature pressure over neck from front or back (Figure 5.48).

The Medical Board concludes that the cause of death in this case is fatal pressure over neck by ligature and same should be corroborated with the circumstantial evidences of the investigation in this case.

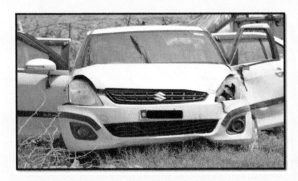

FIGURE 5.46 Dents at the front of the car not consistent with the given history of car rollover.

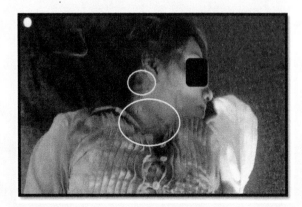

FIGURE 5.48 The ligature mark over the neck seen clearly along with injury near right mastoid process.

The case has been registered by CBI, New Delhi U/S 498 A, 302 and 120 B IPC relating to the death of deceased.

Later the CBI approached the AIIMS Medical Board to comment on the alleged ligature material, one mobile phone charger (Figure 5.49). The injury was correlating with the physical nature of the wire of the charger, and the medical board opined that 'the ligature pressure injury on the neck of the deceased could be produced by the exhibit submitted'.

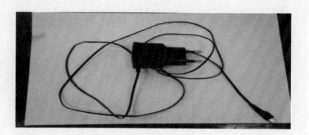

FIGURE 5.49 The mobile charger that was the alleged ligature material recovered by the investigating team.

- **Suicidal** strangulation is not very common but may be attempted by means of a ligature tied around the neck. When a ligature is used, manipulations for committing the act will be evident. A case of self-strangulation by tying a bow-tie has been reported by Rupp (1970). Hocking (1966) came across a case of a woman who tried to commit suicide by hanging but died of accidental strangulation from a ligature tied tightly around the neck before she took the drop. Bhaskar and Shah (1974) have reported a rare case of death from accidental strangulation of a 20-year-old woman while travelling in a rickshaw. Discussed below is a case report from Bengaluru that explains and elaborates the probability and possibility of self-strangulation leading to asphyxia and death.

CASE 2: SELF-STRANGULATION CASE IN BENGALURU

In 2009, a 26-year-old female was found dead in a secluded area near a railway station in Bengaluru (Figures 5.50 and 5.51) with in-situ ligature (cotton cloth string or *naara*) on her neck, which was taken out from her own churidar pajama that she was wearing at that time (Figure 5.52). The scene was undisturbed and her bag was next to her. There were no signs of any theft, and all her belongings were present intact. There were no signs of struggle also seen at the place of occurrence (Figure 5.51). The ligature was encircling the neck twice

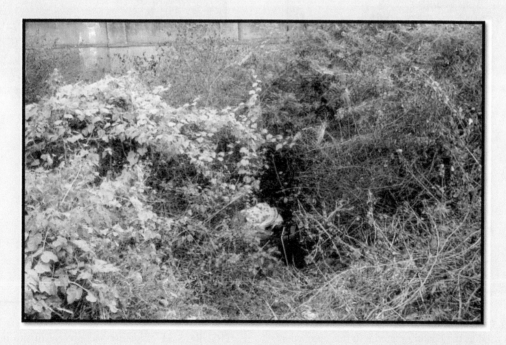

FIGURE 5.50 The deceased was found in a secluded place that was around 40 meters from the railway track. The scene was undisturbed, and her bag was next to her. There were no signs of any theft, and all her belongings were present intact. There were no signs of struggle.

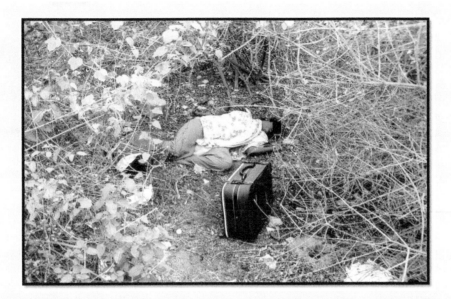

FIGURE 5.51 The deceased was found in the secluded place, and the surrounding and the ground show no signs of any struggle or scuffle before the death. Clothes of the deceased were intact.

(Figure 5.53), with the free ends of the ligature material tied to right hand finger and left hand respectively (Figure 5.54). The case was brought to the public domain as a case of rape and subsequent murder by ligature strangulation. The postmortem examination of the deceased was conducted in a medical college by a well-qualified forensic medicine faculty, and he opined that findings of postmortem are suggestive of ligature strangulation and self-strangulation is ruled out as at a stage of cerebral anoxia, the ligature gets loosened and death does not occur. The Crime Branch, Crime Investigation Department (CB-CID) continued the investigation for

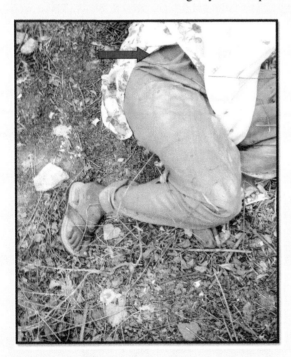

FIGURE 5.52 Naara of the salwar was seen removed, which was used as the ligature material in this case; apart from that, there was no disturbance of the clothes or no tears seen. No injuries of struggle are seen over the foot and legs.

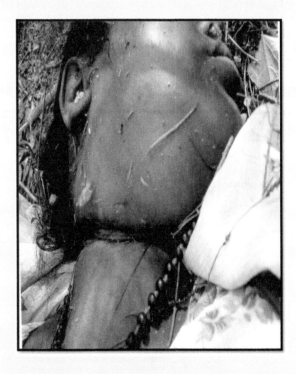

FIGURE 5.53 Ligature was present in situ in the neck, which was the naara of the salwar and the free ends are held in the fingers. The ligature is seen still in tightened state without loosening up.

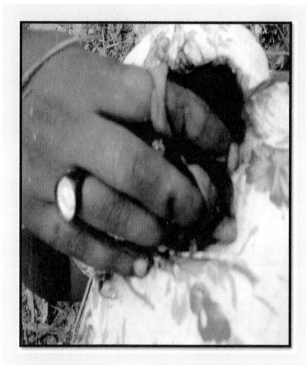

FIGURE 5.54 The one free end of the ligature was found tied to the fingers of the right hand; also some tuft of hair is seen between the fingers along with the ligature. The other free end of the ligature was found in the left hand and was found loosened by grip.

3 years as murder but was unable to find any accused, and the case was referred from CB-CID to CBI by the High Court of Karnataka. CBI also investigated the case as murder thoroughly for more than 1 year but could not find any clue or evidence of murder and then requested AIIMS, New Delhi to give an expert opinion on the postmortem report to intimate the cause and manner of death of the deceased, which was dragged as murder for more than 6 years. AIIMS perused the post-mortem report, photographs of crime scene, inquest papers, videography of postmortem and ligature material. After perusal of various documents/statements, articles and postmortem report, the Board opined that it is a case of death due to ligature strangulation. As per the Textbook *Spitz and Fisher's Medicolegal Investigation of Death*, 4th Edition, strangulation may be homicidal, accidental or suicidal, particularly ligature strangulation. In this case, the postmortem report as well as Forensic Science Laboratory report are negative for any sign of biological evidence of sexual assault. As per the postmortem report, there are no signs of struggle or any defense injury over the body. The Medical Board took into consideration the above information as well as the fact that the ligature material was tied to the right-hand finger and the other end was in left hand. It is also seen that the thyro-hyoid complex was intact in this case. However, in cases of strangulation by assailant, the thyro-hyoid complex is broken due to higher force of injury. However, no injury in thyro-hyoid complex bone in this case was suggestive of light compressive force over the neck. On further perusal of the Textbook *Taylor's Principles and Practise of Medical Jurisprudence*, 13th Edition, it is inconceivable that anyone could die from compression of the neck by his own hand because loss of consciousness would cause relaxation of the constricting fingers. When a ligature is involved, the matter is different. If the ligature is found in situ, suicide is unusual but a distinct possibility.

Self-strangulation involving a ligature is possible in four ways:

1. When the neck is constricted by multiple turns, which are sufficient to maintain constriction without a knot or fewer turns secured either by a half or double knot at a point accessible to the person's own hands.
2. More frequently a rod of some sort is either inserted under a knot or included in it, the neck being compressed by twisting in the fashion of a tourniquet. This, in our experience, is the commonest method used.
3. A running noose with a weight attached to the free end.
4. A running noose with the free end attached to the hand, the weight of the hand and forearm causing compression.

The Medical Board, chaired by the author, perused medical findings of the case and concluded that it is a form of asphyxial death due to self-strangulation; hence, the manner of death is suicidal. The investigative team corroborated all the evidences gathered during 6 years of investigation and the circumstantial findings along with the Medical Board opinion and concluded that it was not a case of murder, but a case of suicide.

- **Accidental:** Accidental strangulations, though rare, can occur among children when they get entangled in the ropes or spokes of their cribs. Fetus may also get strangled around the neck with umbilical cord. In cases where a person falls from any building, the neck may get entangled or trapped in any ladder like object and the person may be accidentally strangled. In many of these cases, the victims can be saved if the incident is witnessed or the mechanism of strangulations fails on its own. Another common scenario is when an individual is intoxicated and his neck gets stuck in any railings or string due to an accidental fall; one such case encountered by the author is illustrated below.

CASE 3: ACCIDENTAL STRANGULATION OF A YOUNG MALE WHO WAS INTOXICATED

A young male was found dead with his neck stuck between the railing and the step. The deceased was an alcoholic, and even on the day of occurrence was seen consuming alcohol and roaming near the place of occurrence. The person was found dead the next morning in the state as shown in Figure 5.55 with his neck stuck between the railing and step, which caused the compression of neck and finally leading to death due to fatal pressure over the neck (Figures 5.56 and 5.57). On autopsy, no injuries suggestive of any forceful compression of neck or the body were seen, and also, no injuries suggestive of any struggle by the deceased were found. Alcohol smell was present in the oral cavity and on dissection from the stomach. Viscera was preserved, and it confirmed the presence of ethyl alcohol. After consideration of the autopsy findings, viscera analysis report and the circumstancial evidences provided by the investigating officer, it was concluded as a case of accidental compression of neck (strangulation) by the iron rod of railing and the step, leading to death. In this case, the deceased, who was intoxicated, was probably walking towards the steps and accidentaly fell and his neck got entangled. Due to his intoxicated state he probably could not free himself from this entanglement, leading to death.

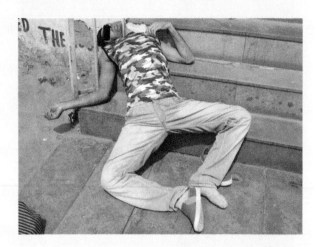

FIGURE 5.56 Front view of the young man, which shows his position, intact clothes and absence of any struggle signs in the scene of occurrence.

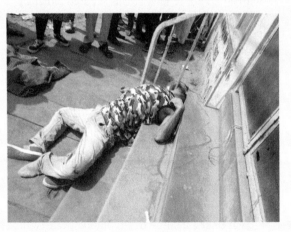

FIGURE 5.55 A young male found dead with his neck stuck between the railing and the step.

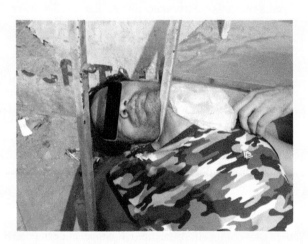

FIGURE 5.57 Closer view of the case, which shows the compression of the neck.

VARIOUS INTERESTING CASE REPORTS

CASE 4: LIGATURE STRANGULATION AND SMOTHERING: CASE REPORT

An elderly female was found dead at her home with evident injuries over her neck and face. The circumstantial evidences were suggestive of a homicide. The case was brought to AIIMS, and the autopsy was performed. External examination revealed ligature mark suggestive of strangulation. The ligature mark was present over the lower half of the neck (Figure 5.58). Multiple reddish dermal contusions were evident over the neck, face, lips and limbs (Figures 5.59 and 5.60). Chest wall injuries were suggestive of traumatic compression. Entire face

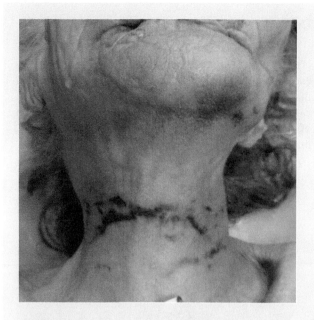

FIGURE 5.58 The ligature mark present in the lower half of the neck. Contusion is also seen over the chin.

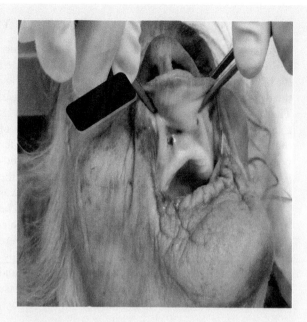

FIGURE 5.60 Contusion present over the inner aspect of the upper lip.

showed congestion and petechiae. Though the lady was edentulous, contusions were present on the inner aspects of the lips. Tongue showed contusions and petechiae. Neck dissection showed multiple subcutaneous and muscle hemorrhages; superior horns of the thyroid

cartilage showed fractures. Fracture and dislocation of the cervical vertebra were present (Figure 5.61). The cause of death was opined as: asphyxia due to combined effect of ligature strangulation, smothering and traumatic asphyxia.

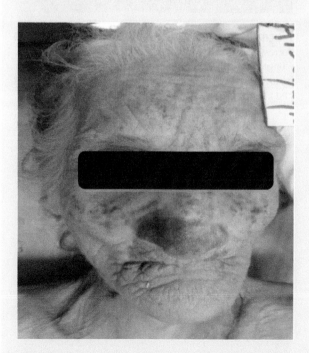

FIGURE 5.59 Multiple petechiae present over the face along with contusion present over the upper lip and the tip of the nose.

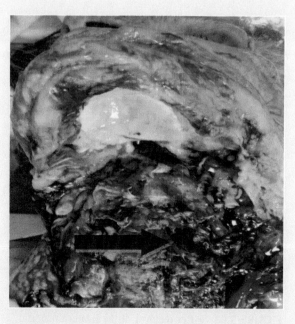

FIGURE 5.61 Fracture and dislocation of the cervical vertebrae in this case of ligature strangulation.

CASE 5: LIGATURE STRAGULATION FINDINGS IN A DECOMPOSED BODY

A 91-year-old male was strangled to death with a ligature by his household worker and his aides. They concealed the body in a refrigerator and later transported and buried the dead body on the same day without anyone's notice. The police started an investigation for the deceased as a missing man case, and within two days, the body of the deceased was unearthed and brought to AIIMS for postmortem examination. The entire body was in a progressively decomposing stage. A cloth, which was the ligature, was not removed by the perpetrators and was found tied tightly around the neck (Figure 5.62). The underlying skin showed a pale band completely encircling the neck (Figure 5.63 and 5.64). Fractures were noted over the hyoid bone and superior horns of the thyroid cartilage (Figure 5.65). Subcutaneous tissues and muscles showed changes of decomposition. The case was concluded as ligature strangulation.

All cases of neck violence, especially when the body is in advanced stage of putrifaction, may not always present with typical textbook description findings. Though the body shows advanced degree of decomposition, a careful external examination and meticulous dissection of the entire neck, including the thyrohyoid complex, may yield some positive findings.

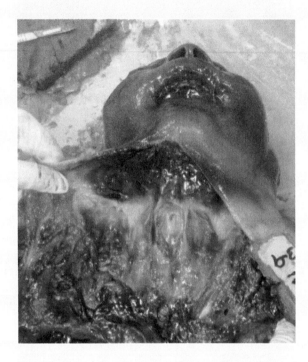

FIGURE 5.64 On dissection of the neck, a pale band corresponding with the external ligature mark was seen. Congestion and hemorrhage were noted above the pale band. Decomposition changes were seen in the muscles and all soft tissues.

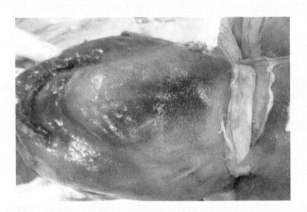

FIGURE 5.62 Ligature material was present tightly tied around the neck.

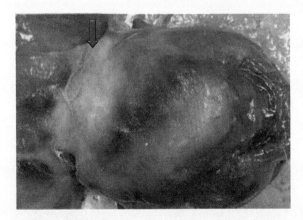

FIGURE 5.63 After removal of the ligature material, a pale band of ligature mark was present, which was completely encircling the neck.

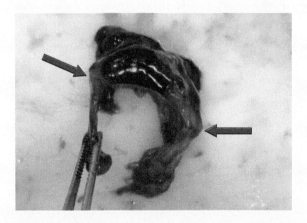

FIGURE 5.65 On dissection of the hyoid bone, bilateral adduction fracture of the greater cornuawas observed with surrounding hemorrhage.

CASE 6: COMBINATION OF LIGATURE STRANGULATION AND SMOTHERING PRESENT IN A CASE PRESENTED AS A NATURAL DEATH

A 35-year-old married lady was found unresponsive at her home. She was suffering from seizure disorder. Initially, it was thought that the death was due to some natural cause of her disease. Postmortem examination revealed small contused abrasions over the inner aspect of lips corresponding to sharp edges of teeth (Figure 5.66). Conjunctivas were congested. Fingernail beds were bluish. Two contusions were noted over the lower jaw. Ligature mark with underlying muscle contusion was present over the lower one third of the neck (Figure 5.67). The ligature mark was transverse in direction. Thyrohyoid complex was intact. Opinion was given as 'Asphyxia due to combined effect of antemortem strangulation and smothering'.

This case points out to the need for meticulous external examination and neck dissection in all cases that come for routine medico-legal autopsy.

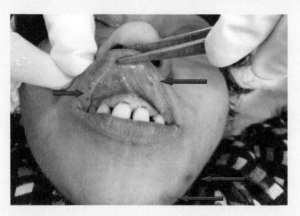

FIGURE 5.66 Multiple contused abrasions corresponding to the sharp edges of the teeth of the upper lip. Multiple contusions seen over the lower jaw.

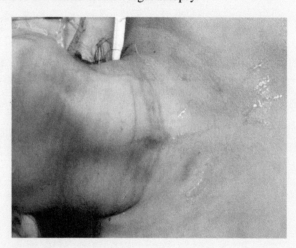

FIGURE 5.67 Ligature mark present over the lower third of the neck.

BIBLIOGRAPHY

1. Häkkänen H. Murder by manual und ligature strangulation. Profiling crime scene behaviors and offender characteristics. In: Kocsis R (ed.). Criminal Profiling: International Theory, Research, and Practice. Totowa, NJ: Humana Press Inc; 2007. pp. 73–88.
2. Sabo RA, et al. Strangulation injuries in children. Part 1. Clinical analysis. Journal of Trauma. 1996;40(1):68–72.
3. Atilgan M. A case of suicidal ligature strangulation by using a tourniquet method. American Journal of Forensic Medicine and Pathology. 2010 Mar;31(1):85–6.
4. Sharma BR, Sharma BR, Harish D, Singh VP, Singh P. Ligature mark on neck: how informative? Journal of Indian Academy of Forensic Medicine. 2005;27(1):10–5.
5. Bohnert M, Marquardt MF, Lutz S, Amberg R, Weisser HJ, Pollak S. Transfer of biological traces in cases of hanging and ligature strangulation. Forensic Science International. 2001;116:107–15.
6. Kanchan T, Atreya A, Raghavendra Babu YP, Bakkannavar SM. Putrefaction, hanging and ligature mark. International Journal of AJ Institute of Medical Sciences. 2014 Nov;3(2).112–7.
7. Mugadlimath AB, Sane MR, Kallur SM, Patil MN. Survival of a victim of Isadora Duncan syndrome: a case report. Medicine, Science and the Law. 2013;53(4):219–22.
8. Bockholdt B, Maxeiner H. Hemorrhages of the tongue in the postmortem diagnostics of strangulation. Forensic Science International. 2002;126:214–20.
9. Pollanen MS, McAuliffe DN. Intra-cartilaginous laryngeal haemorrhages and strangulation. Forensic Science International. 1998;93:13–20.
10. Ramazan A, Ali E, Mahmut SY, Necmi C, et al. A complex suicide by vehicle assisted ligature strangulation and wrist-cutting. Egyptian Journal of Forensic Sciences. 2016;6:534–7.
11. Shields LBE, Corey TS, Jones BW, Stewart D. Living victims of strangulation a 10-year review of cases in a metropolitan community. American Journal of Forensic Medicine and Pathology. 2010 Dec;31(4):320–5.
12. Ma J, Jing H, Zeng Y, Tao L, Yang Y, Ma K, Chen L. Retrospective analysis of 319 hanging and strangulation cases between 2001 and 2014 in Shanghai. Journal of Forensic and Legal Medicine. 2016;42:19–24.
13. Renaud C, Redpath M, Sauvageau A. Mechanism of death in hanging: A historical review of the evolution of pathophysiological hypotheses. Journal of Forensic Sciences. 2010 Sep;55(5):1268–71.
14. Dunsby AM, Davison AM. Causes of laryngeal cartilage and hyoid bone fractures found at postmortem. Medicine, Science and the Law. 2011;51:109–13.

15. Vladislav DK. Pressure on the neck calculated for any point along the ligature. Forensic Science International. 2001;123:178–81.

16. Momin SG, Mangal HM, Kyada HC, Vijapura MT, Bhuva SD. Pattern of ligature mark in cases of compressed neck in Rajkot region: a prospective study. Journal of Indian Academy of Forensic Medicine. 2012 Jan–Mar;34(1): 40–3.

17. Kunnen M, Thomas F, Van De Velde E. Proceedings of the British association in forensic medicine. Semi-microradiography of the larynx on post-mortem material. Medicine, Science and the Law. 1996 Oct;6(4):218–9.

18. Shaikh MMM, Chotaliya HJ, Modi AD, Parmar AP, Kalele SD. A study of gross postmortem findings in cases of hanging and ligature strangulation. Journal of Indian Academy of Forensic Medicine. 2013 Jan–Mar;35(1):971–97.

19. Polson C. Strangulation-manslaughter or murder. The Medico-Legal Journal. 1957;xxv(Part Three).

20. Delbreila A, Gambierc A, Lefrancqd T, Tarisa M, Saint-Martinc P, Sapaneta M. Pathology diagnosis of an atypical thyroid cartilage lesion. Legal Medicine. 2019;36:47–9.

21. Saternus KS, Maxeiner H, Kernbach-Wighton G, Koebke J. Traumatology of the superior thyroid horns in suicidal hanging – an injury analysis. Legal Medicine. 2013;15:134–9.

6 Other Asphyxial Deaths

SMOTHERING

DEFINITION AND CLASSIFICATION

Suffocation is a broad term that includes deaths caused by vitiated atmosphere, smothering and sometimes choking, which are associated with oxygen deprivation. Suffocation is one of the broad classes of asphyxial deaths in the various classifications attempted by different authors, alongside strangulation and drowning. Smothering is included under the broad term of suffocation. Smothering has been defined as an obstruction at the level of the nose and mouth or as an obstruction of the upper airways or obstruction of the external airways by different authors. While Knight B defines it as mechanical occlusion of the mouth and nose, the widely accepted and unified newer classification of asphyxia given by Sauvageau describes it as an obstruction of the air passage above the level of the epiglottis, which includes the nose, mouth and pharynx. However, since the usage of this term for blockage inside the oral cavity and pharynx creates confusion with the term 'gagging', we suggest that the definition of smothering be limited to mechanical obstruction of external respiratory orifices, i.e., the mouth and nose only. This should clear any terminology-related confusion created by the use of more generalized anatomical terms such as 'airways' or 'respiratory passages'. Smothering can be included under the broader classification of suffocation as here there is no confusion in the older as well as newer classifications.

EPIDEMIOLOGY

Infants dying due to accidental suffocation because of heavy bedding is common. Infants can also turn over while asleep, resulting in accidental smothering. This is one of the causes of sudden infant death syndrome (SIDS), and smothering comes under category 2 of the San Diego definition of SIDS. Overlaying by an intoxicated mother can also cause smothering in infants. Children playing with plastic bags are more prone to accidental suffocation. Sometimes, a plastic sheet might adhere to the mouth and the nose due to electrostatic forces, causing accidental smothering. Adults can also get accidentally smothered while involved in acts of bondage, which can also be considered as autoerotic asphyxiation. Adults involved in inhalant abuse such as glue sniffing can also get accidentally smothered. Other than in

the above-mentioned scenarios and in some other rare circumstances, adults commonly are not victims of smothering unless otherwise inebriated or suffering from diseases like epilepsy. Elderly people are more prone to homicidal smothering along with infants and children. Hands, pillows, adhesive tapes, plastic sheets/bags, wet toilet papers, glue, coal dust, sand, mud, grains, etc. are the various means that can be used to cause smothering.

PRE-AUTOPSY

History taking should always be meticulous as is the case in all other kinds of deaths. History regarding the use of inebriants and any history of epilepsy should be carefully elicited in adult and adolescent deaths. A crime scene examination is necessary in every case to verify the history, especially in accidental death cases involving infants, as the autopsy findings will not be prominent in such cases. It also plays an important role in autoerotic asphyxial deaths in adults as the position of the deceased is a vital piece of information in differentiating these from postural asphyxia. Examination of clothes is also mandatory as this may reveal saliva, blood or tissue cells. Any such evidence should be preserved and sent for analysis of the DNA.

POSTMORTEM FINDINGS

EXTERNAL EXAMINATION

- No specific external signs will be present in cases of smothering of infants and old people, especially if soft smothering instruments such as a cushion or a pillow are used. Conjunctival petechiae may be present, and very rarely, petechiae may be seen on the face and oral mucosa. Foreign objects, such as plastic sheets or adhesive tapes, blocking the respiratory passage may be present. These should be carefully removed and sent for chemical examination and DNA analysis. Adhesive tapes can leave residue marks on the face near the nose and mouth, which should also be carefully searched for.
- Circumoral pallor and pallor around the nose are seen and well appreciated in adults, but it is difficult to differentiate these from contact pallor of postmortem lividity in the prone position. Moisture

will be present over the face in cases where plain plastic sheets have been used and inhalants will be present in cases of inhalant abuse. Blood-stained white froth is seen in some cases wherein a struggle had ensued.

- Smothering usually shows a pale face, and the classical signs of asphyxia are absent in most of the cases. The occurrence of petechiae-congestion syndrome is minimal to rare, except in specific circumstances, such as when significant struggle is present. Bluish discoloration of nail beds is also seldom seen.

In cases of rapid deaths due to cardiac arrest, the asphyxial features are classically absent. However, if the death occurs due to slow asphyxia with a significant amount of struggle in adults, all the asphyxial features are severe.

Injuries

Injuries are more common in adults who are not intoxicated as they try to resist the smothering attempt by struggling. Contusions and lacerations of the frenulae and lacerations of the lips are common in people with healthy teeth (Figures 6.1 and 6.2). These occur because of the force exerted by the smothering instrument against the jaw bones bearing intact teeth. It is due to the lack of this that the diagnosis of smothering in infants and elderly is difficult. Abrasions, bruises and laceration may be present on the face, especially around the nose, mouth (Figure 6.2) and sometimes even over the surface of the tongue (Figure 6.3). Fingernail abrasions and small hematomas may also be seen. The front

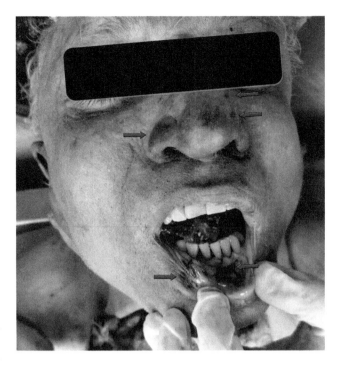

FIGURE 6.2 Contusion of the lower frenulum and the lower lip in a case of smothering. Multiple abrasions and contusions are present over the nose.

teeth may be broken. Other associated neck injuries should also be checked. Homicides will usually be attempted by using multiple methods in young, healthy adults. Hence, strangulation marks and other neck injuries should always be anticipated (Figure 6.4). Posterior neck dissection can be

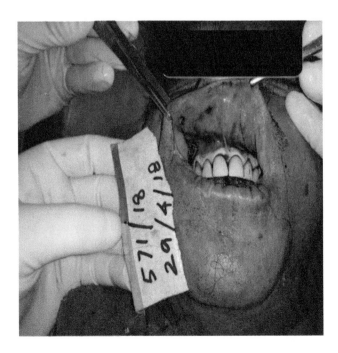

FIGURE 6.1 Lacerations of the inner surface of the upper lip is present in a case of smothering, especially when the deceased has teeth that gives the resistance against compression from the external force.

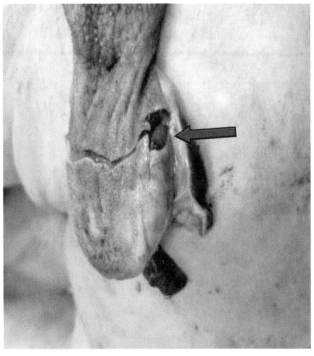

FIGURE 6.3 Laceration and contusion of the tongue in a case of smothering.

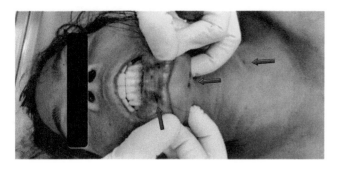

FIGURE 6.4 In homicidal cases involving healthy adults, other methods like strangulation may be attempted along with smothering as in this case showing neck injuries apart from the lip laceration and contusion. Neck examination hence is vital in cases of smothering.

carried out if significant injuries or findings are not present in the face and anterior aspect of the neck. There may be defense injuries in the hands and forearm. Both active and passive defense injuries should be anticipated. Correlation with other injuries on the body is important before concluding the manner of death.

INTERNAL EXAMINATION

Airways may contain blood-stained white froth, and lungs will usually be congested and edematous. Some cases show changes of atelectasis while some show emphysematous changes. The visceral pleura and the epicardium may show petechial hemorrhages. Other internal organs show deep congestion and might also show petechiae. Thymus should not be missed in infants and young children as thymic petechiae and hemorrhages might be the only evident finding in infant deaths due to smothering.

MEDICO-LEGAL IMPORTANCE OF SMOTHERING

- Homicidal smothering is associated with struggle marks over the face and body especially when the victim is conscious and is not completely overpowered by the assailant. Asphyxial signs will be more prominent in such cases due to the period of struggle before death. Usually such homicidal smothering cases have accompanying features of strangulation, so as to cause death of a person with reasonable certainty. A case with similar features is discussed below.

CASE NO. 1: FALL FROM HEIGHT TURNED OUT TO BE A HOMICIDE CASE WITH SMOTHERING AND MANUAL STRANGULATION

In early 2021, the dead body of a young male was found in a dry water channel (nala) near a graveyard by his brother. As per inquest papers, there was an alleged history of the

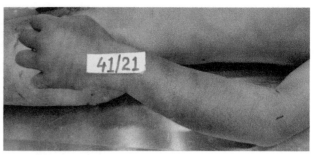

FIGURE 6.5 Contusions present over the left hand and forearm of the deceased.

deceased attempting robbery at a house, following which he was caught and assaulted by the house members. The house members had reported to the police that the thief escaped from their custody, but later the same person was found in an unresponsive state in a deep dry nala on the same day by his brother. He was then taken to a nearby hospital where he was declared brought dead. A medico-legal case was registered, and the dead body was subjected to postmortem examination. On postmortem examination, multiple muscle-deep contusions were noted on all limbs and trunk of the body (Figures 6.5 and 6.6). Contusions were present over the mucosal surface of the upper and lower lip (Figure 6.7). Multiple abraded contusions were present around the mouth and over the neck (Figure 6.8). On dissection of the neck, contusions were present over the sternocleidomastoid muscle and sternothyroid muscle. Fracture of the hyoid bone was present on the right side between the greater horn and body of the hyoid, with infiltration of the surrounding soft tissue. Thyroid cartilage and trachea were intact.

After conducting a thorough postmortem examination and duly considering the available circumstantial evidence, the cause of death was given as 'Asphyxia due to smothering and manual strangulation'. A case of homicide was registered against the house members for the act that resulted in death of a young male.

- Accidental smothering may occur when a person falls over a heap of sand or mud under the influence of alcohol, drugs or during an episode of status epilepticus. It is important to differentiate

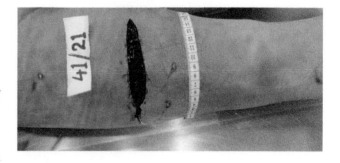

FIGURE 6.6 Contusion present over the right thigh, which was incised during the autopsy to check the depth of the contusion.

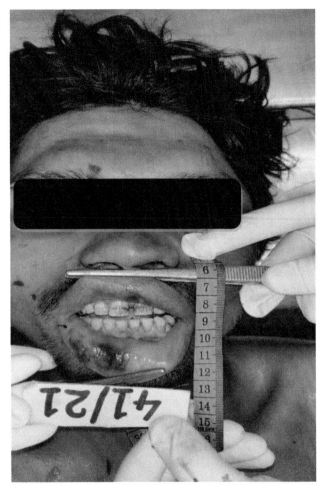

FIGURE 6.7 Contusions were present over the mucosal surfaces of both the upper and lower lip.

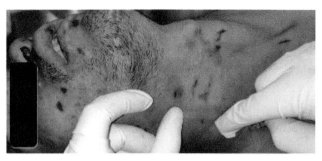

FIGURE 6.8 Multiple abraded contusions present around the mouth and over the neck.

accidental smothering from similarly presenting natural causes of death such as those wherein the deceased is found in a prone position. Such cases should also be differentiated from incidents of postural asphyxia. Loth (1964) has reported a case of death due to suffocation by sand when the deceased fell face down on the ground during an epileptic fit. Smothering can also take place when young inexperienced mothers press their baby too tightly against the breast while suckling or also when the baby accidentally turns prone over the bed. The other situations where babies can get accidentally smothered include pillow or blanket obstructing their external respiratory orifices or when a mother or parent, especially intoxicated, may lay over the baby.

CASE 2: A CASE OF POSTURAL SMOTHERING, AN ACCIDENTAL DEATH CONTESTED AS A CASE OF HOMICIDE DEATH: CLARIFIED BY MEDICAL BOARD UNDER THE CHAIRMANSHIP OF AUTHOR

In 2017, there was a lot of hue and cry among the public after a civil service officer was found unconscious at a roadside in front of the guest house where he was staying (Figure 6.9 a–d). As per history, the deceased was suffering from diarrhea on that day and was on self-rehydration. He was rushed

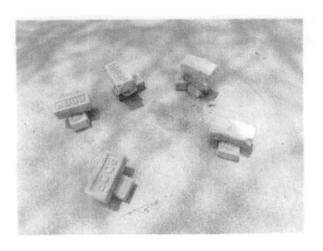

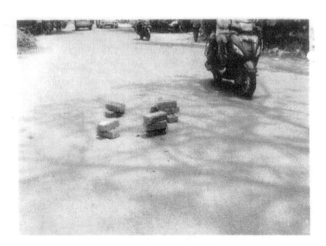

FIGURE 6.9a The scene of occurrence where the deceased was found lying on the road following which he was taken to the hospital. The image shows blood stains over the road.

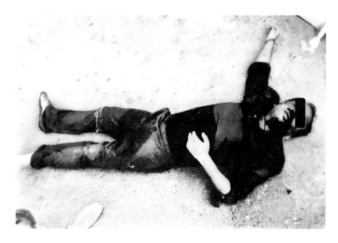

FIGURE 6.9b Deceased found lying unconscious; position was changed from prone to supine.

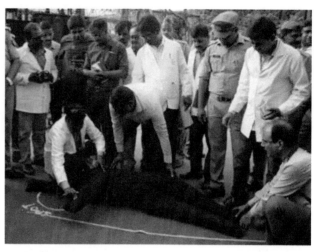

FIGURE 6.9c The crime scene team examining the actual prone position in which the deceased was found by using a dummy.

to the nearby hospital but was declared brought dead. A Medical Board of four doctors conducted the postmortem examination. Viscera analysis revealed nicotine, and the blood sample showed a value of 319 ng/mL. The deceased was a chronic smoker. Histopathological examination of the entire heart preserved did not show any evident pathology. The Board opined that the cause of death was asphyxia; however, the exact reason/cause of asphyxia could not be determined. All injuries were superficial and could be produced

by a fall in prone position. There were no eyewitnesses for the incident, and no evidence of murder could be found. There were many disputes, and a murder case was registered. Later, the case was transferred to the CBI and an expert medico-legal opinion was requested from AIIMS, New Delhi under the chairmanship of the author. Under the author, a Medical Board was constituted at AIIMS, New Delhi.

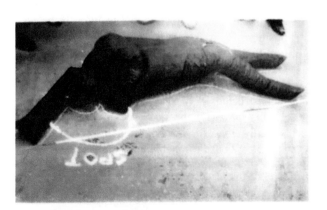

DSC 0619

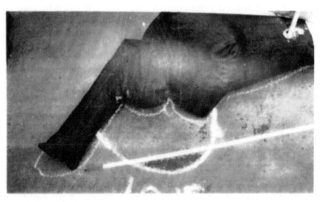

DSC 0620

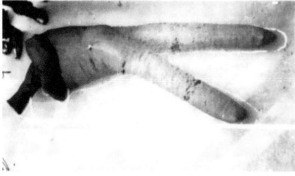

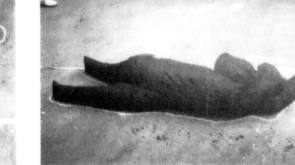

FIGURE 6.9d Crime scene reconstruction by the crime team showing position of the deceased.

QUERIES FOR THE MEDICAL BOARD

1. A holistic opinion into the cause of death of deceased may be opined by constituting a Medical board.
2. Any other opinion which is relevant to the case may be provided.

AIIMS MEDICAL BOARD OBSERVATIONS

i. The dead body of deceased was found on the road in front of State Guest House, local police took him to Civil Hospital where he was declared brought dead.

ii. The deceased was found lying in prone position, with blood stains near nose, chin and adjoining areas of face. Following injuries were observed on perusal of PM report, photograph and videography:

   1. Lacerated wound 2.5 cm × 0.5 cm × muscle deep present on left side of chin.
   2. Lacerated wound 1.5 cm × 0.5 cm × muscle deep present on inner aspect of lower lip in middle.
   3. Abraded contusion 2.5 cm × 1.5 cm present on side of chin just below injury 1.
   4. Abraded contusion 1.0 cm × 1.0 cm present on back of left wrist.
   5. Abraded contusion 1.5 cm × 0.5 cm present on front of right knee joint.
   6. Abraded contusion 1 cm × 1 cm present on left side, 2 cm below and behind left angle of mouth.

iii. Injury no. 1, 2, 3, 4, 5 and 6 (Figures 6.10 a and b) are abraded contusions consistent with ground/low level fall on a rough hard surface like coal tar road, producing blunt force trauma. Injury to chin is below the undersurface of chin, which is due to hitting of underside of chin on a blunt surface with hard impact resulting in split lacerated wound on that region, likely to be due to fall on the hard coal tar road at the scene of crime.

iv. There are no injuries over the body that could suggest scuffle or any alteration of clothing of deceased prior to death. No signs of any vehicular injury could be detected.

v. The presence of split lacerated wound on undersurface of chin and smudged dried blood stains on face area around nostrils, mouth and chin suggests that the face of deceased had an impact with a hard blunt surface compressing the nose, mouth and adjacent face area. In homicidal smothering, usually soft objects like cloth or pillows or hands are used to obstruct the face and nostrils/mouth of the victim; hard objects/surfaces are not preferred by the assailant.

vi. The opinion as to cause of death given by the previous Medical Board was 'Death is due to

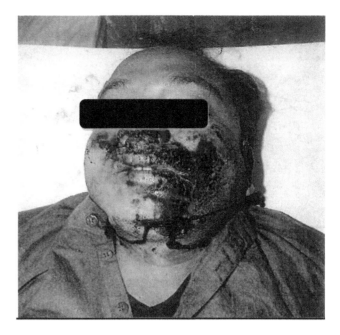

FIGURE 6.10a Face of the deceased showing area of dried smudged blood near mouth, nostril and chin. Also, trickling down of blood from undersurface of chin signifies the deceased might be still alive when body was turned to supine state from prone position.

Asphyxia, as a result of Antemortem Smothering'. Smothering refers to death from mechanical occlusion of mouth/nostrils where either the occluding substance presses down upon the facial orifices, or the passive weight of the head presses the nose and mouth into occlusion, due to body in prone position.

vii. On the basis of inquest papers and statements of witness submitted by CBI, related to the case, the sequence of events prior to death of deceased was reconstructed:

   1. On 17/05/17, the deceased may have allegedly gone for a walk from his room in the guest house (probably for a smoke, as he was

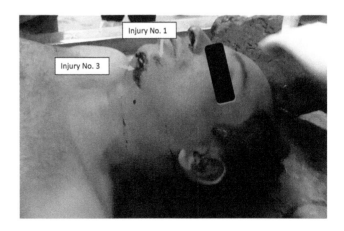

FIGURE 6.10b Injury no. 1 and 3 (injury 1: lacerated wound 2.5 cm × 0.5 cm × muscle deep present on left side of chin; injury 3: abraded contusion 2.5 cm × 1.5 cm present on the side of chin just below injury 1).

a known chronic smoker) and had reached the place where he was allegedly found lying on the road in prone position. The deceased was suffering from Acute Gastro Enteritis (diarrhea) on the day of incident, as per the inquest papers. It was also corroborated by the statement of a witness, who purchased the electrolyte packet for the deceased from the shop and also the presence of electrolyte packet on the room table. It is medically well known that acute diarrhea can produce sudden hypovolaemic syncopal attack and incapacitating weakness due to electrolyte imbalance resulting in sudden accidental fall and unconsciousness. The fall on chin/face on the hard surface resulted in split laceration below his chin, leading to bleeding. It is likely that the deceased could not get up from prone position due to syncopal attack and his incapacitating weakness produced by diarrhea and fall.

2. As the deceased fell in prone position and become unconscious with mouth and nose pressed on the surface, it is likely that it caused positional accidental smothering producing asphyxia leading to death. Such situation is commonly seen in incapacitated/intoxicated person.

viii. If the person falls on ground in prone position and gets injured, bleeding may occur from chin or nose (as face is a highly vascular area and even minimal trauma can produce severe bleeding), which also can obstruct the respiratory passage at the level of mouth and nasal orifice. Dry blood stain pattern over the nose and mouth and area around it is corroborating with the compression of the respiratory passage with head in prone position for prolonged period.

ix. The chemical examination report of the Forensic Science Laboratory reveals presence of Nicotine in concentration of 319 ng/mL, which suggests that the deceased was a chronic cigarette smoker. The report was negative for common insecticides, volatile, metallic/inorganic, alkaloids including nicotine, gaseous and sedative poisons.

x. The histopathological examination report revealed no significant evident pathology of heart. Histomorphology was consistent with normal histology of heart and there was no evidence of any necrosis/infarction, inflammation, thrombosis or atherosclerosis.

AIIMS MEDICAL BOARD OPINION UNDER THE CHAIRMANSHIP OF THE AUTHOR

The Medical Board examined all related evidences/documents/scene visit report, and after perusal of the scientific facts of this case along with examination of scene of crime by the members, the Medical Board unanimously concluded that the cause of death in this case was asphyxia due to positional smothering, consequent upon syncopal fall (due to hemodynamic imbalance subsequent to acute diarrhea) in face down prone position for a significant time.

RARE ASSOCIATIONS AND CASES

Xu-mei Wu et al in 2016 reported a case of domestic violence wherein the woman was found dead at her residence after allegedly being smothered and strangulated by her husband. The husband confessed to having attempted to smother and strangulate his wife, but insisted that she had still been alive afterwards. Autopsy revealed external features of smothering and strangulation along with a massive subarachnoid hemorrhage. After histopathology, a diagnosis of rupture of intravascular malformation was confirmed. The cause of death was given as subarachnoid hemorrhage, but this could have been a possible complication of mechanical asphyxia.

Seon Jung Jang et al in 2013 reported a case of homicidal smothering of an adult wherein a hot steam towel was used as the smothering weapon, probably the only such case in forensic literature. The deceased had been a known case of psychiatric illness for which his mother and a pastoress had tried exorcism on him. He had been physically restrained and the hot steam towel had been kept on his face as part of the exorcism ritual. The autopsy revealed a scalding injury over his face and the cause of death was given as smothering.

RECENT ADVANCES

Qi wang et al in 2012 published a study on intrapulmonary aquaporin-5 (AQ-5) expression in smothering and choking and differentiated it from sudden cardiac deaths. They found that the expression of AQ-5 is suppressed in smothering and choking deaths when compared to sudden cardiac deaths. They proved this using gene expression assay as well as immuno-histochemistry. Hence, AQ-5 should be explored for being a biomarker for smothering.

CASE 3: A TWIN CASE OF HOMICIDE OF TWO FEMALES CAUSED BY SMOTHERING IN DELHI, INDIA ON 15/11/2021 AND POSTMORTEM WAS CONDUCTED IN AIIMS, NEW DELHI UNDER THE SUPERVISION OF AUTHOR

CASE HISTORY

Two women in their early 30's and 40's were found lying dead in a house on the first and second floor of a house. They both were maids working in the same house where they were found dead. The owners lived on the third floor of the house. On the day of the incident, the caretaker of the owners returned to the house from her native place. She tried to contact the maids by calling them, and when no one

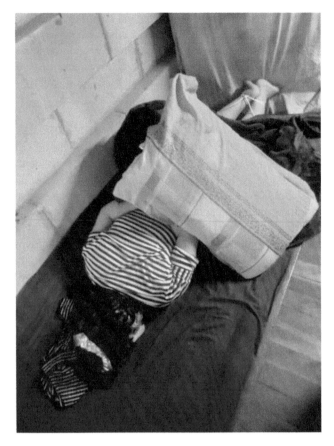

FIGURE 6.11   Victim is placed in prone head down position with hands and legs tied.

responded, finding it fishy, she informed the police regarding the situation. With the help of the police, they entered the locked house to find the first women lying dead on a bed with her hands and legs tied with a nylon rope (Figure 6.11); she was in prone position and a silver tape was wrapped around her face (Figure 6.12).

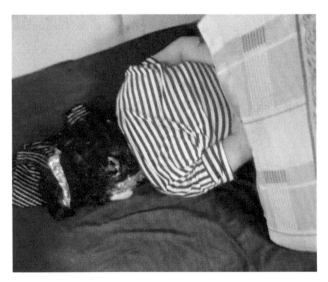

FIGURE 6.12   Silver tape is seen wrapped around the face of the victim.

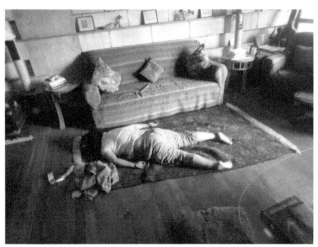

FIGURE 6.13   Second victim found lying in prone position on the floor.

On checking the house further, another maid in her early 40's was found lying dead in the drawing room on the second floor. She was lying in prone position on the floor with face down (Figure 6.13).

The house was a well secured place with advanced security locks and CCTV cameras. None of these locks were broken, and there was no evidence of any forced entry into the house. The police immediately secured the crime scene and informed the crime team to conduct a detailed crime scene analysis. The bodies of the deceased were shifted to AIIMS mortuary for postmortem examination.

AUTOPSY EXAMINATION OF VICTIM 1

External Findings

The dead body of the first female victim in her early 30's was examined. Examination of the clothings worn by the victim showed no tears, and her hands and legs were tied with a nylon rope (Figures 6.14 and 6.15). There were underlying patterned, grooved markings of the rope involving the front and lateral aspects of the left hand, right hand and the left side of lower back across the midline. Both the ankles were tied together with a yellow-colored nylon rope, with two loops, one of which had a fixed knot. The skin beneath the rope showed extravasation of blood along with ligature impression. Reddish brown fluid was seen purging from mouth and nostrils.

Examination of the nylon rope used for tying the hands and feet showed that multiple loops were present and a knot was used to secure the rope in position (Figure 6.16).

The silver adhesive tape was found over the face of the victim, and examination of the tape revealed that it was probably wound to silence the victim. After removal of the tape, it was examined for presence of stains or any other possible foreign material (Figures 6.17 and 6.18).

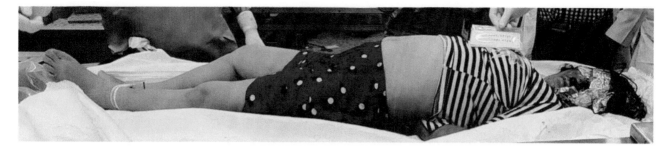

FIGURE 6.14   First female victim with intact clothes and her hands and legs tied with a nylon rope.

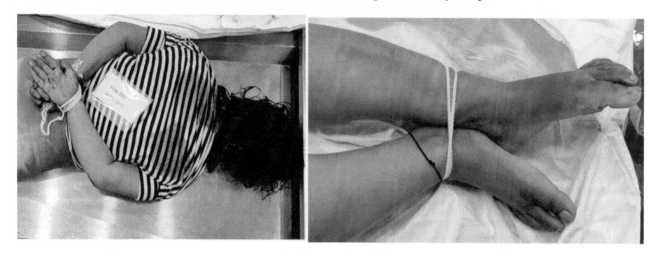

FIGURE 6.15   Both hands tied together at the back and both legs tied with yellow-colored nylon rope.

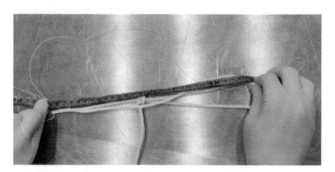

FIGURE 6.16   Ligature examination with knot preservation.

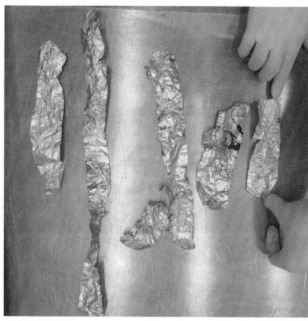

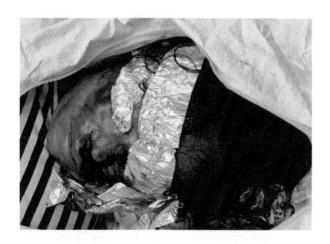

FIGURE 6.17   Silver adhesive tape over the head and face.

FIGURE 6.18   Silver adhesive tape after removal from the face examined for presence of stains or any other foreign material.

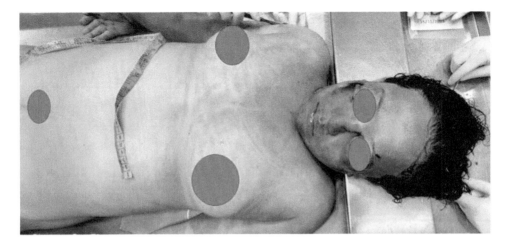

FIGURE 6.19 Postmortem lividity over the face, front of neck, front of shoulders, parts of upper anterior chest with contact pallor over the front of lower chest and abdomen.

On external examination of the deceased, postmortem lividity was present over the face, front of neck, front of shoulders, parts of upper anterior chest with contact pallor over the front of lower chest and abdomen corresponding to the position of the victim at the crime scene (Figure 6.19).

Examination of the eyes showed bilateral subconjunctival hemorrhages and petechial hemorrhages over the palpebral conjunctivae with severe congestion (Figure 6.20). Bluish discoloration of fingernail beds and palms (Figure 6.21) was noted. Bluish discoloration of lips with multiple reddish blue contusions along with skin peeling were present over the inner aspect of both upper and lower lips (Figure 6.22). Tongue was clenched between the teeth.

Multiple injuries were present over the forehead and face. Reddish abrasions were present around the nose and over the right side of the face (Figure 6.23). A bluish red contusion was present at the front of the right arm and tip of the shoulder. A reddish abrasion was also noted at the front of the right knee. No other injuries were present over the neck (Figure 6.24).

Internal Findings

Scalp was intact. On reflection, multiple subscalp petechial hemorrhages were present. The brain was intensely congested. Larynx was congested and edematous with presence of reddish froth; postmortem computed tomography (CT) examination prior to autopsy also showed features of laryngeal edema (Figures 6.25 and 6.26). Tracheal mucosa was congested and edematous with presence of reddish froth (Figure 6.27) along the entire tracheobronchial tree. Both the lungs were congested and edematous (Figure 6.28). Subpleural petechiae were present over the surface of both lungs. The cause of death was concluded as asphyxia due to ante-mortem smothering based on the observations.

AUTOPSY EXAMINATION OF VICTIM 2

Postmortem lividity was present over front of shoulders, parts of chest and abdomen and over the back except over pressure areas, and was fixed. Face, neck and upper and lateral part of chest were congested and showed multiple petechiae and ecchymoses (Figure 6.29).

Bilateral eyes were congested, and subconjunctival hemorrhage was present over the right eye. Bluish discoloration of fingernail beds and palms (Figure 6.30) was noted. Bluish discoloration of lips with laceration and multiple reddish blue contusions were present over inner aspect of both upper and lower lips (Figure 6.31).

Multiple reddish contusions were present over the inner aspect of upper and lower lips at places (Figure 6.32). Multiple reddish abrasions and abraded contusions were present over the forehead and lower part of the face (Figure 6.33). Multiple contusions were present over the right scapular region (Figure 6.34). Subscalp contusion and pericranial hemorrhage was present over mid frontal region. Larynx and tracheal mucosa were congested and edematous

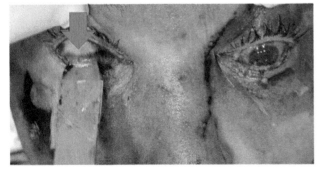
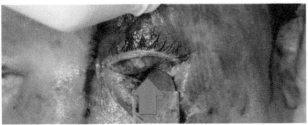

FIGURE 6.20 Congested eyes and petechial hemorrhages over palpebral conjunctivae.

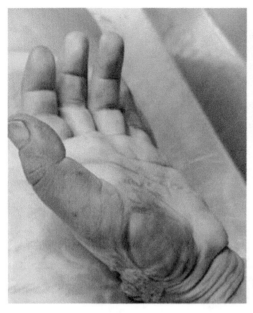
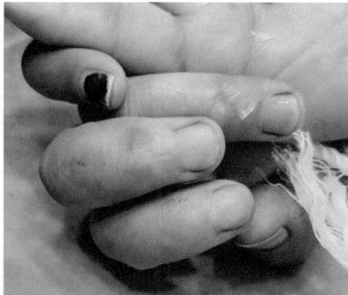

FIGURE 6.21 Bluish discoloration of nailbeds and palms.

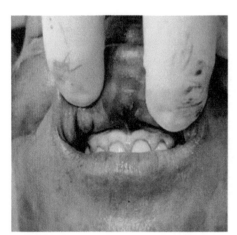
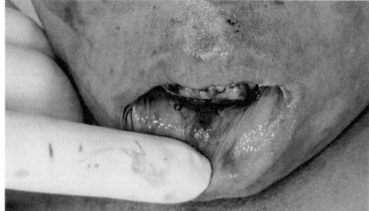

FIGURE 6.22 Contusions and mucosal peeling of upper and lower lips.

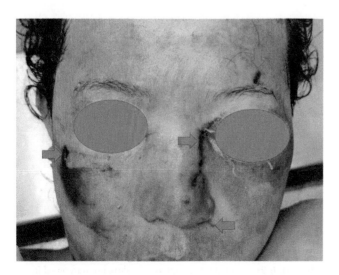

FIGURE 6.23 Multiple injuries over forehead and face.

(Figure 6.35). The cause of death was concluded as asphyxia due to ante-mortem smothering based on the observation.

PECULIARITIES OF BOTH THE CASES

The novelty behind these cases was the ways by which the act was committed and the injuries interpreted. These cases may be a simple smothering, but the scenario in which it was accomplished makes it a novel occurrence. The position of the victim in both the cases may be similar, but in the first case, the victim was made to lie on a mattress while the victim in the second case was lying on the carpet spread on the floor. This led to the difference in the pattern and severity of the injuries found on the corresponding bodies. There were injuries like abrasion and contusions found over the face of both the victims. The lip laceration was seen only in the second victim but not in the first due to the difference in the surface in which smothering was accomplished.

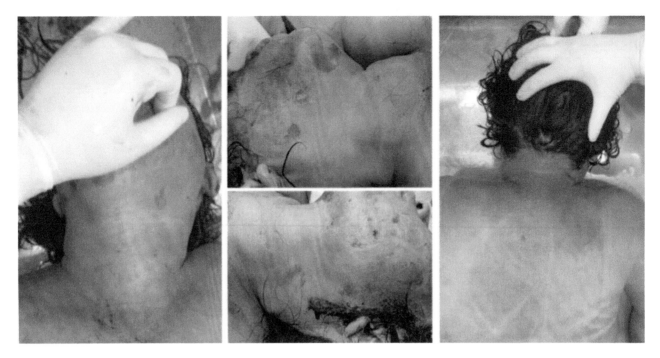

FIGURE 6.24 There were no external injuries over the neck.

The methods used by the accused to incapacitate the victim also differed in both the cases. There was usage of chloroform to make both the victims unconscious, which was confirmed in the confession by the accused. The victim's hands and legs were tied with a nylon rope to control the movements during the act in the first victim, while the second victim was not tied. The second victim had an injury in the form of subscalp contusion as a result of blunt surface impact, i.e., the floor. The victim also had injuries on the scapular region of the back of the chest, suggesting the possibility of the accused applying force to control the movement of the victim. This type of injuries was not seen in the first victim as the hands and legs were tied. This explained that to smother a victim on a soft surface, more amount of force and effort in the form of restraining the victim is required as the victim tries to fight back to the maximum. The act of smothering on a hard surface doesn't require much force as a single impact of the surface makes the victim lose consciousness.

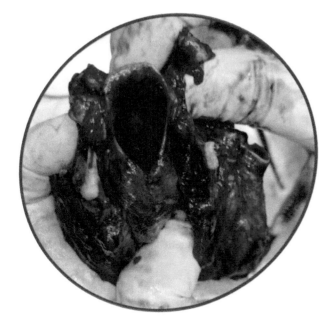

FIGURE 6.25 Laryngeal congestion, edema and reddish froth in inlet.

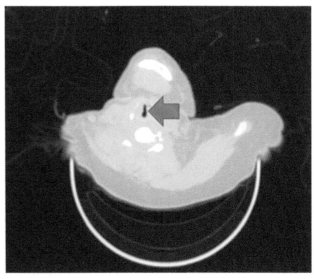

FIGURE 6.26 The axial image of CT showing narrowed laryngeal inlet suggestive of laryngeal edema.

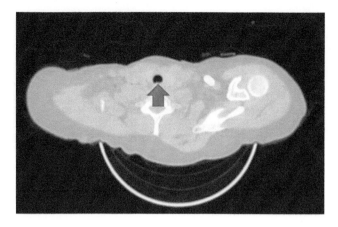

FIGURE 6.27 Axial image of CT depicting the presence of edematous tracheal mucosa and narrowing of tracheal lumen.

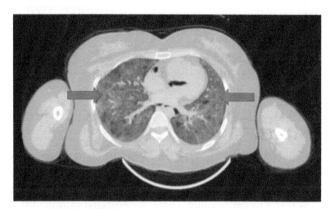

FIGURE 6.28 Axial image of CT depicting the congested lungs.

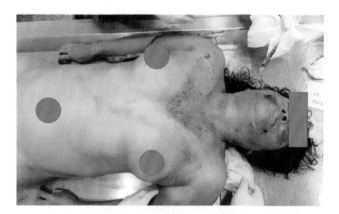

FIGURE 6.29 Postmortem lividity over the face, front of neck, front of shoulders, parts of upper anterior chest with contact pallor over the front of lower chest and abdomen.

SEQUENCE UNVEILED BY INVESTIGATIVE AGENCY

The act of twin smothering was a planned dacoity; unfortunately, it became a twin smothering. It was confirmed through the investigative agency that the accused was planning for more than a month. The accused was a relative of the previous maid who was working in the same home 2 years back. The act was committed by the said relative

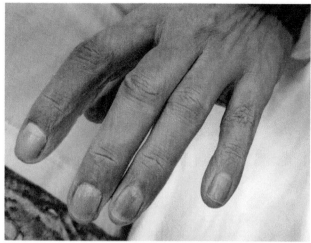

FIGURE 6.30 Bluish discoloration of nailbeds.

who led a crew of four other people known to him and they knew the working system of the locks. This was the reason of absence of forced entry into the building as the locks were intact as they knew the procedure to unlock the advanced locking system of the house. The assailant knew very well about the installed CCTV and hence removed the digital video recorder (DVR) of the CCTV after entering the building. Their main intention was dacoity; however,

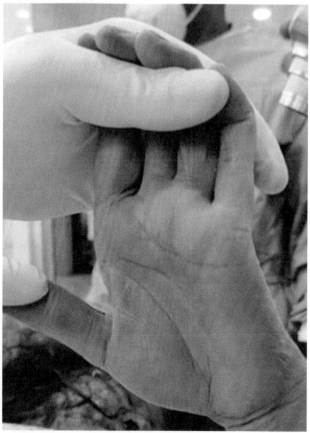

FIGURE 6.31 Bluish discoloration of palm.

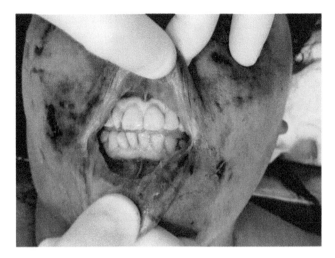

FIGURE 6.32 Multiple contusions and lacerations over the upper and lower lips.

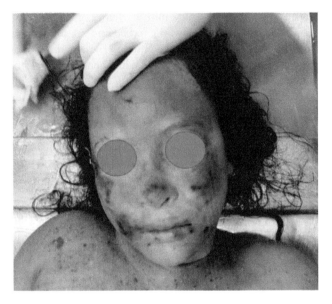

FIGURE 6.33 Multiple abrasions and contusions over the face and forehead.

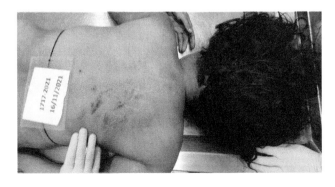

FIGURE 6.34 Multiple contusions present over the back.

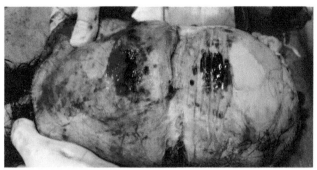

FIGURE 6.35 Subscalp contusion and peri-cranial hemorrhage present over mid frontal region.

they were mentally prepared to commit murder of the person who creates hindrance during the act. The police had also recovered chloroform, rope, cutter, punch, DVR of CCTV of the house, bike used in crime and seven mobile phones from them. It was known from the investigation that the victims tried to shout and hence they killed them in order to accomplish the dacoity successfully.

CASE 4: A CASE OF COMBINED SMOTHERING AND STRANGULATION OF A FEMALE

A 35-year-old female was found unconscious in her residence in a vessel washing place with her head and right hand inside the bucket containing water (Figure 6.36). She was taken to the hospital where her husband informed that she was suffering from epilepsy for many years, and while working in sitting position, she had an epileptic attack and became unconscious and fell into the bucket containing water. She was declared brought dead at the hospital and the case was registered as medico-legal. Postmortem was conducted at AIIMS under the supervision of the author.

Autopsy revealed multiple injuries around the mouth and over the neck, and there were features of asphyxia over the body. Following injuries were observed:

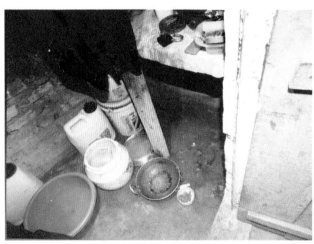

FIGURE 6.36 Scene of occurrence where the woman was found dead in her residence.

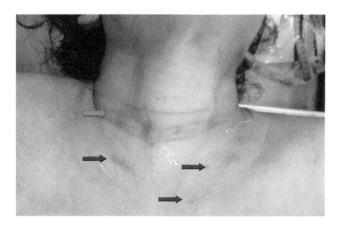

FIGURE 6.37   Horizontal pressure abrasion over the lower third of neck (blue arrow) with multiple contusions (red arrows).

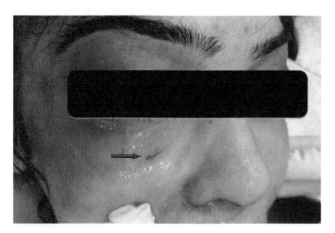

FIGURE 6.38   Hemorrhage in the subcutaneous tissue corresponding to the pressure abrasion.

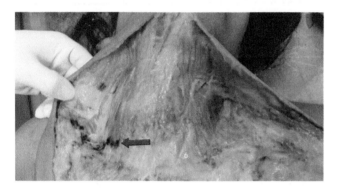

FIGURE 6.39   Abraded contusion seen below the right eye.

A red-colored pressure abrasion was seen in the lower one third of the neck below the thyroid cartilage along with multiple contusions on the right and left side of the lower neck (Figure 6.37). On dissection, the underlying subcutaneous tissue showed hemorrhage corresponding to the pressure abrasion (ligature mark) (Figure 6.38). The blood vessels and thyrohyoid complex were intact, and tracheal mucosa was congested. A reddish contused abrasion was found below her right eye (Figure 6.39), and multiple

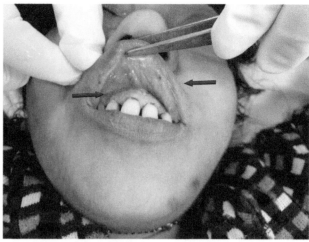

FIGURE 6.40a   Multiple abrasions seen on the inner surface of the upper lip.

contused abrasions were present over inner mucosa of the upper lip (Figure 6.40 (a)). Reddish abraded contusions were present over left side of the chin and mandible (Figure 6.40 (b)).

Based on the autopsy observations and circumstantial evidences, it was concluded as a case of asphyxial death resulting from the combined effect of smothering and strangulation.

CASE 5: MATERNAL FILICIDE BY SMOTHERING, MANUAL STRANGULATION AND HEAD INJURY; AUTOPSY CONDUCTED AT AIIMS, NEW DELHI UNDER THE SUPERVISION OF AUTHOR

CASE HISTORY

On the fateful day, a young mother was attempting to commit suicide by hanging when her child started crying. In the

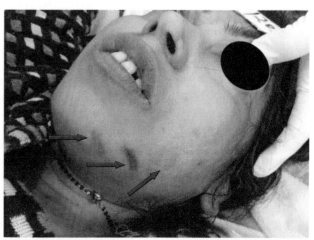

FIGURE 6.40b   Multiple abraded contusions seen over the left side of the chin and mandible.

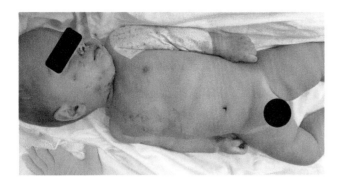

FIGURE 6.41   An average-built child with dried blood stains seen over the face and chest.

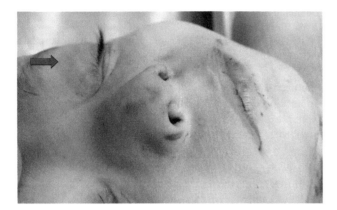

FIGURE 6.42   Left-sided peri-orbital ecchymosis seen in the case.

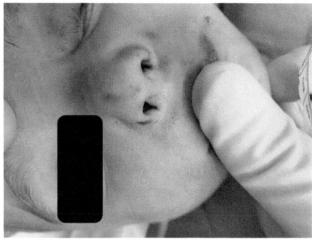

FIGURE 6.43   Multiple abrasions over and around the nose.

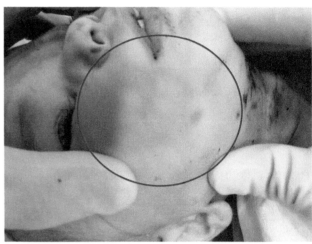

FIGURE 6.44   Multiple contusions seen over the right cheek.

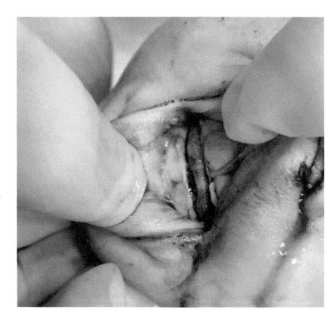

FIGURE 6.45   Lower lip inner surface showing contusion.

process of silencing the crying child, the mother smothered, strangled and threw the baby on the floor. The child was brought to AIIMS where he was declared 'brought dead' and the body was sent for medico-legal autopsy.

At autopsy, the body was that of a 11-month-old child of average built. External examination of the deceased body showed the entire face and front of upper chest was smeared with dried and wet blood stains (Figure 6.41). Peri-orbital echymosis was seen on the left side (Figure 6.42). Dried blood stains were present inside the ear canals.

Multiple small reddish abrasions were present over the bridge of nose and alae of nose (Figure 6.43). Soft tissues of cheeks and under chin areas showed multiple contusions (Figure 6.44). Inner aspect of the lower lip showed a contusion, and a lacerated wound was seen on the right angle of the mouth (Figure 6.45). Upper lip showed lacerated frenulum-associated blood extravasation (Figure 6.46). Multiple abraded contusions were seen on the front side of the neck (Figure 6.47). A scalp contusion along with underlying fissure fracture of the skull were present over the right fronto-temporao-parietal region (Figure 6.48) associated with subdural hemorrhage.

Based on all autopsy observations, it was concluded that the cause of death was asphyxia due to the combined effect of smothering and manual strangulation coupled with head injury due to blunt force trauma to the head.

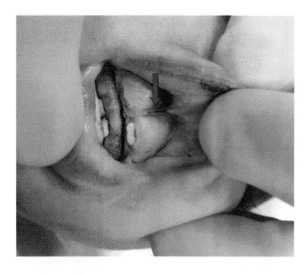

FIGURE 6.46 Upper lip frenulum laceration along with extravasation seen.

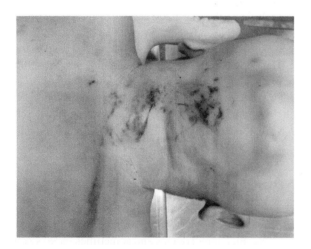

FIGURE 6.47 Multiple abraded contusions over the front of the neck.

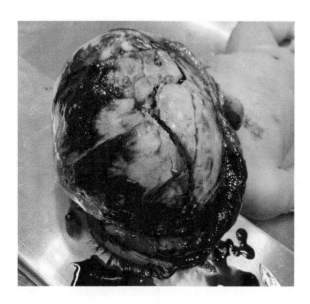

FIGURE 6.48 Subscalp hematoma with fissured fracture of right side of the head.

BIBLIOGRAPHY

1. Nixon JW, Kemp AM, Levene S, Sibert JR. Suffocation, choking and strangulation in childhood in England and Wales: epidemiology and prevention. Archives of Disease in Childhood. 1995;72:6–10.
2. Shkrum MJ, Ramsay DA. Asphyxia. In: Karch SB (series ed.). Forensic pathology of trauma: common problems for the pathologist. Totowa, NJ: Humana Press; 2007. pp. 65–179.
3. Spitz WU. Asphyxia. In: Spitz WU, Spitz DJ (eds.). Spitz and Fisher's Medicolegal Investigation of Death: Guidelines for the Application of Pathology to Crime Investigation, 4th ed. Springfield, IL: Charles C Thomas; 2006. pp. 783–845.
4. Walker A, Milroy CM, Payne-James J. Asphyxia. In: Payne-James J, Byard RW, Corey TS, Henderson C (eds.). Encyclopedia of Forensic and Legal Medicine, vol. 1. Oxford, UK: Elsevier Academic Press; 2005. pp. 151–7.
5. Oehmichen M, Auer RN, Kçnig HG. Forensic types of ischemia and asphyxia. In: Oehmichen M (ed.). Forensic Neuropathology and Associated Neurology. Berlin: Springer-Verlag; 2005. pp. 293–313.
6. Knight B, Saukko P. Knight's forensic pathology, 4th ed. Boca Raton. Taylor & Francis Group, LLC; 2016. p. 359.
7. Sauvageau A, Boghossian E. Classification of asphyxia: the need for standardization. Journal of Forensic Sciences. 2010 Jun 17;55(5):1259–67.
8. Bajanowski T, Vennemann M. Sudden infant death syndrome (SIDS). In: Siegel JA, Saukko PJ (eds.). Encyclopedia of Forensic Sciences. Waltham: Academic Press; 2013. pp. 63–9.
9. Mehdi A, Nimkar N, Darwish N, Atallah R, Usiene I. Distinguishing suicidal attempt from autoerotic asphyxiation. Psychiatric Annals. 2015 Jun 11;45(6):285–9.
10. Das S, Jena MK. Homicide by a combination of three different asphyxial methods. Egyptian Journal of Forensic Sciences. 2016 Sep 1;6(3):298–302.
11. Viero A, Cecchetto G, Boscolo-Berto R, Viel G, Montisci M. Suicidal smothering by rubber latex gloves and handkerchief. Journal of Forensic Sciences. 2015 Aug 6;61(1):268–70.
12. Saint-Martin P, Bouyssy M, O'Byrne P. An unusual case of suicidal asphyxia by smothering. Journal of Forensic and Legal Medicine. 2007 Jan 1;14(1):39–41.
13. Wu X, Zhang X, Yun L, Liu M, Yi X. Sudden death from ruptured intracranial vascular malformations during mechanical asphyxia. American Journal of Forensic Medicine and Pathology. 2017 Mar;38(1):35–8.
14. Jang SJ, Park JH, Kim YJ, Ham SH, Jo NY, Ha H. Death by homicidal smothering using hot steam towel: a case report. Korean Journal of Legal Medicine. 2013;37(2):90.
15. Wang Q, Ishikawa T, Michiue T, Zhu B-L, Guan D-W, Maeda H. Intrapulmonary aquaporin-5 expression as a possible biomarker for discriminating smothering and choking from sudden cardiac death: a pilot study. Forensic Science International. 2012 Jul;220(1–3):154–7.

GAGGING

Gagging is a form of asphyxia produced by forcing a foreign object into the mouth and/or throat. It is usually resorted to as a means of preventing the victim from shouting for help, and the resultant death is usually not intentional. Hence, sometimes the victim's hands and legs may also be found tied so as to prevent him or her from removing the gag and escaping. However, at times, the gagging may be homicidal, particularly in the cases of infants, individuals incapacitated by alcohol or other drugs, the elderly and infirm, etc. The commonly encountered gagging materials include rolled-up clothes, papers, ties, scarves, etc., but other unusual items such as false dentures are also known to have been used as a gag. Some authors do not consider gagging to be a separate category of asphyxial death in its own right and prefer to include it as a type of smothering or, sometimes, choking.

The gag not only blocks the mouth, but it also prevents the passage of air coming in via the nostrils, through the back of the throat. Once in place, the gag quickly gets moistened by saliva, mucus and edema fluid, and it may also get sucked in further with inspiratory gasps, thus progressively resulting in complete obstruction. The size and position of the gag play a role in its pathophysiology; either there is direct occlusion of the nasopharyngeal space by the gag itself or it occurs due to the upwards displacement of the base of the tongue caused by it. For gagging to cause death, there must be complete obstruction of the upper airways, namely the oral and the nasal cavities, both of which converge at the pharynx. Hence, the gag should reach up to the posterior wall of the pharynx for causing fatal obstruction; this is referred to as complete gagging. By contrast, in incomplete gagging, the gag forced into the oral cavity does not reach up to the posterior pharyngeal wall, and since the airway behind the gag remains patent, death usually does not occur immediately. However, especially since most of the materials commonly used as gags tend to be fluid absorbents, the gag absorbs saliva and other secretions and swells up with the passage of time, such that complete obstruction occurs, which then leads to death.

Up to 100 mL of volume obstruction by the gag may be tolerated by an individual, but if it obstructs 150–200 mL or more, it will result in the closure of the internal airways and cause asphyxia due to respiratory obstruction. Deaths due to gagging commonly occur due to pharyngeal obstruction. Apart from this, if nasal respiration is also blocked more proximally by the gag, it may create the fatal situation earlier.

The autopsy findings will depend upon the intensity of the struggle to breathe and at times may be negligible to absent. If the gagging material has subsequently been removed, blunt mucosal injuries, viz., bruising, abrasions or lacerations may be evident on the lips, soft palate and/ or over the pharynx, individually or in varying combinations. Injuries like peri-oral abrasions and gag marks on the angles of the mouth and over the cheeks may also be seen if adhesive tapes were used to fix it in position. There may even be traces of the gag in the mouth and between the teeth, which can be analyzed by taking smear samples from the oral cavity as these may at times yield evidence of the textile material used for gagging.

To check whether a particular material has been employed in the process of smothering or gagging, it may be examined for the presence of buccal epithelial cells. The normal saliva contains around 200–2000 buccal epithelial cells per cubic mm, and these cells may be demonstrable if the material has been in contact with the mouth.

There are, however, instances when the gagging material is just affixed to the face or only partially occludes the oral cavity but is still sufficient to cause death. In such cases, the gag is initially porous and admits air, but later due to the absorption of saliva, the material becomes impervious and expands. The nasal cavity further becomes narrower due to the pressure effect and development of mucosal edema. Some authors have even reported cases where only an adhesive tape was applied to the mouth, leaving the nasal orifices patent, yet the development of oedema in the nasal mucosa led to occlusion of the airways, causing death due to asphyxia. Other situations where gagging has been documented include suicides, usually in combination with other methods to ensure fatality, and in sexual asphyxias.

Forensic analysis in deaths due to gagging usually includes assessment of the gagging material to determine its proprietorship, especially if it cannot be traced to the victim and analysis of the gag for volatile poisons, foreign DNA, etc. Sometimes even fingerprints can be recovered from the material, especially if adhesive tape has been used to fix the gag. Hence, the gagging material should be removed with care to avoid any destruction of potential evidence.

The mode of death in the majority of these cases is asphyxia, but in some cases, the death may occur due to reflex vagal inhibition.

POSTMORTEM EXAMINATION FINDINGS IN GAGGING

On external examination during autopsy, the classical signs of asphyxia, viz., congestion, especially over the face, cyanosis, petechial hemorrhages and sometimes facial swelling may be seen. The petechial hemorrhages are usually pinpoint, scattered and present over the sclerae and conjunctivae, as well as other parts of the face. These are more commonly seen when the victim is elderly and are uncommon in young individuals. However, these findings are non-specific and may be seen in any type of asphyxia, as well as in other non-asphyxial causes of death. On examination of the oral cavity, the gag will usually be present inside, and after checking for completeness of occlusion, the gagging material must be carefully removed, examined and described in detail and then be sent for analysis to the forensic science laboratory. Besides this, the oral cavity may also show mucosal congestion and petechiae, commonly over the soft palate. The oral and nasal cavities and orifices should be examined for injuries such as abrasions, contusions and sometimes even mucosal lacerations and nasal bone fractures, which could have occurred during the forceful insertion of the gag inside the mouth or its tight application over the face.

- The gag itself may be found in the oral cavity or in the oropharynx.
- Injuries over lips, hard and soft palates, tongue or oral mucosa.

- Injuries over the peri-oral region and nostrils.
- Petechial hemorrhages and hemorrhages over the base of the tongue and the auxiliary muscles of respiration, along with facial congestion, which are general and non-specific signs of asphyxia, are usually seen.

DISSECTION METHOD FOR GAG IN SITU

If the gag is present in situ and is left as such during autopsy after describing and photographically documenting the facial injuries, an incision can be made, starting from the corners of the mouth and transversely extending until the cheeks on both sides, so as to expose the oral cavity and nasopharynx to ascertain the extent of gagging and thus help in confirming whether or not it is the cause of death.

MEDICO-LEGAL IMPORTANCE

- Gagging is mostly homicidal in manner and is not an uncommon method for committing infanticide. Materials such as rolled papers or rags are frequently forced down the throats of victims to prevent them from shouting.
- It may be suicidal such as when one stuffs the gag into one's own mouth to stifle the cries of pain and prevent any potential rescue attempts.
- Can be seen in combined suicides, wherein it is one of the different modalities used.
- Rarely, it is seen as a part of autoerotic asphyxial deaths.

BIBLIOGRAPHY

1. Aggrawal A. Asphyxia. In: Textbook of Forensic Medicine and Toxicology, 1st ed. New Delhi: Avichal Publishing Company; 2014. pp. 363–72.
2. DiMaio D, DiMaio VJ. Asphyxia. In: Forensic Pathology. London: CRC Press; 2001. pp. 247–56.
3. Saukko P, Knight B. Suffocation and 'asphyxia'. In: Knight's Forensic Pathology, 4th ed. London: CRC Press; 2016. pp. 353–68.
4. Kannan K, Modi. A Textbook of Medical Jurisprudence and Toxicology, 25th ed. Haryana: LexisNexis; 2016.
5. Dolinak D, Matshes E, Lew EO. Asphyxia. In: Forensic Pathology: Principles and Practice. China. Elsevier; 2005. pp. 202–20.
6. Spitz WU, Spitz DJ, Fisher RS (eds.). Spitz and Fisher's Medicolegal Investigation of Death: Guidelines for the Application of Pathology to Crime Investigation. Illinois. Charles C Thomas Publisher; 2006. pp. 783–99.
7. Zanjad NP, Dake MD, Bhosle SH, Godbole HV. Homicide by gagging: a case report. Journal of Indian Academy of Forensic Medicine. 2014;36(3):320–1.
8. Tyagi A, Kumar-Vashisht Y, Panchal K, Haneef-Beg M. Gag deadens but doesn't mute the crime: a case series of homicidal gagging. International Journal of Medical Toxicology and Forensic Medicine. 2015;5(4):222–6.
9. Bhosle SH, Zine KU, Niturkar GD, Wasnik RN. Death due to gagging by an onion: a case report. Journal of Forensic Medicine, Science and Law. 2016;25(1).

CHOKING

Choking refers to the blockage of the internal respiratory passages, usually somewhere between the pharynx and the bifurcation of the trachea, by a solid/semi-solid material. The common agents causing such an obstruction may be pieces of food such as lumps of meat or kernels of corn, false teeth, coins, buttons, marbles, hemorrhages, aspirated vomitus, etc. The highest rates of choking deaths are commonly reported at the extremes of age with young children and elderly people being the usual victims. Data from 'Injury Facts 2017' shows that choking is the fourth leading cause of unintentional fatal injuries, and out of the 5,051 people who died from choking in 2015, 2,848 had been elderly aged more than 74 years. Choking should be considered as one of the possible causes of death in situations where death occurs while the person is having food.

Choking by food materials or bolus deserves a special mention. Food may be drawn into the larynx, either while passing down through the mouth during the act of swallowing or it may be regurgitated from the stomach. Undigested food may also be found in the air passages. This is usually seen in old and/or mentally impaired persons, but it can occur in any age group. In certain cases, when the food bolus is too large, it may get stuck in the posterior hypopharynx and thereby cause obstruction of both the esophagus and glottis. In such cases, sometimes only exhalation of air is possible and the person is not able to inhale due to the obstruction. If the bolus is smaller and passes through the glottis, it will generally get lodged either in the trachea or the bronchi.

The presence of any neurological deficits like epilepsy, brain tumors, dementia, cerebrovascular accidents, multiple sclerosis, mental retardation, organic brain syndromes, cerebral palsy or any condition with anatomical and/or physiological difficulty related to swallowing like dysphagia, pharyngeal tumors, laryngeal cancers and esophageal dysmotilities increase the risk of choking.

Ingestion of unmasticated or uncrushed materials by infants and young children especially in whom only the incisors have emerged and the molar teeth, which are the main masticators, are absent results in an increased risk of asphyxial choking incidents, and the simultaneous presence of upper aerodigestive structural abnormalities such as Treacher–Collins syndrome, which presents with cleft palate and mandibular hypoplasia, also further increase this risk.

The stomach contents and any food particles found in the respiratory tract need to be thoroughly examined to determine whether the food entry into the respiratory tract occurred during the process of swallowing or was due to regurgitation of stomach contents. The first step in this process is to check whether the particles are partially digested food material mixed with gastric acid or not. This can be done by examining the pH of the contents as respiratory secretions have a slight basic pH while gastric contents are acidic. Knight (1975) in his study found that 25% of deaths from various causes revealed the presence of gastric contents in the air passages. Gardner deduced that the presence of gastric contents in the bronchi, or even in the alveoli, cannot be accepted as evidence of ante-mortem aspiration unless precautions are taken in the immediate postmortem period while handling the dead body, so as to prevent the possible spillage of gastric contents to the lungs. He also showed that microscopic differentiation between postmortem and ante-mortem aspirations is very difficult due to continued cellular reactions in the lungs (until molecular death) even after somatic death has occurred.

Food material may be found in the respiratory passage due to the following reasons:

i. Food entering the larynx during swallowing.
ii. Ante-mortem regurgitation just prior to or considerable time before death, leading to aspiration pneumonia (Mendelson's syndrome).
iii. Agonal reflux during the process of death or the peri-mortem period.
iv. Passive spillage of gastric contents into the air passages during the postmortem period.

CLASSIFICATION BASED ON THE SITE OF OBSTRUCTION

- *Obstruction of the larynx (bolus death):* The bolus material lodged in the throat triggers the reflex by impacting the larynx.
- *Obstruction of the trachea and bronchi:* Asphyxiation due to obstruction of the trachea and/or bronchi is caused by aspiration of a material either originating within the body or by a foreign body.

CAUSES OF CHOKING

1. **Accidental**
   a. **Foreign bodies:**
      - Children and mentally retarded individuals place various objects such as small toys, gags, meat, dummies, etc. in their mouths.
      - Occasionally adults will also do the same by accident.
   b. **Food material:**
      - Food may be drawn into the larynx by different mechanisms:
        - *While passing down from the mouth during the act of swallowing:* This situation might be misinterpreted, as whole undigested food material may be found in the air passages and there is usually a history of death taking place while eating.
        - *Regurgitated from the stomach:* This is most commonly encountered in old persons, mentally impaired and in intoxicated persons.
        - *Cafe coronary syndrome:* Term coined by Haugen in 1963.

A sudden, unexpected, accidental death of an individual due to food bolus obstructing the upper airway and causing choking is often referred to as a 'cafe coronary'. The term was coined by Dr. Roger Haugen in 1963, who belonged to the Office of the Broward County Medical Examiner, where they investigated nine such cases over a period of several years, which had been reported by the attending physicians as natural deaths, probably due to coronary artery disease. Dr. Haugen reported of these in his paper entitled 'The Cafe' Coronary Sudden Deaths in Restaurants'. Original observation by Haugen was that most of the times victims were well-nourished, healthy individuals, who died suddenly and unexpectedly, usually during a party, with no signs of respiratory distress or any of the 'classical' signs of asphyxia. Previously, such deaths used to be misdiagnosed as having occurred due to coronary heart disease, but later, autopsies revealed boluses of food lodged in the pharynx or larynx. A contributory role of alcohol has also been established because it has an activating effect on the parasympathetic nervous system and an inhibitory effect on the sympathetic system, and a relatively large proportion of the subjects have been known to have consumed alcohol during the bolus event (Patzelt 1992). He considered these cases as accidental deaths occurring as a result of asphyxiation due to obstruction of the airway by food and considered alcoholism, poor dental status and bad table manners as being some of the contributory factors for the victims who died in such a pattern, which mostly comprised middle-aged or elderly persons. While the original study considered alcohol to be an important contributory factor in most cases of cafe coronary deaths due to the suppression of gag reflex by it, recent studies have shown many other drugs like psychotropic medications, particularly sedative/hypnotic drugs, anticholinergic and dopaminergic medications to also have a similar effect in increasing the risk of choking.

   c. **Iatrogenic:**
      - *Dentures and hemorrhage:* false teeth (especially partial plates), large extracted tooth, blood clots and frank hemorrhages following dental or ear, nose and throat surgical procedures such as tonsillectomy.
      - *Acute obstructive lesions:* lesions of the glottis or other parts of the larynx, such as the edema of acute hypersensitivity to a drug or other agents.
      - *Obstructive airway lesions:* lesions of the glottis larynx or upper respiratory tract, such as the edema or inflammatory response to infective conditions, the most dangerous of which are diphtheria and Haemophilus influenzae epiglottis in children.
   d. **Insect stings**
      - *Acute obstructive lesions:* Due to sudden hypersensitivity reaction to insect stings, there may be development of edema over glottis or larynx.

e. **Accidental inhalation**
  - Accidental inhalation of irritant vapors and hot gases can also cause edema of upper respiratory tract, resulting in obstruction.

2. **Suicidal:**
   - There have been a few published cases wherein individuals have died by suicidal choking; in one such case, the individual had pushed a closed pill bottle into his pharynx.
   - Forster and Schulz (1964) documented a case of self-inflicted gagging by a schizophrenic subject, which evidently triggered death by choking by bolus mechanism.

3. **Homicidal:**
   - Elderly or handicapped patients with dysphagia have been, at times, wrongly or hastily fed solid food, which has caused a bolus death. These may be considered as negligent acts resulting in the death of an individual.
   - Cases of homicidal choking of an adult have been reported; one such case of death at a mental hospital with a tissue paper thrust inside his mouth is also reported (Kurihara et al). Upon further investigation in that case, it was found that he was choked to death by another male in-patient, his roommate, who had thrust a large amount of tissue paper into his mouth after making him semiconscious by applying pressure over his neck.

4. **SIDS:** The possibility of negligence should be ruled out before considering an accidental manner. In this scenario, parents may mislead themselves into thinking it was some negligence on their part, e.g., them failing to observe vomiting, which may have caused death of their infant.

5. **DIDS:** Talbert described the term 'dysphagic infant death syndrome' as "the consistent intracranial venous hypertension resulting from feed aspiration, violent coughing, or a high intrathoracic pressure which is necessary in attempted cardiopulmonary resuscitation following apnea'.

PRESENTATION OF CHOKING

- Difficulty or inability to speak
- Difficulty in breathing
- Vomiting
- Person may begin clutching the throat
- Cyanosis
- Person may become unconscious and die

* Choking can be ruled out as a diagnosis during a sudden collapse if there is coughing, as for coughing to occur, one requires an open airway, which is not possible in a case of choking.

MECHANISM

The usual expected mechanism of death in choking cases is mechanical asphyxia as there is obstruction of the respiratory passage and there are clear features of hypoxia with large foreign bodies getting impacted in the pharynx and closing the larynx causing death due to hypoxic hypoxia or anoxic anoxia. In many cases, witnesses of choking deaths have reported that the victim did not struggle much while dying, and in some cases, the crime scene examination has implied that the victim merely died while sitting without any evident signs of struggle. The mode of death possibly explains there is reflex neurogenic cardiovascular failure causing cardiac arrest and the possible pathway responsible for triggering this mechanism is stimulation of tenso-receptors in the wall of respiratory passage by the obstructed food material resulting in increased vagal outflow to the medulla and these overlapping impulses to the cardiovascular and respiratory centers, causing bradycardia, dysrhythmia and/or bronchospasm. Another postulated mechanism is impacted foreign material at the bifurcation of the trachea causing irritation, resulting in parasympathetic cardiac inhibition. Even when the food material only partially obstructs the laryngeal lumen, the irritant nature of the impacted material has been observed to trigger complete obstruction by laryngeal spasm.

MANAGEMENT OF CHOKING

- For a conscious choking victim, one should give him or her an encouragement to cough.
- If victim is unable to cough, one should place blows over the back or on the sternum as this may cause coughing and thus expulsion of the impacted foreign material.
- If the victim still isn't relieved, one should give abdominal thrusts (Heimlich maneuver).
- Abdominal thrusts are not possible in cases where the victim is obese or pregnant and hence chest thrusts should be given.
- In case of an unconscious choking victim, cardiopulmonary resuscitation (CPR) should be initiated.
- Failing this, the foreign body should be removed from the hypopharynx with one's middle and index fingers or using forceps.

Autopsy Finding

Soiling wearing apparels with vomit and gastric content.

1. **External findings:**
   - Vomit stains around nostrils and mouth.
   - Petechiae only occur very rarely in the conjunctivae or not at all.

2. **Internal findings:**
   - Thickening of the epiglottis and aryepiglottic folds due to jelly-like edema and inflammatory tissue will be found occluding the laryngeal inlet.

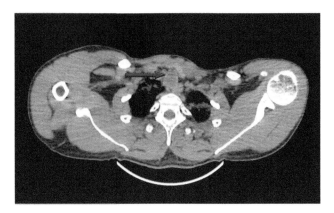

FIGURE 6.49 Postmortem CT examination of the case shows complete occlusion of the trachea due to aspiration of the gastric contents.

- *Gastric contents in the air passages (Figures 6.49 and 6.50):* Identification and distinguishing the origin of gastric content (i.e., whether freshly swallowed or regurgitated) is an important and difficult task. Identifying the origin is best guided by the available history unless the material found is obviously partially or fully digested. In case of doubt, the smell and acidic reaction to pH indicators may be useful. The dissection has to be done carefully as there is a risk of dislodgement of the food bolus during handling and dissection of the organ blocks (Figures 6.49 and 6.50). Knight, however, observed that this may also be due to agonal or postmortem spillage as he found that 25% cases out of 100 consecutive autopsies on both adults and children contained some gastric contents in the air passages.

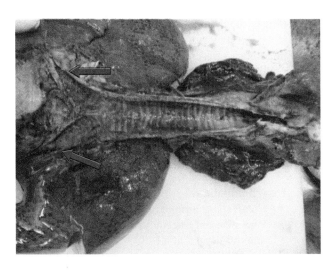

FIGURE 6.50 Presence of gastric contents in the respiratory passage occluding the main bronchus on both sides. Disparity of the PMCT and gross findings shows possible dislodgement of the obstruction due to handling of the organ block during dissection.

HISTOPATHOLOGICAL FINDING

Certain studies revealed massive emphysematous areas with rupture of septa in the lungs, peri-bronchial alveoli embedded with erythrocytes and hemosiderophagic histiocytes in certain cases. Abundant cellular debris, comprising degenerated epithelial lining and mucus, were also identified in the terminal branches of the bronchi and bronchioles.

BIOCHEMICAL MARKER

- Studies show intrapulmonary aquaporin-5 expression in asphyxial death cases where the AQP-5 mRNA expression was found to be significantly lower in both smothering and choking groups than it was in the control and strangulation groups, in which there was no such significant difference in the expression of AQP-5 mRNA.

CAUSE OF DEATH

- In hypoxia due to occlusion of airway, all the asphyxial signs, such as congestion, cyanosis and perhaps even petechiae, may be present as the victim struggles to breathe over a significant period of time.
- In a majority of the cases, death occurs suddenly before the appearance of any of the possible hypoxic manifestations. These fatalities may be caused by neurogenic cardiac arrest, which may be accelerated due to the excess catecholamine release resulting from an adrenaline response.
- In some cases of cafe coronary, the mode of death is clearly cardiac arrest, presumably resulting from an overactivity of the parasympathetic nervous system due to stimulation of the laryngeal or pharyngeal mucosa, i.e., the so-called 'vasovagal reflex' or 'reflex cardiac inhibition'.

RADIOLOGICAL FINDING

- In an experiment conducted by Gardner wherein barium was placed in the stomachs of recently expired hospital patients and X-rays were performed after they were first moved to the mortuary and then again when they were shifted into the autopsy room, barium was found to be present in the tracheobronchial tree in most of the cases, thereby proving that the phenomenon of postmortem over-spilling being very common.
- Lino M et al conducted a postmortem CT study on upper airway obstruction by food. They could localize the position of food precisely in all the 14 cases.

MEDICO-LEGAL IMPORTANCE

- Accidental choking is the most common. Suicidal and homicidal choking are very rare.
- Accidental choking occurs most commonly in children below 5 years. Elderly, persons under the

influence of alcohol, drugs and cases of status epilepticus also get choked due to the aspiration of the gastric contents. However, these may reach the bronchi even after death. If the aspiration is antemortem, unexplained diffuse hemorrhagic areas in the dependent parts of the lung, perhaps with interstitial emphysema and signs of asphyxia, will also usually be evident and microscopy will show alveoli filled with debris, red cells, macrophages and a few polymorphs (Gardner, 1958).

- Occasionally, inhalation of food into the air passage may bring about sudden death from reflex cardiac inhibition. These cases may be mistaken for death from coronary disease and are called as 'cafe coronaries'.

BIBLIOGRAPHY

1. Dettmeyer R B, Marcel A, Verhoff, Harald F. Schutz. Forensic Medicine Fundamentals and Perspectives. Springer-Verlag, Berlin, Heidelberg; 2014. pp. 237–40.
2. Dolkas L, Stanley C, Smith AM, Vilke GM. Deaths associated with choking in San Diego county. Journal of Forensic Sciences. 2007 Jan;52(1):176–9.
3. National Safety Council. Choking prevention and rescue tips. Available from: https://www.nsc.org/home-safety/safety-topics/choking-suffocation
4. Dolinak D, Matshes E, Lew EO. Asphyxia. In: Forensic Pathology: Principles and Practice. China. Elsevier; 2005. p. 206.
5. Mittleman RE. Fatal choking in infants and children. American Journal of Forensic Medicine and Pathology. 1984;5:201–10.
6. Jacobs S, Papperman SM. Studies on the pH of the respiratory tract. American Review of Respiratory Disease. 1960 Sep;82(3):416–7.
7. Knight BH. The significance of the postmortem discovery of gastric contents in the air passages. Forensic Science. 1975 Nov 1;6(3):229–34.
8. Vij K. Textbook of Forensic Medicine and Toxicology: Principles and Practice, 6th ed. New Delhi, Elsevier India; 2014. pp. 112–3.
9. DiMaio VJ, DiMaio D. Asphyxia. In: Forensic Pathology, 2nd ed. Boca Raton, FL: CRC Press; 2001. pp. 229–77.
10. Haugen RK: The cafe coronary: sudden deaths in restaurants. Journal of the American Medical Association. 1963;186:142–3.
11. Berzlanovich AM, Fazeny-Dörner B, Waldhoer T, Fasching P, Keil W. Foreign body asphyxia. A preventable cause of death in the elderly. American Journal of Preventive Medicine. 2005;28:65–9.
12. Jacob B, Wiedbrauck C, Lamprecht J, Bonte W. Laryngologic aspects of bolus asphyxation—bolus death. Dysphagia. 1992;7:31–5.
13. Hunsaker DM, Hunsaker JC. Therapy-related cafe´ coronary deaths. Two case reports of rare asphyxial deaths in patients under supervised care. American Journal of Forensic Medicine and Pathology. 2002;23:149–54.
14. Hsieh HH, Bhatia SC, Andersen JM, Cheng S-C. Psychotropic medication and nonfatal cafe coronary. Journal of Clinical Psychopharmacology. 1986;6:101–2.
15. Saukko P, Knight B. Fatal pressure on the neck. In: Knight's Forensic Pathology, 4th ed. London: CRC Press; 2016. pp. 369–72.
16. Madea B (ed.). Handbook of Forensic Medicine. West Sussex: John Wiley & Sons; 2014.
17. Taylor AS, Mant AK. Taylor's Principles and Practice of Medical Jurisprudence. Edinburgh: Churchill Livingstone; 1984.
18. Berzlanovich AM, Muhm M, Sim E, Bauer G. Foreign body asphyxiation—an autopsy study. American Journal of Medicine. 1999;107:351–5.
19. Edwards GA. Mimics of child abuse: can choking explain abusive head trauma? Journal of Forensic and Legal Medicine. 2015;35:33–7.
20. Talbert DG. Paroxysmal cough injury, vascular rupture and 'shaken baby syndrome'. Medical Hypotheses. 2005;64(1):8–13.
21. Sharma L, Sirohiwal BL, Paliwal PK. Choking due to fruit drink aspiration. 2013 Jan 5;1(1):1–3.
22. Kurihara K, Kuroda N, Murai T, Shinozuka T, Yanagida J, Matsuo Y, Nakamura T. 5. A Case of Homicidal Choking Mistaken for Suicide. Medicine, Science and the Law. 1992 Jan;32(1):65–7.
23. Talbert DG. Shaken baby syndrome: does it exist? Medical Hypotheses. 2009;72(2):131–4.
24. Talbert DG. Pyloric stenosis as cause of a venous hypertensive syndrome mimicing true shaken baby syndrome. Journal of Trauma and Treatment. 2011;1(1):102.
25. Gardner AN. Aspiration of food and vomit. Quarterly Journal of Medicine. 1958;27:227–42.
26. Wang Q, Ishikawa T, Michiue T, Zhu BL, Guan DW, Maeda H. Intrapulmonary aquaporin-5 expression as a possible biomarker for discriminating smothering and choking from sudden cardiac death: a pilot study. Forensic Science International. 2012 Jul 10;220(1–3):154–7.

POSTURAL ASPHYXIA

INTRODUCTION

Postural asphyxia is defined as a type of mechanical asphyxia wherein it is the particular position of an individual that compromises his or her ability to breathe. There are various positions that may impede respiration by multifarious mechanisms. The documented positions that can cause such deaths include the head down position, prone or face down position, orthograde suspension and jack-knife position. In rare cases, even supine position has caused death and a case of fatal hyperflexion of the neck in supine position has also been reported. Any position in which an incapacitated individual gets stuck in a confined place can also lead to death by positional asphyxia since the expansion of chest is affected. Postural asphyxia is different from traumatic asphyxia in the sense that for traumatic asphyxia, a heavy weight compressing the chest is needed, whereas postural asphyxia needs just the inhibition of chest expansion without any necessity of this being caused by an external heavy object. Postural asphyxia is largely a diagnosis of exclusion, and it may be considered in cases where the body of the deceased was recovered in any of the positions mentioned above as these could potentially have caused difficulty in the expansion of chest or blocked the airway. An underlying pathology may have been responsible for making the deceased fall into the abnormal position in the first place, and hence as a rule of thumb, obvious natural causes of death should be ruled out in such cases. Viscera should also be preserved for toxicological analysis in all these since such a condition is commonly associated with an incapacitated state. The final diagnosis should be made based on circumstantial evidence, history, any asphyxial features seen on autopsy and the toxicological analysis report after excluding all the other possible causes of death.

EPIDEMIOLOGY

Epidemiologically, postural asphyxia peaks in infancy, early childhood and old age. Infant deaths are usually accidental as their fall from bed on the wall end while sleeping at home may go unnoticed. Death may happen in children and young adults too in case of physical or intellectual disability. Deaths in adolescents and young adults are commonly associated with one form of intoxication or another, with ethanol intoxication being the commonest. Epilepsy can also predispose adults to postural asphyxia, and an epileptic fit even if not fatal by itself may incapacitate the individual and facilitate postural asphyxia. Old-age deaths are commonly associated with underlying chronic cardiovascular diseases. Pre-existing heart failure, coronary artery atherosclerosis and chronic myocarditis can themselves be fatal and can also predispose one to reach an incapacitated state that facilitates postural asphyxia.

PRE-AUTOPSY

Crime scene investigation by a forensic medicine specialist becomes important in such cases because police officers are often not well trained to handle such rare circumstances of positional deaths and may even fail to recognize the importance of not altering the position in which the body is found before proper photographs have been taken. Presence of legal or illegal drugs and drug paraphernalia should be checked properly. Before starting the autopsy, detailed history including personal history, history of any pre-existing illnesses and family history should be meticulously taken. Clothing examination is also mandatory as this can reveal the presence of stains from the possible intoxicants that the deceased might have taken.

EXTERNAL EXAMINATION

The position of postmortem lividity could explain more about the position of the body at the time of death in the absence of proper crime scene examination. Postmortem lividity is expected to be present over the head, neck and upper chest areas in most of the cases of head down position; in incidents of orthograde suspension, a stocking pattern can be observed. Presence of lividity on either of the sides would indicate the position of the body wherein the deceased was stuck in a confined place. External injuries should be checked to rule out the possibility of a homicide followed by an attempt to conceal the actual manner of death by throwing the body into a confined space. Other possible injuries that can be expected would be those occurring in the peri-mortem period due to the fall. Petechiae-congestion syndrome will be present and be more pronounced over the face, neck and upper chest with bilateral sub-conjunctival hemorrhages. The bluish discoloration will be more prominent in lips and oral mucosa than in the fingernail beds. External signs of torture may be present in suspicious cases where the body is found in the jack-knife position.

INTERNAL EXAMINATION

There will be marked brain congestion due to the accumulation of blood in the head and neck. Heart and lungs should be thoroughly examined to rule out possible natural causes of death. Sub-epicardial petechial hemorrhages might be seen. Stomach contents should be grossly analyzed to rule out alcohol intoxication, but irrespective of one's findings, viscera should be preserved for toxicological analysis. Viscera samples for histopathology can be preserved in obscure deaths such as suspected epilepsy, diabetic ketoacidosis and concealed trauma.

HEAD-DOWN POSITION

Death in head-down position is a rare phenomenon. Literature shows that such deaths are observed commonly in older people, especially those with pre-existing cardiovascular diseases. The mechanism of death in this position has been studied using experimental animals, and it predominantly revealed asphyxial features. However, observations in humans have revealed other possible pathophysiologies of death such as the occurrence of heart failure due to increased workload, derangement of carotid sinus reflex due to increased stroke volume and cardiac output, and cerebral hypoxia due to disproportionately increased venous blood flow compared to the arterial supply reaching the brain. Cerebral hypoxia can also be justified by the Bayliss effect, which states that veins show vasodilation in conditions with increased intracranial pressure, but arteries show vasoconstriction. Predominantly, the mechanisms as mentioned above can all cause death in human beings, and postural asphyxia due to the abdominal viscera hindering respiration by pushing diaphragm upwards is only one of the mechanisms by which death can happen in head-down position. The manner of death is almost always accidental in such cases. This condition is also a diagnosis of exclusion since deaths due to natural diseases or alcohol intoxication are more common in circumstances where the body is recovered in the head-down position.

PRONE FACE-DOWN POSITION

Prone face-down position can cause impairment of respiration by multiple mechanisms. The expansion of the chest is prevented, causing decreased oxygen supply. This posture, if encountered in situations such as restraint in the hog-tied prone position, increases adrenaline levels, which in turn increases oxygen demand, worsening the situation. Finding blockage of external orifices in this position points more towards a smothering incident than towards a death due to postural asphyxia. Natural diseases should be looked into in detail as the individual may have fallen unconscious into the observed position due to some other underlying disease. Viscera should be preserved to rule out alcohol or any other drug intoxication. The possibility of shallow water drowning should also be ruled out by crime scene examination and toxicological analysis. The manner of death may well be accidental in infants found dead in such positions, but a co-existing component of accidental smothering should also be considered in these, along with the observed postural asphyxia. The homicidal or accidental manner is also seen in cases of custodial restraints, where the deceased may have been shackled in the hog-tied prone position. Postmortem findings as well as circumstantial evidences and statements of any eyewitnesses should be considered before concluding the manner in such circumstances. Autoerotic sexual practices like bondage can also lead to accidental deaths due to postural asphyxia if the bondage is tied in the prone position.

SUPINE POSITION

Supine position can cause asphyxial death only when the deceased is stuck in a position that can block his airway such as a hyperextended neck combined with an incapacitated state. The manner of death in these cases will mostly be accidental. There are rare case reports like the elephant man who had a combination of neurofibromatosis type 1 and Proteus syndrome and spent 26 years of his life sleeping in sitting position. When he eventually tried to sleep in the supine position, he died due to blockage of the trachea because of the unusually heavy weight of his head.

JACK-KNIFE POSITION

This position is seen in victims who encounter torture in custody. The knees and thighs are flexed over the chest, thereby causing difficulty in the expansion of the chest. Other signs of torture and defense injuries may be encountered in such cases. The manner of death can be homicidal as well as accidental.

ORTHOGRADE SUSPENSION

Suspension of the body from above with the head up, legs down and arms raised above the head can cause death. Road traffic accidents on hill stations can cause the person to be thrown out of the vehicle and get stuck in branches of trees where he or she may hang on with only the hands. For

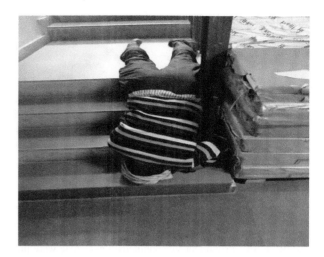

FIGURE 6.51 Body was found with the head in dependent position on the stairs.

respiration in such circumstances, one would have to raise one's entire body, and after a point of time, one's respiration would get hampered due to fatigue, eventually resulting in death. Stocking pattern of postmortem lividity will be seen on autopsy, and history and circumstantial evidence will play the main role in diagnosis here.

CASE REPORT 1: POSITIONAL ASPHYXIA

A 45-year-old man was found dead in the head-down prone position on the stairs of his home (Figure 6.51). He was a known alcoholic with alleged history of having consumed a large amount of alcohol the previous night. The body underwent postmortem examination at AIIMS, New Delhi. The entire face was covered with dried blood stains and two small superficial injuries were noted over the face. The entire face and the front of the neck and upper chest showed congestion, petechiae and fixed postmortem staining (Figure 6.52). Multiple petechiae were also present over these areas. The lips and extremities showed bluish discoloration, and sub-conjunctival hemorrhages were present

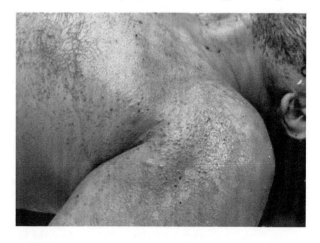

FIGURE 6.52 Fixed postmortem staining and postmortem hypostatic petechiae due to the body being in that position for a long time.

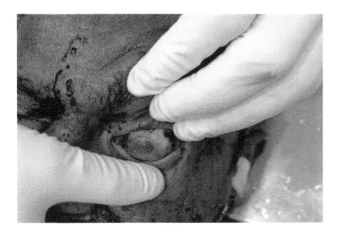

FIGURE 6.53 Prominent subconjunctival petechiae were present bilaterally.

bilaterally (Figure 6.53). There was no other significant injury present over the body. On internal examination, both the lungs were congested and edematous, and the smell of alcohol was detected in the stomach. Routine viscera were preserved in this case and sent to Forensic Science Laboratory for further chemical analysis.

This case is a typical presentation of death due to positional asphyxia. Usually such cases show an associated intoxication or another cause of physical incapacitation, which could be age or pathology.

BIBLIOGRAPHY

1. Sauvageau A, Boghossian E. Classification of asphyxia: the need for standardization. Journal of Forensic Sciences. 2010 Jun 17;55(5):1259–67.
2. Doberentz E, Madea B. Positionale Asphyxie–Tod in Kopftieflage nach Treppensturz. Archiv fur Kriminologie. 2012;230:128–36.
3. Treves F. The elephant man and other reminiscences. Рипол Классик; 1923.
4. Chaudhari VA, Ghodake DG, Kharat RD. Positional asphyxia: death due to unusual head-down position in a narrow space. American Journal of Forensic Medicine and Pathology. 2016 Jun 1;37(2):51–3.
5. Byard RW, Wick R, Gilbert JD. Conditions and circumstances predisposing to death from positional asphyxia in adults. Journal of Forensic and Legal Medicine. 2008 Oct;15(7):415–9.
6. Belviso M, De Donno A, Vitale L, Introna F. Positional asphyxia: reflection on 2 cases. American Journal of Forensic Medicine and Pathology. 2003;24:292–97.
7. Amanuel B, Byard RW. Accidental asphyxia in bed in severely disabled children. Journal of Paediatrics and Child Health. 2000;3:66–8.
8. Padosch SA, Schmidt PH, Kroner LU, Madea B. Death due to positional asphyxia under severe alcoholisation: pathophysiologic and forensic considerations. Forensic Science International. 2005;149:67–73.
9. Bell MD, Rao VJ, Wetli CV, Rodriguez RN. Positional asphyxiation in adults. A series of 30 cases from the Dade and Broward County Florida Medical Examiner Offices from 1982 to 1990. American Journal of Forensic Medicine and Pathology. 1992;13:101–7.
10. Madea B. Death in a head-down position. Forensic Science International. 1993;61(2–3):119–32.
11. Yamazaki F, Matsumura N, Nagata J, Ando A, Imura T. Spontaneous arterial baroreflex control of the heart rate during head-down tilt in heat-stressed humans. European Journal of Applied Physiology. 2001;85:208–13.
12. Bosone D, Ozturk V, Roatta S, Cavallini A, Tosi P, Micieli G. Cerebral haemodynamic response to acute intracranial hypertension induced by head-down tilt. Functional Neurology. 2004;19(1):31–5.
13. Schafer AT. Death in a head-down position. In: Tsokos M (ed.). Forensic Pathology Reviews, vol. 3. Totowa, NJ: Humana Press; 2005. pp. 137–54.
14. Glatter K, Karch SB. Positional asphyxia: inadequate oxygen, or inadequate theory? Forensic Science International. 2004;141:201–2.
15. Chan T, Vilke G, Neuman T, Clausen J. Restraint position and positional asphyxia. Annals of Emergency Medicine. 1997;30:578–86.
16. Stratton SJ, Rogers C, Brickett K, Gruzinski G. Factors associated with sudden death of individuals requiring restraint for excited delirium. American Journal of Emergency Medicine. 2001 May 1;19(3):187–91.
17. Blanchard R, Hucker SJ. Age, transvestism, bondage, and concurrent paraphilic activities in 117 fatal cases of autoerotic asphyxia. British Journal of Psychiatry. 1991 Sep 1; 159(3):371–7.
18. Benomran FA. Fatal accidental asphyxia in a jack-knife position. Journal of Forensic and Legal Medicine. 2010 Oct 1; 17(7):397–400.
19. Patscheider H. Die Todesursache beim freihängenden, am Rumpf suspendierten Menschen. Beitrage zur gerichtlichen Medizin. 1961;21:87–93.

TRAUMATIC ASPHYXIA

The term 'traumatic asphyxia' in forensic practice represents asphyxia following mechanical fixation of the chest wall, resulting in restriction of respiratory movements. A considerable amount of mechanical force is involved in most of the circumstances leading to such deaths, and hence the term 'traumatic asphyxia' was adopted for these. Many alternative terminologies are in use to denote this particular type of asphyxial death, including Olivier's syndrome, Perthes' syndrome (named after the pioneers who recognized the entity), compression cyanosis, crush asphyxia and cervicofacial cutaneous asphyxia. Traumatic asphyxia is the subgroup of asphyxial deaths that presents with the most vivid demonstration of the repeatedly described 'classic signs' of asphyxia. Many circumstances have been identified that are unique to this type of asphyxial death.

CIRCUMSTANCES

In most of the instances, heavy and unyielding materials compress the chest and upper abdomen of the victim persistently, making him or her unable to expand the thoracic cavity for inspiration. This mechanical fixation also curtails the inspiratory movement of the diaphragm. Circumstances of traumatic asphyxia usually include motor vehicle accidents wherein the individual might get trapped beneath an overturned vehicle, gym accidents, railway track accidents, accidental burial under collapsed buildings or the remnants of an avalanche, mining or other industrial mishaps and entrapment between two hard and unyielding surfaces like in case of fall of a vehicle over the body of a mechanic following slippage of the jack. Though the face of the victim is usually outside the area directly under the compressing material, the trapped individual dies in a matter of minutes if not rescued immediately. If the face of the victim is also compressed, it results in complete blockage of the mouth and nostrils as well, and the death is thus caused by a combination of accidental smothering and traumatic asphyxia. Stampede in a crowd can cause traumatic asphyxial deaths. The pressure over the chest may itself be intermittent, but its effects can be long lasting and fatal. Mass disasters involving human pile deaths happen from time to time, and most of the victims show signs of traumatic asphyxia along with other associated injuries. Stampede by animals have also been reported. Though rare, overlaying can also cause some unfortunate deaths due to 'traumatic asphyxia' in which children are the usual victims. Young children are more prone to this type of accidental death as they may get stuck between two hard surfaces while playing. In all doubtful cases, the scene of occurrence examination and interaction with the first responders helps in reaching a conclusion regarding the circumstances of the death. Cases of fatal traumatic asphyxia have also been reported among adults while performing certain sexual acts. Usually in these scenarios, at least one of the individuals involved is incapacitated due to the consumption of alcohol or other drugs.

MECHANISM

The chest comes to be in a compressed and mechanically fixed state. This persistent chest compression makes the person unable to inspire, resulting in generalized tissue hypoxia. Being thinner and more superficially placed, the right side of heart also gets compressed, thereby causing an increased back pressure in the great veins. Since the jugulars are valveless, the congestion due to this venous back pressure dominates the face, neck and uppermost portion of chest, including the shoulders. The upper limbs are generally spared, and this phenomenon can be explained by the presence of valves in the subclavian veins that prevent the venous back flow. The combination of asphyxia due to the inability to inspire and venous congestion due to cardiac compression intensifies the cerebral hypoxia, which results in the death of the victim if not rescued swiftly. Fatalities due to an isolated 'traumatic asphyxia' mechanism are rare as practically, most of these cases show many other associated injuries that contribute to the death. As mentioned earlier, accidental smothering by the same compressing material is frequently seen in deep buried individuals.

EXTERNAL FEATURES

The external features are diagnostic in most of these cases. The body shows the features of 'masque ecchymotique', i.e., red or purple discoloration of the skin over the face, neck and upper chest, which is a classical external appearance in these, along with marked congestion, cyanosis, petechial hemorrhages and edema of the face, neck and upper trunk. A line of demarcation is often seen between the congested upper region and pale trunk. This line does not have any relation with the shape or extent of the external compressing object and may sometimes reach up to the level of third rib and rarely beyond that. Intense congestion and hemorrhagic bulges are seen in the conjunctivae. Multiple petechiae and ecchymoses are seen on the face. Hemorrhages from nostrils and mouth are also seen due to the rupture of congested small blood vessels. The friction between the body and the unyielding compressing surfaces may directly produce multiple blunt injuries such as abrasions and contusions.

INTERNAL FEATURES

Traumatic asphyxia cases show marked congestion and petechiae of scalp, brain, pharynx and larynx. Internal examination usually reveals congestion and petechiae at thoracic structures, including lungs, pleurae and pericardium. Bones of chest wall, including clavicles, ribs and sternum, show multiple fractures in many cases. A persistent high compressing force for a reasonably long duration causes internal soft tissue injuries, including lung lacerations, hemo-pneumothorax, acute emphysema of lung parenchyma, mediastinal injuries and intra-abdominal injuries. Other associated injuries like fractures of spine, limbs or pelvis have to be anticipated and recorded.

MANNER OF DEATH

Traumatic asphyxial deaths due to suicidal or homicidal acts are extremely rare. As already discussed, most of the cases in this category are accidental in nature. The diagnosis is usually made by identifying the above-mentioned external and internal features and correlating these with the available circumstantial evidences. Statements of the first respondents, photographs of the scene of occurrence and a scene of incident visit by the forensic pathologist are useful in determining the manner of death. Viscera analysis of the victim for the presence of any intoxicating drug has to be done in all cases. Before giving his opinion regarding the cause and manner of death, the pathologist should rule out all the other possible causes of death in the case.

CASE REPORT: TRAUMATIC ASPHYXIA AT WORKPLACE

A 25-year-old man was working under heavy machinery, a portion of which suddenly collapsed over him (Figure 6.54). Rescue attempts were made by his co-workers,

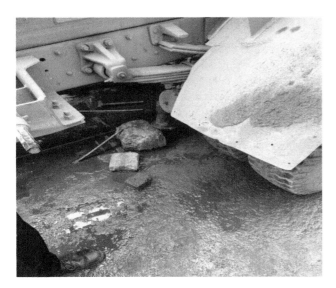

FIGURE 6.54 The heavy machinery under which the victim got compressed.

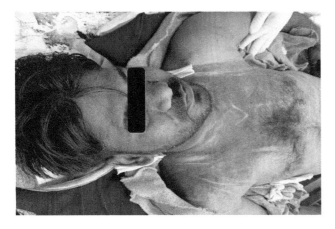

FIGURE 6.55 Facial and front of chest showed intense congestion and petechiae with sparing of upper limbs.

but by the time they rushed him to the hospital, he died. Postmortem examination was carried out at AIIMS, New Delhi, and it revealed intense congestion and petechiae over the face, including the bilateral conjunctivae, the neck and the front of upper chest and shoulders (Figure 6.55). The lower line of demarcation was not very clearly identifiable over the trunk, but it reached up to the level of fourth rib. Rib fractures and underlying lung injuries were also present. This was a case of a combination of blunt trauma to chest resulting in hemorrhage along with the compression of chest causing traumatic asphyxia.

BURKING

Burking is a unique type of homicidal death named after the notorious serial killer of Edinburgh of the early 19th century, William Burke. It represents a combination of traumatic asphyxia and smothering. Here, the assailant sits or kneels over the upper torso of the victim and smothers him

or her to death. Death happens due to the combined effect of smothering and impaired chest expansion due to the external compression, i.e., traumatic asphyxia. Findings of both the modalities along with counter-pressure abrasions over the dependent projecting surfaces can be appreciated in most of the cases.

BIBLIOGRAPHY

1. Colville-Ebeling B, Freeman M, Banner J, Lynnerup N. Autopsy practice in forensic pathology—evidence-based or experience-based? A review of autopsies performed on victims of traumatic asphyxia in a mass disaster. Journal of Forensic and Legal Medicine. 2014 Feb;22:33–6. Available from: http://dx.doi.org/10.1016/j.jflm.2013.11.006.
2. Domènech MS, Alcázar HM, Pallarès AA, Vicente IG, García JC, Gutiérrez CV, et al. The murderer is the bed: an unusual case of death by traumatic asphyxia in a hotel folding bunk bed. Forensic Science International. 2012 Jul;220(1–3):e1–4. Available from: http://dx.doi.org/10.1016/j.forsciint.2012.01.031.
3. Byard RW, Wick R, Simpson E, Gilbert JD. The pathological features and circumstances of death of lethal crush/traumatic asphyxia in adults—a 25-year study. Forensic Science International. 2006 Jun;159(2–3):200–5. Available from: http://dx.doi.org/10.1016/j.forsciint.2005.08.003.
4. Pathak H, Borkar J, Dixit P, Shrigiriwar M. Traumatic asphyxial deaths in car crush: report of 3 autopsy cases. Forensic Science International. 2012 Sep;221(1–3):e21–4. Available from: http://dx.doi.org/10.1016/j.forsciint.2012.04.011.
5. Jumbelic MI. Traumatic asphyxia in weightlifters. Journal of Forensic Sciences. 2007 May;52(3):702–5. Available from: http://dx.doi.org/10.1111/j.1556-4029.2007.00429.x.
6. Hitchcock A, Start RD. Fatal traumatic asphyxia in a middle-aged man in association with entrapment associated hypoxyphilia. Journal of Clinical Forensic Medicine. 2005 Dec;12(6):320–5. Available from: http://dx.doi.org/10.1016/j.jcfm.2005.05.010.
7. Byard R, Hanson K, James R. Fatal unintentional traumatic asphyxia in childhood. Journal of Paediatrics and Child Health. 2003 Jan;39(1):31–2. Available from: http://dx.doi.org/10.1046/j.1440-1754.2003.00067.x.
8. Gill JR, Landi K. Traumatic asphyxial deaths due to an uncontrolled crowd. American Journal of Forensic Medicine and Pathology. 2004 Dec;25(4):358–61. Available from: http://dx.doi.org/10.1097/01.paf.0000147316.62883.8b.
9. Taff ML, Boglioli LR. Homicidal traumatic asphyxia associated with pebble impaction of the upper airway. American Journal of Forensic Medicine and Pathology. 1992 Sep;13(3):271. Available from: http://dx.doi.org/10.1097/00000433-199209000-00023.
10. Cappelletti S, Cipolloni L, Piacentino D, Aromatario M. A lethal case of hoarding due to the combination of traumatic and confined space asphyxia. Forensic Science, Medicine and Pathology. 2018 Dec 10;15(1):114–8. Available from: http://dx.doi.org/10.1007/s12024-018-0056-x.
11. Boghossian E, Tambuscio S, Sauvageau A. Nonchemical suffocation deaths in forensic setting: a 6-year retrospective study of environmental suffocation, smothering, choking, and traumatic/positional asphyxia. Journal of Forensic Sciences. 2010 May;55(3):646–51. Available from: http://dx.doi.org/10.1111/j.1556-4029.2010.01351.x.

12. Kumar Khalkho S, Kumar Pathak M. Death due to traumatic asphyxia in Varanasi region, India. International Journal of Medical Toxicology and Forensic Medicine. 2019 Oct 30;9(2):51–6. Available from: http://dx.doi.org/10.32598/ijmtfm.v9i2.24129.

13. Howannapakorn J. Traumatic asphyxial death from two-wheel 'Walking Behind' tractor. Asian Archives of Pathology. 2015;11(3):80–85.

14. Sah B, Yadav BN, Jha S. A case report of traumatic asphyxia. Journal of College of Medical Sciences-Nepal. 2014;10(3).

15. Richards EC, Wallis ND. Asphyxiation: a review. Trauma. 2005;7:37–45.

SEXUAL/AUTOEROTIC ASPHYXIA

INTRODUCTION

Sexual asphyxia or autoerotic asphyxia is a condition wherein an individual attempts to enhance his or her sexual responses with asphyxia. It is also known as asphyxiophilia, hypoxyphilia, breath control play, terminal sex, sex hanging or erotized repetitive hanging and has been clearly described as a type of paraphilic disorder under the Diagnostic and Statistical Manual of Mental Disorders (DSM–5) classification. If the death of an individual occurs during such an act of sexual gratification, it is termed an 'Autoerotic death/Autoerotic Asphyxial death'. By definition, an autoerotic death refers to 'the death of an individual which occurs during a sexual activity, usually in solitary, during which a device, apparatus or prop which was used to enhance the sexual stimulation in some way caused unintended death of the individual'. This broad definition encompasses case fatalities from various kinds of asphyxia such as by ligature, plastic bag, aqua eroticum (autoerotic drowning) or inhalation of chemicals, etc. and even some non-asphyxial deaths from methods like electrocution, hyperthermia, etc. Death in such autoerotic conditions is usually a misadventure rather than an intentional suicide attempt. In these cases, usually the drive to experience a more pleasurable act may push the individual to take greater risks in their act, which can result in the loss of control over their assembled apparatus, and the subsequent lack or failure of the reversal mechanism leads to death.

Autoerotic deaths are usually less encountered due to the misconception and also misdiagnosis of such circumstances. The main reason for this is the social stigma surrounding such practices due to which the parents, spouses or relatives of the deceased usually hide important details while giving history. Many cases are reported where the wives have been aware of their husbands being involved in such practices, but have not reported the same to the investigators. The other main issue resulting in the under-reporting of these cases is the lack of awareness among the police and doctors regarding the existence of such behaviors. Resnik, in his attempt to psycho-dynamically explain this condition, which he referred to as 'Sex hanging syndrome' or 'erotized repetitive hanging syndrome', described ten elements of these deaths, which included the following:

1. Evidence of repetitive autoerotic behaviour and practice
2. The presence of access to pornographic material at the scene
3. The neck constricting material being one that can be controlled voluntarily or having an in-built self-rescue mechanism
4. Lack of any suicidal intention
5. Practiced as a solitary act
6. Circumstantial evidence of masturbation
7. The victim being an adolescent or a young adult male
8. The body being found in a state of nudity (partial or complete)
9. Associated bondage of the body, extremities and genitals
10. Presence of female attire.

Hazelwood et al considered the first five points of the above-mentioned elements as the criteria for determining death during dangerous autoerotic practice.

MECHANISM

Oxygenated blood to the brain is carried by the carotids that get easily compressed by acts like strangulation or hanging, and this causes a sudden loss of oxygen supply to the brain, and as a result, carbon dioxide concentration increases. This hypoxic state creates a feeling of giddiness, lightheadedness and pleasure, all of which will heighten masturbatory sensations. Later when that pressure is released and blood along with oxygen starts to flow again, the person may feel another type of high due to a release of pleasure inducing substances like dopamine, serotonin and endorphins that can cause extreme excitement.

PSYCHIATRIC AND PSYCHOLOGICAL PERSPECTIVE

From a psychiatric point of view, sexual asphyxia is discussed under 'sexual masochism' as 'hypoxyphilia', i.e., a dangerous form of sexual masochism involving sexual arousal by oxygen deprivation that may be achieved by means of chest compression, ligatures, plastic bags, masks or chemicals, which may be a volatile substance, such as nitrite, that causes a temporary decrease in brain oxygenation by peripheral vasodilatation. Here it is important to note the difference between paraphilias and paraphilic disorders. Paraphilias are defined as sexual practices that are atypical but not necessarily rise to the level of being called disorders. On the other hand, paraphilic disorders are clinically diagnosable diseases, which cause distress, impaired functioning and/or entail a risk of harm to one's own self or to others (DSM5). Sexual asphyxia is usually achieved by neck compression by a ligature, most frequently by hanging, followed by strangulation and suffocation. The deceased in such cases are almost exclusively males, mainly adolescent or young adults. There are often pornographic or sadomasochistic literatures or pictures within view and mirrors or cameras near the victim for observation purposes found during the autoerotic ritual. Moreover, many cases involve other associated paraphilias such as transvestism, bondage, fetishism, sadism, masochism and narcissism and the presence of various fantasy props at the scene. Such paraphilias and the presence of erotic objects at the scene of death are more common in males than in cases involving females. Even the nearest relatives are usually not aware of the victim's autoerotic activities. In a few cases, the victim's wife has been aware of the deceased's transvestism habit, bondage or possession of female clothing.

The person who practices such autoerotic asphyxiation can display psychological characteristics of having academic successes or overachiever at their workplace with the general notion among the public about them being highly intelligent individuals. They are often considered as religious and introverted with usually a neat and physically fit appearance. Practitioners of such activities may, on the other hand, also have a history of clinical depression that may have manifested in their past as history of previous suicidal attempts or there may be a history of them having been victims of sexual molestation in their childhood. Important evidence corroborating such history could be the presence of old hesitation marks/cuts on external examination, and such findings could point towards the possible mental state of the individual.

Such individuals usually have some distorted erotic fantasies in the beginning, which then get entangled with reality, resulting in the actual practice of autoerotic activity. Autoerotic asphyxia falls under the purview of hypoxiphilia, whose central essence is a desire to reach a cerebral hypoxic state by mechanical or chemical asphyxiation, leading to heightened sexual pleasure. Transvestophilia or Eonism is also seen in such participants, where the individual gets the sexual excitement while wearing the attire of opposite sex like female bras, panties and/or various other items of female clothing, especially the intimate wear. Sanitary pads, wigs and make-up may also be used. A few cases also have elements of ligottism, cordophilia, masochism or bondage, wherein the individuals experience sexual excitement by being humiliated, bound or restrained, or enforcing such acts on their partners. Here the victim may tie one's wrists and ankles together with a chain, rope or wire. The victim may also blindfold oneself. Evidences of self-mutilation like burns or cuts can also at times be found on the body. Clamps or pincers may be attached to genital or breasts. In such conditions, the participant's feeling of helplessness due to the physical restraints increases the excitement. Pictophilia, i.e., the practice of one getting their sexual arousal by watching pornographic pictures or movies, may be implied by the presence of such materials at the scene of death. In rare cases, Pygmalionism, i.e., the practice of individuals having a sexual attraction towards statues, dolls or mannequins, may also be seen with autoerotic asphyxia. Pedophilia is another paraphilic condition that

may co-exist among practitioners of autoerotic asphyxia. Investigation of the death may uncover evidences that provide proof of masturbation/Onanism/ipsation having been practiced by the participant during the act of sexual asphyxia.

EPIDEMIOLOGY

The true picture of the actual incidence of sexual asphyxia is difficult to determine due to the highly secretive nature of this condition, and such cases usually come to light when there is a fatal outcome. Even the deaths are commonly misinterpreted as suicides due to the lack of awareness among the attending police and doctors. Epidemiological studies done in Canada show an incidence rate of 0.2–0.5 cases per million inhabitants per year, and United States data show the incidence in their country to be between 2–4 cases per million per year without there being an epidemiological study to prove these figures, which are usually considered to be an overestimate. Data from Scandinavian countries shows an incidence of 1–2 cases per million inhabitants, while Australian and Swedish national data review show incidences of 0.3 and 0.14 cases per million inhabitants per year, respectively. Apart from these few developed regions, there is a need for systematic studies to be conducted to better understand the prevalence of such practices as changes in geographical, socioeconomic, cultural or ethnic variables have a significant impact on the occurrence of this condition.

Cases of autoerotic death are more common in western countries and are more prevalent among the younger male population, especially among those in their early thirties. Cases reported in literature show a range of 9 years to 87 years, though the incidence in people aged above 65 years is uncommon and accounts for less than 1% of the total cases. Cases of autoerotic fatalities among females are rare but not entirely unreported, and these also pose a challenge to the investigators due to the frequent absence of expected pornography material or sadomasochistic devices at the scene. Most of the female cases reported in the literature are identical, and not all cases designated as accidental autoerotic deaths fulfilled the set criteria, part of which by definition requires such deaths to be an accidental, solitary event caused by asphyxiophilia.

The occurrence of autoerotic deaths has no significant relation to the time of the day, but when it comes to the seasonal aspects, they are more common in summers. In the category of geographical distribution, they are seen more commonly in urban areas than among the rural population.

LOCATION OF DEATH

The secretive nature of the act results in such cases being mostly found indoors, in secluded locations such as basements, bedrooms or bathrooms as these individuals usually keep the knowledge of them participating in such acts away from even their family members. Some other locations where individuals may be found practicing such acts include hotel rooms, living rooms, garages and rarely even outdoor bushes shielded from public view. The place may have some pornographic pictures or literature, female clothing, electric wiring and equipment, handcuffs, mouth gags, ropes, cords, mirrors, videorecorders, etc.

TYPES OF AUTOEROTIC CASES

Most cases of autoerotic deaths employ typical asphyxia means like hanging, ligature, plastic bags, chemical substances or a mixture of these, which together account for around 90–95% of these cases. Atypical methods of autoerotic activity leading to death accounts for the remaining 5–10% of cases and includes means like electrocution (3.7%), overdressing/body wrapping (1.5%), foreign body insertion (1.2%) and atypical asphyxiations (2.9%). Other uncommonly reported means of achieving auto-eroticism include aqua-eroticum, severe hemorrhage, peritoneal sepsis, air embolism, hyperthermia or heat exposure.

AUTOPSY AND TOXICOLOGICAL FEATURES

On autopsy, usually, marked congestion of face and neck with petechial hemorrhages present over the skin of face and neck and in the conjunctival linings are observed. Petechial hemorrhages may also be seen over the pleural and pericardial surfaces. Brain swelling and pulmonary edema may also be seen in such cases. Though a ligature may sometimes be present over the neck, usually there is accompanying padding material to avoid the formation of a ligature mark and bruising. Foreign bodies (like threads, cords, pens, ping pong balls, metallic objects, rings, etc.) may be seen around the genitals, with the ones like rings possibly tied around the shaft of penis and other foreign materials inserted into anus or vagina. In atypical cases, there may be presence of joule burns or thermal burns in electrocution cases, thermal burns in heat exposure cases, puncture marks in air embolism cases and the presence of water in the respiratory track in aqua-eroticum cases.

Toxicological analysis shows the presence of alcohol, methadone, diazepam, olanzapine, methyl amphetamine or cocaine, etc. in some cases. Alcohol is the commonest intoxicant seen in such cases.

CAUSE AND MANNER OF DEATH

Manner of death in autoerotic cases is always accidental as by definition these are 'unintended deaths'. While there are ongoing debates on various case reports presented as homicide or natural deaths in autoerotic scenarios, these manners are clearly ruled out by definition. Autoerotic death needs to be differentiated from cases where death occurs from cardiovascular or any other systematic disease exacerbated by the sexual activity, as in such cases the manner of death is natural. Baber Y et al presented a rare case wherein a 69-year-old male was found dead in a typical autoerotic setting but the autopsy revealed an acute pulmonary embolism along with deep vein thrombosis. Here the forensic pathologist linked the possibility of this natural pathology arising out of repeated autoerotic activity and related the death to it. In such scenarios, the manner of death is natural, while by definition to be considered as an autoerotic death, the manner needs to be accidental. Suicidal or homicidal manner of death don't qualify for autoerotic deaths, though some literature presents cases where the sexual activity was done with a partner and death occurred, but all the criteria of autoerotic death clearly rule these out as the condition's very nature needs it to have occurred in a solitary setting with failure of the rescue mechanism.

The typical cause of death is asphyxia, caused accidentally by hanging, smothering, suffocation or drowning, etc., when the safety measures employed by the victim fails. Other possible causes of death could be stimulation of carotid sinus or vasovagal shock following the insertion of foreign object into vagina or anus. In atypical cases, deaths can also occur due to chest compression, inhalation of chemicals or electrocution, depending on the method employed. In electrocution cases, the act may actually cause death by precipitating cardiac dysrhythmias or chest wall paralysis due to low voltage electrocution.

BIBLIOGRAPHY

1. Byard RW. Asphyxia: pathological features. Encyclopedia of Forensic and Legal Medicine, 2nd ed. 2016. pp. 252–60.
2. Byard RW, Bramwell NH. Autoerotic death: a definition. American Journal of Forensic Medicine and Pathology. 1991;12(1):74–6.
3. Shields LB, Hunsaker DM, Hunsaker JC. Autoerotic asphyxia: part I. American Journal of Forensic Medicine and Pathology. 2005 Mar 1;26(1):45–52.
4. Resnik HL. Erotized repetitive hangings: a form of self-destructive behavior. American Journal of Psychotherapy. 1972 Jan;26(1):4–21.
5. Hazelwood RR, Burgess AW, Groth AN. Death during dangerous autoerotic practice. Social Science & Medicine. Part E: Medical Psychology. 1981 May 1;15(2):129–33.
6. Lloyd EL. Points: hallucinations, hypoxia, and neurotransmitters. British Medical Journal (Clinical Research ed.). 1986 Mar 29;292(6524):903.
7. American Psychiatric Association. Desk reference to the diagnostic criteria from DSM-5®. American Psychiatric Pub; 2014 Oct 3.
8. Holmes ST, Holmes RM. Sex Crimes: Patterns and Behavior. Thousand Oaks: Sage Publications; 2002.
9. Jobes DA, Berman AL, Josselson AR. The impact of psychological autopsies on medical examiners' determination of manner of death. Journal of Forensic Sciences. 1986;31:177–89.
10. Litman RE. 500 psychological autopsies. Journal of Forensic Sciences. 1989;34:638–46.
11. Hazelwood RR, Dietz PE, Burgess AW. Autoerotic fatalities. Lexington: D.C. Heath and Company; 1983.
12. Money J. Lovemaps. New York: Irvington; 1986.
13. Litman RE, Swearingen C. Bondage and suicide. Archives of General Psychiatry. 1972;27:80–5.

14. Sauvageau A. Autoerotic deaths: a 25-year retrospective epidemiological study. American Journal of Forensic Medicine and Pathology. 2012 Jun 1;33(2):143–6.

15. Byard RW, Winskog C. Autoerotic death: incidence and age of victims—a population-based study. Journal of Forensic Sciences. 2012 Jan;57(1):129–31.

16. Byard RW. Autoerotic death: a rare but recurrent entity. Forensic Science, Medicine, and Pathology. 2012;8(4): 349–50.

17. Burgess AW, Hazelwood RR. Autoerotic asphyxial deaths and social network response. American Journal of Orthopsychiatry. 1983;53:166–70.

18. Innala SM, Ernulf KE. Asphyxiophilia in Scandinavia. Archives of Sexual Behavior. 1989;18:181–9.

19. Sauvageau A, Racette S. Autoerotic deaths in the literature from 1954 to 2004: a review. Journal of Forensic Sciences. 2006;51(1):140–6.

20. Byard RW. Female autoerotic asphyxial death-features and issues. Forensic Science, Medicine and Pathology. 2017;13: 107–9.

21. Behrendt N, Buhl N, Seidl S. The lethal paraphiliac syndrome: accidental autoerotic deaths in four women and a review of the literature. International Journal of Legal Medicine. 2002 Jun 1;116(3):148–52.

22 Laws DR, O'Donohue WT, editors. Sexual Deviance: Theory, Assessment, and Treatment. Guilford Press; 2008: pp. 250.

23. Sauvageau A, Racette S. Aqua-eroticum: an unusual autoerotic fatality in a lake involving a home-made diving apparatus. Journal of Forensic Sciences. 2006 Jan;51(1):137–9.

24. Byard RW, Eitzen DA, James R. Unusual fatal mechanisms in nonasphyxial autoerotic death. American Journal of Forensic Medicine and Pathology. 2000 Mar 1;21(1):65–8.

25. Modelli ME, Rodrigues MS, Castro BZ, Corrêa RS. Self-induced fatal air embolism: Accidental autoerotic death or suicide? Journal of Forensic Sciences. 2013 Jan;58:S261–3.

26. Baber Y, Bott E. Natural death in the setting of autoerotic practice. Forensic Science, Medicine, and Pathology. 2016 Jun 1;12(2):174–7.

ASPHYXIA BY HEAD POLY BAG

Polythene bag asphyxia occurs in a scenario where the polythene bag is placed over the head and entangling it leads to decreased oxygen concentration for the individual to breath or physical obstruction of the external air passage (mouth and nose). The theory behind this is stimulation of the sympathetic nervous system, terminating in fatal ventricular fibrillation and other types of arrythmias. This gives the reason for the absence of post-mortem findings in such type of asphyxia deaths. It is very rare to find the potential asphyxia findings as follows: cutaneous and conjunctival petechial hemorrhages, facial congestion, edema and cyanosis.

The polythene bag asphyxia death mostly occurs in a suicidal manner; however, there are case reports of accidental deaths, especially autoerotic asphyxia. Homicidal asphyxia may also be concluded as a suicide or natural if the perpetrator removes the plastic bag from their victim after death. Thus, for classifying a polythene bag asphyxia in either manner, a thorough history evaluation in addition to scene

of crime analysis are mandatory. The main reason is lack of specific external and internal findings at postmortem, supplementary to the misguidance of the bystanders. Distortion of the death scene by friends or family members may mislead investigators. The decedent's family member may alter the scene in an autoerotic asphyxia death due to the social stigma associated with this type of death. In addition, an individual who selects to end their life by polythene bag asphyxia may leave evidence at the scene such as the polythene bag, drugs, the ideology or the source from where they had learnt this type of death, suicide note, etc., to intimate others that they are seeking the option to leave the life. Thus, the police personnel have a major role in securing the crime scene to the maximum post-incident and intimating the forensic professionals at the earliest to get the scene examined. Hence, in cases of equivocal deaths, the psychological autopsy is essential to conclude the manner of the death.

Based on the literature analysis, a suicidal death in such a scenario may mostly have the following findings: most common in people nearing the old age, i.e., > 50 years, the deceased would have suffered from a medical or psychiatric illness, suicide note presence may be common, he/she would have expressed suicidal intent or presence of previous history of suicidal attempt, the findings will be equivocal of a natural death, history of drug abuse and postmortem blood toxicology may have high alcohol level. The author happens to witness a case at his institute, which is detailed below.

CASE HISTORY

A 25-year-old man was found unconscious inside a white-colored transparent polythene bag. He was lying in the right lateral position in the bathroom of his rented apartment (Figure 6.56a). An empty, red-colored CO cylinder was found inside the polythene bag, tied and secured with the fittings of the bathroom (Figure 6.56b). The room was locked from the inside. A suicide note recovered from his trouser pocket mentioned his hopelessness for life and the intention to undergo a painless death. The victim was a graduate in web designing and out of work for the past few months. Investigation concluded that 10 days before the incident, the victim had ordered a CO cylinder by e-mail and received it five days before the incident. The reason he stated for procuring was 'it will be used for his research project on the environment'.

AUTOPSY FINDINGS

The body was that of a 25-year-old man of average build with face and eyes deeply congested. Both eyes showed subconjunctival hemorrhages. Multiple bright cherry red-colored petechiae were present diffusely over the abdomen, the back and the posterior surface of the thighs. Nasal and oral mucosae were of bright cherry red. Internally, all solid organs were congested and were of cherry red. Frothy edematous fluid was present in the respiratory tract reaching the terminal bronchioles (Figure 6.57a). The pleural cavities

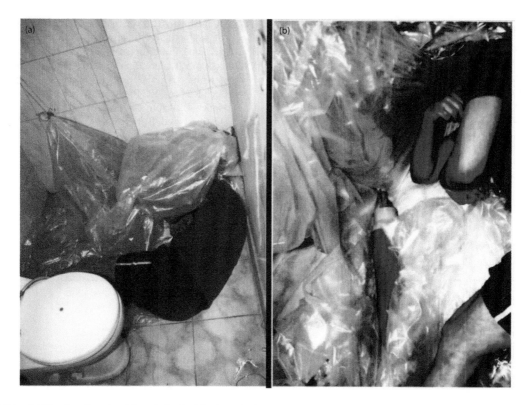

FIGURE 6.56 (a) Head and neck of the victim inside the polythene bag. (b) Carbon monoxide cylinder inside the polythene bag.

contained about 200 mL of bloody transudation. The lungs were edematous. Histopathology examination of the brain showed red neurons, suggestive of hypoxia. Edema and hemorrhage were remarkably seen on pulmonary microscopy. The liver portrayed dilated sinusoids with focal macrovesicular steatosis. Congestion of the white pulp was seen in the spleen. Kidney microscopy was within normal limit. Hoppe-Seyler's qualitative test for carboxyhemoglobin was positive (Figure 6.57b). Hence, the cause of death was concluded as asphyxia as a result of CO poisoning.

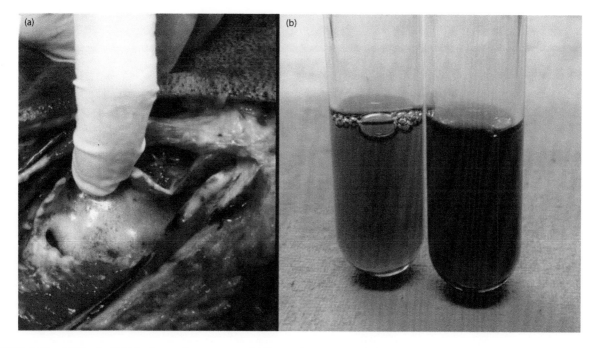

FIGURE 6.57 (a) Frothy fluid in the respiratory tract. (b) Hoppe-Seyler's qualitative test showing positive for carboxyhemoglobin.

BIBLIOGRAPHY

1. Byard RW, Simpson E, Gilbert JD. Temporal trends over the past two decades in asphyxial deaths in South Australia involving plastic bags or wrapping. Journal of Clinical Forensic Medicine. 2006;13(1):9–14.
2. Jaffe FA. Petechial hemorrhages. A review of pathogenesis. American Journal of Forensic Medicine and Pathology. 1994;15(3):203–7.
3. Jones LS, Wyatt JP, Busuttil A. Plastic bag asphyxia in southeast Scotland. American Journal of Forensic Medicine and Pathology. 2000;21(4):401–5.
4. Saint-Martin P, Prat S, Bouyssy M, O'Byrne P. Plastic bag asphyxia: a case report. Journal of Forensic and Legal Medicine. 2009;16(1):40–3.
5. Saukko P, Knight B. Suffocation and 'asphyxia'. In: Saukko P, Knight B (eds.). Knight's Forensic Pathology, 4th ed. Boca Raton: CRC Press; 2016. pp. 353–68.
6. Madea B. Asphyxiation, Suffocation, and Neck Pressure Deaths, 1st ed. Boca Raton: CRC Press; 2021.

7 Drowning Deaths

Opining the cause and manner of death in the case of a corpse recovered from a water collection or washed ashore, where the fatal event was not witnessed, generally becomes a difficult task for any practicing forensic surgeon. The changes due to putrefaction make this exercise even tougher. Though it is one of the areas where extensive studies have been carried out, clear diagnostic criteria for drowning deaths for practical use do not exist. The term 'drowning' in forensic context represents asphyxial death following occlusion of respiratory orifices or air passages by water or any other fluid. Since immersion of the nose and mouth for a sufficient period can cause death, complete submersion of the individual is not necessary for drowning. Deaths in shallow water can cause unbelief among relatives, which is often followed by controversies and litigations, resulting in a reinvestigation. Another description of the term drowning is 'suffocation and death resulting from filling of the lungs with water or other fluid so that gas exchange becomes impossible'. From this perspective, deaths due to 'laryngeal spasm' and 'vagal mediated reflex cardiac inhibition- immersion syndrome' are not covered by 'drowning' in a strict sense. Hence, the existence of 'dry lung' drowning deaths has been challenged by many researchers during the past few decades. Conventionally, the term 'near drowning' stands for both nonfatal incidents and delayed deaths following an episode of submersion. These delayed deaths are also of forensic importance. Though most of these cases give a clear picture about the final event, many forensic surgeons still consider drowning as a diagnosis of exclusion.

INCIDENCE

It occurs more commonly among males than in females, with predominance during the summer season. Children and young adults are the most commonly involved age group.

PATHOPHYSIOLOGY OF DROWNING

When someone falls into water, the momentum of fall initially takes him to a certain depth under water. Along with this momentum, specific gravity of the body of that individual plays a role in the duration and depth of submersion. The victim sinks up to a level where the momentum

of fall and the upward thrust on the body by the medium reach equilibrium. The individual then begins to rise back to the surface due to the natural buoyancy and the body movements of struggling. During his desperate efforts and struggle to stay afloat, the victim who does not know swimming usually drinks and aspirates some amount of water. This stage is followed by sinking, where the victim vigorously struggles to resurface with a closed mouth – the breath holding spell. The period of breath holding is negligible in many cases where the victim is incapacitated by drugs, alcohol or injury, or if there is a deliberate attempt to inhale water as in some suicide cases. Other factors influencing the duration of the breath holding spell include temperature of the drowning media and mental preparedness of the victim. As hypoxemia and hypercapnia progress beyond a level, the breath holding breaks, and the medium rushes into the respiratory tract. Sudden influx of fluid into the airway immediately results in laryngospasm and closure of glottis as a protective measure to restrict foreign material from reaching the lower airways. This entire breath holding and laryngospasm episode intensifies hypoxemia and hypercapnia, resulting in respiratory and metabolic acidosis. Continuing respiratory movements result in inhalation of the fluid medium into the alveoli, resulting in lack of air for efficient gas exchange. The victim loses consciousness, which is followed by a phase of tonic-clonic seizures due to cerebral hypoxia, and then death.

Aspirated hypotonic media also causes surfactant dysfunction, atelectasis and reduced lung compliance. These ventilation-perfusion changes result in decreased oxygenation of hemoglobin and cerebral hypoxia. Hypertonic media results in dysfunction of pulmonary surfactants by attracting fluid from plasma into the alveolar cavity, eventually resulting in atelectasis and end-organ hypoxia. Older animal studies showed electrolyte imbalances in blood due to trans-membrane osmosis of the drowning medium. Newer studies on blood samples of immediate survivors of nonfatal submersion incidents are not supportive to this 'electrolyte imbalance - cardiac arrhythmia' theory. Many newer studies do not consider electrolyte imbalance as the main mechanism in drowning deaths.

Drowning of swimmers due to fatigue follows a similar mechanism as discussed in terminal stages, and generally takes a longer time. If a swimmer sinks and drowns, possibility of an underlying natural disease, any injury or drug

DOI: 10.1201/9780429026317-7

intoxication that could incapacitate the individual while swimming should be evaluated.

Deaths in bathtubs and other shallow water collections may not follow the exact mechanism always. Commonly, these deaths show association with some degree of incapacitation in the form of alcohol or drug intoxication, presence of any debilitating disease or an act of suicidal or homicidal intent. In deaths due to any natural causes where the victim was at or near a water body, aspiration of water happens as a terminal event, which is practically very difficult to differentiate from the features of drowning.

STAGES OF DROWNING

- **Stage 1**: **Surprise** – lasts 5 to 10 seconds, basically inactive, may inhale once or twice.
- **Stage 2**: **1st stage of respiratory arrest** – lasting about 1 minute. Vigorous attempts to resurface. Mouth is shut.
- **Stage 3**: **Deep respiration** – lasting about 1 minute. Takes deep breaths and expels white foam to surface. Agitation ceases. Eyes and mouth open. May swallow a few times.
- **State 4**: **2nd stage of respiratory arrest**, lasting about a minute. Hypoxic convulsions may set in. Pupils are markedly dilated.
- **Stage 5**: **Terminal gasps**, lasting for about 30 seconds (about three or four respiratory movements). Hypoxemia Acute Respiratory Distress Syndrome (ARDS) set in.

TYPES OF DROWNING

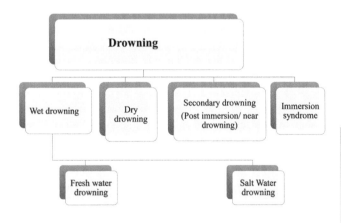

WET DROWNING

In the majority of cases, irrespective of whether they are fresh water or saltwater drowning, enormous amount of water enters the lungs. Respiratory struggles of the victim produce a mixture of water, mucous, proteinaceous material, surfactant and trapped air, resulting in a peculiar foamy material by churning effect. Many forensic surgeons consider this foam as a pathognomonic sign of drowning. When the victim is healthy and not incapacitated,

he exhibits a great amount of struggle for survival, and these violent respiratory movements produce a churning effect in alveoli and respiratory bronchi. Entrapped air in alveoli keep the lungs in inspiratory position, and during this violent respiratory struggle, emphysematous distension of many alveoli occurs, resulting in ballooning out of the lungs. This peculiar lung finding is termed *emphysema aquosum* by some authors. Lungs are water-logged, crepitant, voluminous, ballooned out and doughy. Anterior border of each lung crosses the midline, resulting in overlapping. Airways, including small bronchioles, contain this fine, lathery, tenacious white froth, all the way till the external orifices. This foam subsides with the passage of time and is not detectable in many cases where the bodies are recovered after a few hours or if there is prolonged time gap before examination. In cases of putrefaction, corresponding volume of pleural effusion is seen along with collapsed lungs.

- Fresh water is hypotonic to human plasma and intracellular fluid of alveolar epithelial cells. Meanwhile, sea water is usually hypertonic in this regard. Based on this concept and on experiments conducted on submerged animals, two separate tissue-level mechanisms were postulated for fresh water and sea water drowning. Hypotonic medium reaches alveoli, penetrates the capillaries through the alveolar epithelial cells by osmosis, which results in hypervolemia in circulatory system along with a drop in tonicity of plasma. Hypotonic atmosphere at alveoli and adjacent capillaries results in bursting of cells, which release the intracellular K^+ ions. This ion leak results in an altered Na^+/K^+ ratio, a potential stimulant for cardiac arrhythmia that can cause ventricular fibrillations. Evidence-based supportive results in human studies are not available for this postulation and are even contradictory in many instances. Nowadays, asphyxia due to the inability to exchange gas is considered as the main mechanism of death by many forensic surgeons.

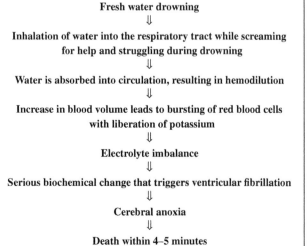

- In case of hypertonic medium like sea water, tissue level fluid movement is in reverse direction, i.e., towards alveoli and Na^+ and Cl^- ions follow an influx into microcirculation along the concentration gradient. Oozing of fluid out of blood vessels results in hemoconcentration at pulmonary microcirculation level and crenates red blood cells. Lungs will be more waterlogged than in case of freshwater drowning. Based on these postulations, it was explained that death supervenes earlier in freshwater drowning. However, later studies conducted on the histological alteration of lung architecture and biochemical alteration of composition of plasma negate the above hypothesis. Now it is generally accepted that time of survival and pathology of both these types of drowning mainly depend on the degree of cerebral hypoxia due to obstructed gas exchange by the barrier created by fluid. Many studies, based on evidence from treatment of survivors, do not support the ventricular fibrillation theory of death in freshwater drowning. Moreover, it is established that redistribution of fluid and electrolytes happens fast as the body responds in these situations. Absorption of sea water from the intestine, which was consumed during the struggle, can also cause spurious increase in Na^+/Cl^- concentrations.

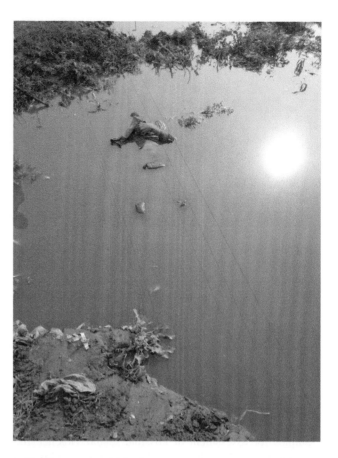

FIGURE 7.1 A middle-aged man found dead in the shallow water of a pond, which usually happens when an individual enters the water in an incapacitated or intoxicated state.

Sea water drowning

⇓

Inhalation of water into the respiratory tract while screaming for help and struggling during drowning

⇓

Due to higher saline content of water, plasma is drawn from the circulation and enters the alveolar spaces, producing hemoconcentration in the pulmonary circulation and pulmonary edema

⇓

Due to hemoconcentration, red blood cells get crenated

⇓

Hemoconcentration and crenation of red blood cells leads to myocardial anoxia

⇓

Death within 8–12 minutes

- Cases of drowning in different mediums like beer, sewage and petroleum products have been reported in literature. The local changes of these uncommon mediums follow unique tissue-level mechanisms according to their chemical and microbial contents, but asphyxia due to the lack of gas exchange will be the most important factor in determining the immediate fatal outcome. In cases of immediate survival following submersion, properties of the medium play a great role in deciding the management of the victim and the final outcome. For example, a medium that is highly contaminated with microorganisms usually results in fulminant pneumonia in the following days.

- **Shallow water drowning:** In daily forensic practice, cases come with dead bodies recovered from shallow water collections, which do not show any signs other than that of drowning. Death in these cases creates confusion for the investigating agencies due to the genuine doubt as to how drowning is possible in a knee or hip height of water column. Lung and respiratory tract findings in these cases are generally not of the typical *emphysema aquosum*. Sign of vigorous respiratory efforts in terms of typical foam is rarely seen. In most of these cases, it is believed that the victim is in an incapacitated state at the time of entering the water (Figure 7.1). Drugs, alcohol, head injury, sudden mental shock or other natural diseases may be the precipitating factors for lack of vigorous struggle. Persistent laryngospasm is another possible contributing factor. In such cases, the quantity of water that enters the airway is less than that in a typical wet drowning, and this lesser waterlogged airway appearance is termed *edema aquosum* by many authors.

Case Report 1: Shallow Water Drowning in Goa

The dead body of a young foreign national lady was found in a semi-naked state at a beach in Goa (Figure 7.2). The corpse underwent postmortem examination at a nearby

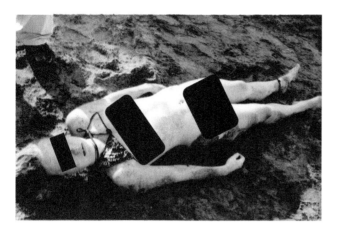

FIGURE 7.2 Body of a young lady found ashore in semi-naked position.

medical college. Six minor ante-mortem injuries were present over the body. Fine, white, lathery and tenacious froth was seen at her mouth and nostrils. Fingernail beds were bluish. Trachea contained froth and beach sand particles. Both lungs were heavy (837 g and 828 g), voluminous and crepitant, with prominent rib markings. Froth and beach sand particles were present within the airways. Specimens for toxicological analysis and test for diatoms were preserved and sent to Forensic Science Laboratory. Samples for assessment of possible sexual violence like vaginal and oral swabs were also preserved. Opinion as to the cause of death was given as 'drowning in the beach sand water'. After autopsy, the body was embalmed and kept under refrigeration. About three weeks later, a second autopsy was carried out by a board of three doctors who identified about 50 external injuries that were minor dermal injuries. Most of them were categorized as postmortem injuries. Inner aspect of the lower lip showed a small contusion that was ante-mortem in nature. Lungs were voluminous and crepitant. Bronchi on both sides contained sand particles. The hymen showed a tear at 6 o'clock position. The board of doctors preserved tissue bits for microscopic evaluation. Chemical examination of the visceral organ samples preserved during the first autopsy showed presence of ethyl alcohol, cocaine and morphine. Diatom test was negative.

The case was transferred to the CBI and expert medicolegal opinion regarding few issues related to the case were requested by the investigating officer. The AIIMS Medical Board was provided with all available materials, including videos of postmortem examination, multiple photographs, copy of inquest proceedings, both postmortem reports and the Forensic Science Laboratory examination reports. The Medical Board opined it as a case of ante-mortem drowning. The Medical Board observed that all the ante-mortem injuries mentioned in both the post-mortem reports are insufficient to cause death of a person in the ordinary course of nature. Though no positive finding of foreign DNA was found in all the samples preserved, sexual violence against the deceased lady was not completely ruled out. This is a

typical example of shallow water drowning under the influence of incapacitating drugs.

DRY DROWNING

Routine autopsy practices fail to demonstrate evidence of entry of water into the airway in about 15% of drowning cases. These cases have been termed 'dry drowning' due to the dry status of the lungs. Protracted laryngospasm following the first bolus of influx is the main postulated reason for these cases. Persistent laryngospasm and closure of glottis obstruct air entry to lower respiratory tract, resulting in asphyxia and death. However, many newer studies have demonstrated fluid entry into the lungs in almost all cases of drowning and challenge this postulation of laryngeal spasm resulting in 'dry drowning'.

HYDROCUTION, IMMERSION SYNDROME

A healthy individual suddenly enters a cold water body, and without any evidence of struggle becomes motionless and sinks. This phenomenon has been observed on many occasions, and vagal-mediated reflex cardiac inhibition has been opined as the mechanism behind it by many authors. This mechanism is impossible to prove on an individual case basis. Some risk factors are identified, which include sudden immersion of upper portion of body, very low temperature of the medium, full stomach, alcohol and drugs. Multiple potentially sensitive areas and afferents pathways can play a role as the initial point of this fatal and abnormal neural stimulation. Sensory pathways originating from eyeballs, ears, upper airway and skin of the front of the trunk are the usual sites of origin, although proving the same in a case is virtually impossible.

SECONDARY DROWNING, NEAR DROWNING, POST-IMMERSION SYNDROME

Individuals survive an episode of submersion when there is timely rescue and resuscitation. If the victim survives for a minimum duration of 24 hours after an episode of submersion, it is generally termed near drowning. Here, the individual either succumbs to the sequelae of entry of fluid into the respiratory tract or may survive. Hypoxic encephalopathy is one of the serious complications among immediate survivors of submersion. Primary alveolar dysfunction is seen in many cases. Cardiac arrhythmias and electrolyte imbalances are relatively rare. Commonly, about three-fourths of the survivors develop symptoms within 7 hours of submersion. Central nervous system functions are impaired in most cases, ranging from agitation to coma. Cyanosis can be demonstrable in most of the cases, which implies ineffective oxygenation. There are frequent coughs with production of pinkish frothy sputum. Heart rate and respiratory rate are increased in most of the cases. Mild increase in body temperature is common. Wheeze is evidently present in most of the cases and rhonchi are demonstrable.

TREATMENT

Not all individuals who appear dead during rescue operations are actually dead. Some of them are only in a stage of suspended animation. They may remain in that state for periods up to half an hour or more (Payne 1940). These people can be brought back to life by timely resuscitation. Treatment of drowning consists mainly of the following:

- **Artificial respiration** combined with **external cardiac massage**. These measures should be applied immediately and continued until natural breathing and rhythmic heartbeat have commenced. Neither postural drainage nor external pressure on the chest will bring out any significant amount of water from the lungs. The water that flows out of the mouth during artificial respiration actually comes from the stomach, as a result of external compression.
- In the hospital, an **external defibrillator** should be applied to the chest of an individual drowned in fresh water if the pulse is imperceptible. If the sinus rhythm is restored, respiration should only be assisted.
- In sea water, if the heart is still beating, the treatment should be aimed at getting oxygen into the blood. **Tracheal intubation**, repeated suction and artificial respiration with oxygen are the best means of achieving this.
- Meanwhile, hemoconcentration should be tackled by the **infusion of hypotonic fluids**. The treatment is maintained or modified based on the hematocrit values and plasma sodium levels. Those who recover from an accident of near drowning do not show evidence of impairment of pulmonary function and arterial oxygenation (Butt et al 1970).
- Attempts should then be made to **correct electrolyte disturbances** and to replace the lost red blood cells.
- One should always guard against **tubular necrosis** (hemoglobinuria nephrosis) from free hemoglobin in the plasma. If anuria becomes evident, it must be treated on conservative lines.

POSTMORTEM FINDINGS

EXTERNAL

- Clothes remain wet for some time after removal from water, and the wetness may persist longer. Clues about the medium of immersion may be evident from traces present on the clothes and will be useful in situations where the site of drowning is disputed.
- The entire face shows some congestion, but it is practically difficult to differentiate from the hypostatic pooling of blood due to the dependent position of head. Subconjunctival petechiae

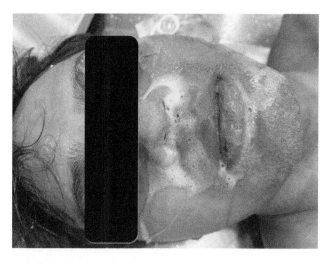

FIGURE 7.3 Fine froth seen oozing from the nostrils and mouth.

of asphyxial deaths are rarely seen in drowning, although congestion of conjunctivae is common. Inlets of respiratory openings commonly show smudging with mud or pieces of aquatic vegetations. Teeth of corpses recovered from water show a pinkish discoloration in many instances. This is observed generally when the body was in water for considerable duration. This may be due to increased venous pressure due to the depended position of teeth followed by hemolysis. No diagnostic value can be attributed to this finding.

- Fine **froth** (Figure 7.3), occasionally blood-stained (Figure 7.4), may be seen at the mouth, nostrils or both. The froth is the result of the churning of air, mucous and water, by the process of respiration and is diagnostic of drowning. Froth formation is facilitated by a lipoprotein, surfactant, normally present in the alveolar walls. It is impossible to obtain a persistent froth from any material other than a proteinaceous fluid. The froth may disappear as a result of cleaning the face and in the process of removal of the body from the water but reappears on applying pressure on the chest or with the onset of rigor mortis and putrefaction.

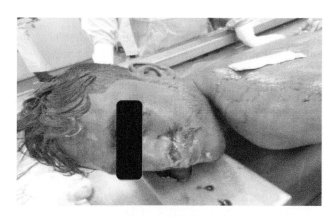

FIGURE 7.4 Blood-stained froth seen oozing from the nostrils.

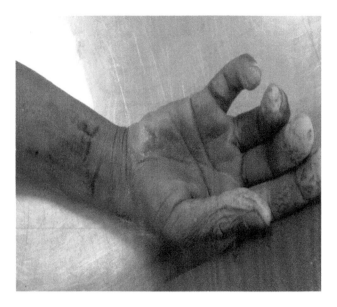

FIGURE 7.5   Wrinkling of the skin of palms in a case of drowning.

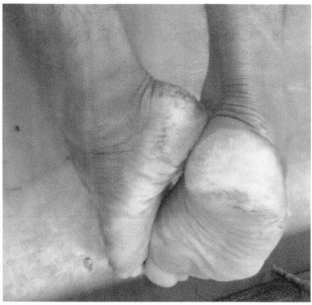

FIGURE 7.6   Wrinkling of the skin of soles in a case of drowning.

This sign is time dependent, and in many cases is not present a few hours after death. Shallow water drowning and dry drowning do not exhibit this persistent froth. Similar frothing is seen in many different scenarios like carcinogenic pulmonary edema and opioid poisoning.

- Fingertips and nail beds commonly show bluish discoloration, but it's not considered a reliable sign of asphyxia by many authors. Imbibing of water into the superficial layers of skin gives a peculiar sign commonly observed when the body was in the water for a minimum of few hours. This water-imbibed palms and soles give a sodden, bleached and wrinkled appearance of the thick epidermal layer and is called washerwoman hands and feet.
  - Wrinkling of the skin – **couple of hours** (Figures 7.5 and 7.6).
  - Bleaching of the cuticle – **12 hours**.
  - Bleaching, corrugation and soddening – **24 hours** (Figures 7.7 and 7.8).
  - Cuticle begins to separate from the palm and hands, soles of feet – **48 hours**.

Keeping hands and feet immersed in water results in the same findings even in living people, and hence is not of much use in the diagnosis of ante-mortem nature of submersion. If the body stays in water for a prolonged duration, this soaked layer of epidermis will start detaching and will slip off, commonly in a 'glove and stocking' pattern. Since the time taken for every step of these skin changes varies according to many factors, a precise calculation of time of submersion is not possible by such analysis.

- **Cutis anserina** or goose-skin may be present. It is due to the contraction of involuntary muscles (erector pilae) of the skin, which elevates the hair

follicles above the surface. In living people, these changes can be caused by a cold wind or even fear. The penis and scrotum may be retracted. The presence of **cutis anserina** and the retraction of the penis and scrotum in a dead body show that **molecular life** was present at the time of submersion. Therefore, a body submerged in water soon after death will also show these phenomena. Cutis anserina may also be produced by rigor mortis of erector pilae muscles.

- Postmortem staining possesses some relevance in drowning cases. Colour of the postmortem staining is pinkish in most of the cases, which

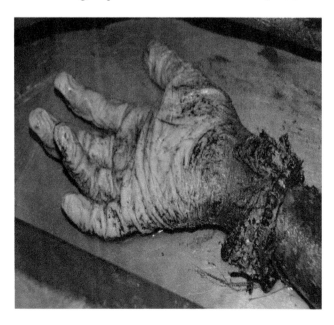

FIGURE 7.7   Typical skin changes of the palm after imbibing water, showing bleaching, corrugation and soddening.

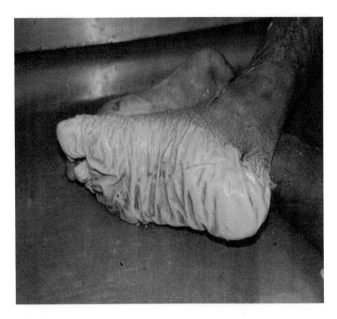

FIGURE 7.8 Typical skin changes of the sole after imbibing water, showing bleaching, corrugation and soddening.

resembles the color in prolonged refrigeration or carbon monoxide poisoning. Relatively cold temperature of water results in the decrease in deoxygenated hemoglobin, which is the reason for this pinkish discoloration. After death, the immersed human body assumes a prone posture in which relatively heavier portions like the head and limbs take the lowermost position, and postmortem staining commonly appears over the face, neck, front of upper chest and distal portions of limbs. This pattern of postmortem staining is commonly seen in bodies found in static water collections. Postmortem staining established in any other pattern in corpses recovered from static water bodies must be interpreted with caution. Intensive postmortem staining on the face and neck may mimic injuries. Conversely, some minor, but fatal, injuries like those of smothering and strangulation may be overlooked.

- Putrefactive changes take more time to establish in corpses in water mainly due to two reasons, decreased temperature and limited access to air/oxygen, and hence, interpreting the time since death needs caution. As a rule of thumb, Casper's dictum can be used. Speed of putrefaction gets accelerated after removal from the water body. Many factors have been postulated as reasons for this phenomenon, which include increased water content of the body due to imbibition and extrinsic organisms that have gained access to skin, respiratory and gastrointestinal systems.

- **Postmortem artefacts**: Corpses recovered from water collections show many artefacts. In case of flowing water bodies like rivers, postmortem injuries are common. Since water washes out the blood

and lyses the blood cells, differentiation between ante-mortem and postmortem injuries is practically difficult in many cases. Another common artefact is the postmortem tissue loss by aquatic animal activity. Lips, eyes and nose are common sites of this artefact, which may alter findings of homicide cases like those of smothering. As discussed above, intensive postmortem hypostasis on the face and front of neck creates difficulty while interpreting soft tissue injuries of possible trauma to neck and smothering. It is difficult to differentiate superimposed blunt impact injuries from discoloration of postmortem hypostasis when putrefaction sets in. Artefacts due to machineries like boat propellants, hooks and ropes should be interpreted with caution.

Case Report 2: Accidental Drowning with Postmortem Artefacts Misinterpreted as Homicide

In December 2020, three adolescent boys who were relatives and on a visit to one of their relative's home for a marriage ceremony went to roam around and collect some berries. Since they did not come back by the evening, the families started searching for them in the nearby forest and villages. A complaint was lodged at nearby police station. During their search, clothes of these boys were identified near a pond that was in an undisturbed condition (Figure 7.9). Later, corpses of all the three boys were recovered from that pond and were sent for postmortem examination to a nearby hospital. The medical officer who issued postmortem reports opined all those deaths were due to 'Shock and haemorrhage due to ante-mortem injuries'. A first information report (FIR) was registered as murder cases by the state police. An expert medico-legal opinion was requested from AIIMS and all related documents, photographs, video recording of the postmortem examination, etc. were made available for perusal.

Postmortem reports recorded multiple injuries that caused hemorrhage and, thereafter, death of the children. The AIIMS Medical Board, after examining the available documents, photos and video recording of the postmortem examination, came to a conclusion that cadaveric spasm was observed in the corpses immediately after recovery, with postmortem staining present over the front of the body, face and lower aspects of the upper limbs due to the prone

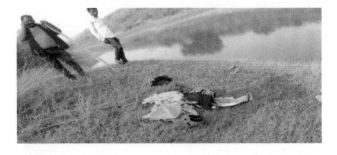

FIGURE 7.9 Clothes of the victims found near the pond in an undisturbed condition.

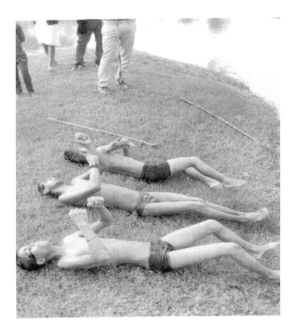

FIGURE 7.10   Victims were wearing only undergarments, the bodies showed cadaveric spasm and postmortem staining was found over the front of the body, face and lower part of the limbs.

position of the cadaver in water with suspended upper limbs and head (Figure 7.10). Most of the findings over the face of the victims that were interpreted as injuries were postmortem artefacts due to scavenging activity of aquatic animals (Figure 7.11). Internal examination revealed clear picture of wet drowning. Froth typical of drowning was present at the airways (Figure 7.11). After detailed perusal of the case, the AIIMS Medical Board opined the cause of death in all the three cases as 'asphyxia due to ante-mortem drowning, which is accidental in manner. The Investigating officer may correlate the same with the circumstantial evidences'.

INTERNAL EXAMINATION IN DROWNING CASES

Lungs and Pleural cavity

- Lungs and respiratory passages show many changes due to replacement of air by a fluid medium. In the majority of cases, lungs are

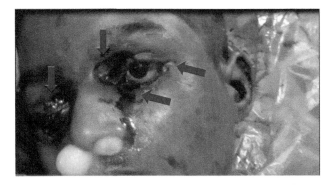

FIGURE 7.11   Froth of drowning is evident at the nostrils. Postmortem aquatic animal scavenging near the eyelids and eyes misinterpreted as ante-mortem injuries by the autopsy surgeon.

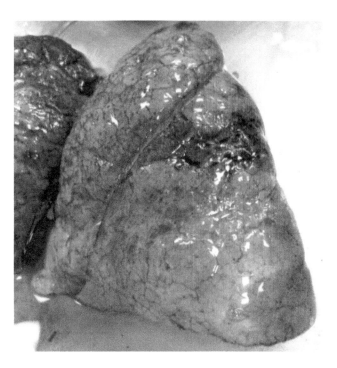

FIGURE 7.12   Voluminous, hyperinflated, ballooned-out lung.

over-inflated, ballooned out, doughy, crepitant, waterlogged and heavier – **emphysema aquosum** (Figure 7.12). Anterior margins of both lungs overlap at midline. If the examination is conducted within a few hours of death, the froth is present throughout the respiratory passages (Figure 7.13).

- Rupture of alveoli results in minute red mottled areas over the lung surfaces. These sub-pleural hemorrhages, commonly denoted as **Paltauf's spots/hemorrhages** (Figure 7.14), are not specific for drowning. Lungs on sectioning show grittiness and frothy fluid oozes out from the sectioned

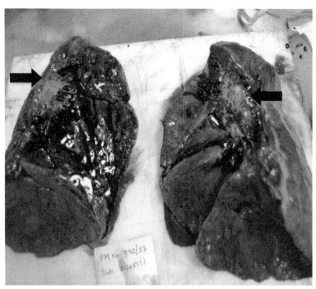

FIGURE 7.13   Froth seen oozing from both bronchi.

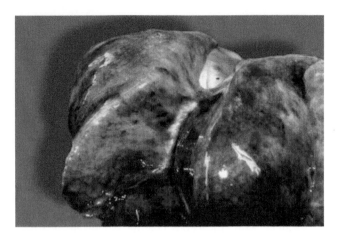

FIGURE 7.14 Paltauf's hemorrhages seen in the interlobar fissure of the lung.

surfaces. Respiratory tract commonly shows the medium of drowning in abundance. This fluid shows mud and pieces of aquatic vegetations in many cases.

- Postmortem immersion gives similar findings in the airway, and the lung is called as **hydrostatic lung** because water enters the lung due to sheer hydrostatic pressure. In this case, depth of submersion in terms of pressure and the duration under water plays a vital role for the passive percolation of water into the tracheo-bronchial tree.
- In 'shallow water drowning' cases, where the victim did not show severe respiratory struggle during death, although the lungs show some waterlogging, typical voluminous-hyperinflated lung picture is not present. The size of the lungs matches with the size seen in other cases during autopsy. Some authors use the term **edema aquosum** for describing this lung finding.
- In case of 'dry drowning', where the postulated mechanism is laryngospasm or vagal inhibition, water entry may not be demonstrable in the entire lower respiratory tract. Some studies that demonstrate evidence of water entry into the airway in almost all cases of their series challenge the validity of these mechanisms.
- Pleural effusion is commonly associated with drowning deaths, and the volume of the same keeps increasing with postmortem duration. Due to the ambiguity of the total amount of water that enters the lungs in each case, quantification of pleural fluid does not have much diagnostic value in calculating postmortem duration. In cases of putrefaction, the lungs collapse, the water escapes and gets collected in the thoracic cavities.

Gastrointestinal Tract

- The upper gastrointestinal tract shares a direct connection with and is in the immediate proximity of the upper respiratory tract. Examination reveals findings useful for the conclusion of many drowning cases. Victims of drowning, during their struggle to inspire, swallow variable amounts of water. The collapsed esophagus shows mud particles and portions of aquatic vegetations in many cases. Stomach is distended with swallowed water in many cases. Many experimental studies prove the possibility of postmortem passive percolation of water in the stomach in cases of postmortem submersion, which makes this postmortem sign unreliable in opining a case of drowning. But the quantity of water, type of contaminants in the form of mud and aquatic vegetations will give a clear narrative for evaluation and for an experienced forensic surgeon in reaching a logical conclusion. At the same time, the stomach does not show water entry in many 'typical' drowning cases.

Sinuses

- Cranial sinuses are bony cavities directly connected to the upper airway. Drowning medium enters these sinuses. **Svechnikov sign**, i.e., detection of fluid in frontal and sphenoid sinus, is positive. However, studies show that water collection in sinuses is only suggestive of drowning, not confirmatory. Cases of postmortem immersion also showed this finding during many experimental studies.

Middle Ear

- Middle ear shows collection of water in many cases, which is explained by influx through the eustachian tube during the struggle for life. Increased venous pressure during the violent asphyxial phase explains the mastoid hemorrhages, a common associate of drowning.

Heart

- The right chambers of the heart are full of dark, fluid blood and the left side is usually empty. The fluidity of the blood is in part due to the release of the plasminogen activator, from the damaged endothelium of the pulmonary microvasculature, which causes fibrinolysis (Nopanitaya et al 1974).

Spleen

- Spleen of drowning victim shows some degree of shrinkage, and some indices have been postulated based on the weight of spleen. Drowning index (DI) is one of them, which is the ratio of weight of lungs and pleural effusion to the weight of spleen. Variability in the weights of these organs makes this method to assess drowning unreliable, and the same has been questioned by many systematic studies.

Circulatory System

- Many cases of freshwater drowning show hemodilution and hemolysis. Blood maintains its fluidity, and clot formation is commonly absent. Vessel walls show reddish pigmentation. Right side of the heart is commonly completely distended. All these findings are subjective interpretations, nonspecific and have been challenged by many systematic studies.

Laboratory Diagnosis

The classical signs of drowning are absent in most cases. Several laboratory methods have been used from time to time to arrive at a definite diagnosis. Some of them are as follows:

1. **Specific gravity of blood**: Determination of the specific gravity of blood from each side of the heart has been used to diagnose drowning. In a study of 92 cases, Durlacher and associates (1953) found that the specific gravity of the left atrial plasma was lower than that of the right atrial plasma. The reverse was seen in non-drowning control cases. The salinity of the drowning medium did not seem to influence the results. Chiaravilio and Wolf (1963) suggested that the estimation of total plasma solids between the right and left chambers of the heart by refractometry was useful in diagnosing drowning, especially freshwater drowning.

2. **Chloride estimation (Gettler's test)**: Gettler in 1921 studied the differences in the chloride content of blood in both sides of the heart in cases of drowning. According to him, **a difference of more than 25 mg/100 mL** in the chloride content of **whole blood** indicated drowning. Normally, the chloride content is almost equal on both sides of the heart and is about 600 mg/100 mL. The chloride content of the left side was found to be increased in saltwater drowning and decreased in freshwater drowning. This has been confirmed by Foroughi (1971). The chloride value is liable to be altered by putrefactive changes, but Fisher (1967) was of the view that advanced putrefaction does not affect the result always. When death takes place from vagal inhibition as in dry drowning, the electrolyte changes are absent. Likewise, the test is of no value in the presence of abnormal communication between the left and right sides of the heart.

3. **Magnesium content (Mortiz)**: The estimation of plasma magnesium content between the right and left sides of the heart has been employed to diagnose saltwater drowning. Normally, there is a difference of 0.0 mg–0.9 mg of magnesium/100 mL of blood between the two sides. A difference of more than 1.25 mg/100 mL is diagnostic of drowning (Jetter and Moritz 1943). The results are affected by putrefaction and hence not of much significance. Strontium concentration evaluation initially showed promising results in case of seawater drowning cases. This area needs more systematic studies.

4. **Aquaporins:** They are a family of homologous water channel proteins whose study by immunohistochemical methods in organs like lung, brain and kidney have shown potential positive results in differentiating ante-mortem and postmortem drowning and also freshwater drowning from saltwater drowning.

5. **Presence of diatoms:** Diatoms are microscopic algae with siliceous coating. There are nearly 15,000 types of diatoms, of which half are found in fresh water and the rest in sea water. They may be ribbon-like, stellate or fan-shaped and can be seen singly or in groups. In a victim of drowning, the diatoms in the drowning medium are absorbed into the blood and get deposited in the viscera and bone marrow. The demonstration of their presence in the lungs, kidneys and bone marrow is believed to be diagnostic of death from drowning. Several methods are described for their detection in tissues and water.

   A. **Detection of diatoms in water:** One or more long bones are extracted from the body. All attached soft tissues are cut off and the bones scrubbed thoroughly. Halfway along the shaft for a distance of a couple of centimeters, a layer of bone is cut out to a depth of about 2 mm by means of a machine tool. Alternatively, one can also perform the procedure at two different places near the epiphyses. This procedure effectively prevents the contamination of the bone marrow. The shaft is then sawn through at the sites marked out by the machine tool. The bone marrow can be collected by means of a gynecological curette of adequate size. Experience teaches that 15–45 g of marrow can thus be recovered. The marrow is placed in a Kjeldahl flask in which it is chemically digested by adding small quantities of nitric acid at a time. Sulfuric acid is contraindicated because it produces precipitates that completely obscure the microscopic picture. Heating is best done with an ordinary Bunsen burner. The procedure lasts 1–2 hours and yields a transparent yellow fluid with a supernatant disc of fat. The yellow fluid is centrifuged, and the deposit (hardly visible to the naked eye) is poured on to a slide and examined for diatoms while still wet under a cover glass.

   B. **Limitations of the test**: Diatoms may not be present in the drowning medium. Similarly, diatoms can be demonstrated in bodies that died from causes other than drowning, possibly derived from vegetables, shellfish, crustaceans, etc. used as food. Workers in industries in which Kieselgur (diatomaceous earth) is made use of may inhale it. Contamination of diatoms containing dusting powder used for lubricating gloves is another source of error. Rushton (1961) found the detection of diatoms useful in the diagnosis of drowning. Notwithstanding the disadvantages, the identification of diatoms in experienced hands provides a very reliable proof of drowning (Timperman 1969). When the postmortem features are atypical, or when the body is highly decomposed, the diatom test will provide supportive evidence for the diagnosis of drowning.

6. **Role of Virtual Autopsy in Diagnosis of Ante-Mortem Drowning:** Direct detection of bronchospasm, hemodilution and water in the paranasal sinus is possible with virtual autopsy, which is rather complicated or impossible with classical autopsy. A study was done by Kawasumi Y et al on the 'Assessment of the relationship between drowning and fluid accumulation in the paranasal sinuses on post-mortem computed Tomography'. They retrospectively investigated 151 subjects, 39 drowning and 112 non-drowning cases, and found that fluid accumulation in the maxillary or sphenoidal sinuses was associated significantly with drowning, along with changes in the trachea and bronchi, pulmonary parenchyma, emphysema, pulmonary edema and bronchoconstriction.

Author, in his experience, has found the following virtual autopsy findings useful in cases of drowning:

- Fluid in paranasal sinuses (Figure 7.15).
- Fluid or mud particles in respiratory tract (Figures 7.16 and 7.17).
- *Lung changes:* Ground glass opacities seen in the lung parenchyma due to drowning (Figure 7.18).

MEDICO-LEGAL ASPECTS OF DROWNING

Opining the manner of death in cases of victims recovered from water bodies is important from the medico-legal point of view (Table 7.1). The forensic surgeon should take into consideration the circumstantial evidences, including descriptions of witnesses, before reaching a conclusion. Approaching a case solely based on these background data provided by investigating agencies and witnesses is also not advised, since in each case, there is a chance of foul play.

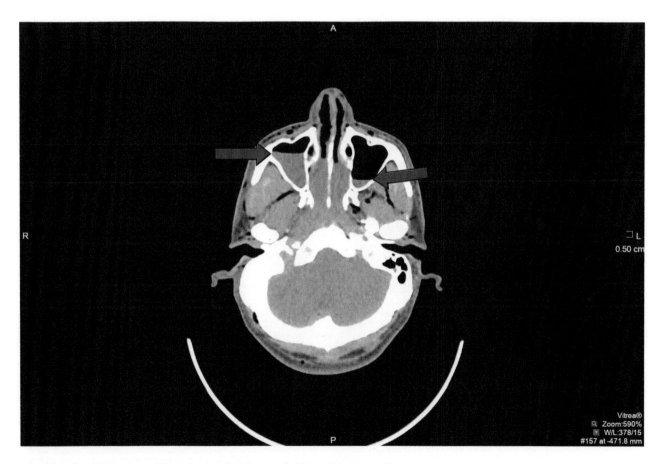

FIGURE 7.15 Bilateral maxillary sinuses showing air-fluid level in a case of drowning.

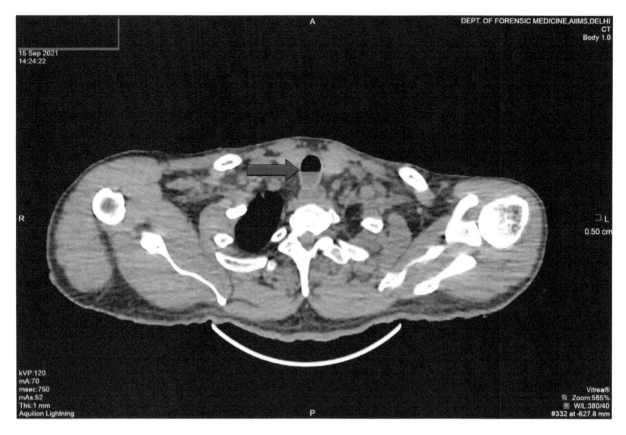

FIGURE 7.16   Trachea showing air-fluid level in a case of drowning.

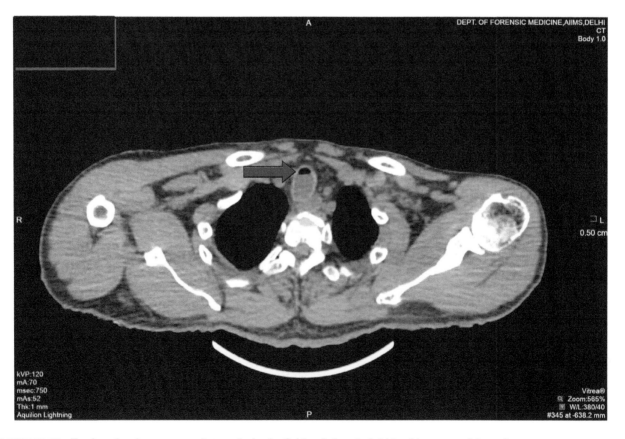

FIGURE 7.17   Trachea showing near complete occlusion by fluid and also air-fluid level in a case of drowning.

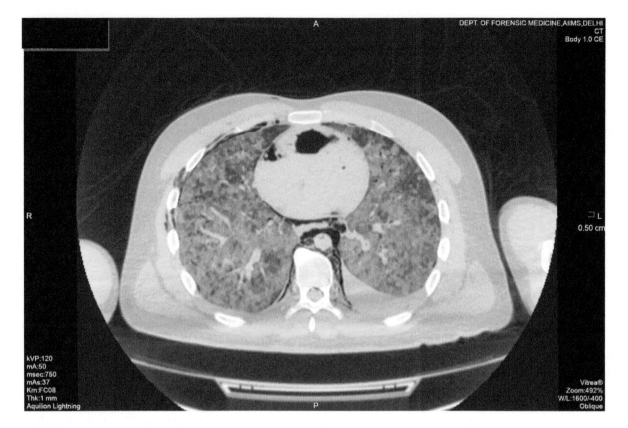

FIGURE 7.18 Ground glass opacities of the lung seen in cases of drowning.

All possible precautions have to be taken before reaching a conclusion. Nowadays, video surveillance system has proven to be of much use in this scenario.

Besides the problem of establishing identity, various other questions may be raised, such as:

- Was death due to drowning?
- Was drowning due to suicide, accident or homicide?
- How long was the body in water?

Ascertaining the Cause of Death

When a dead body is found in water, it is not safe to assume that death was due to drowning, because the bodies of victims of murder may be thrown into the water to avoid detection of the crime. The diagnosis of drowning is easy when the classical signs are present in autopsy but difficult when the signs are absent or when the dead body has undergone decomposition. Even after using the available methods of investigation, the cause of death may remain uncertain.

TABLE 7.1

Difference between Ante-Mortem Drowning and Postmortem Drowning

S. no.	Ante-Mortem Drowning	Postmortem Drowning
1.	Froth from mouth and nostrils is present. The froth is fine and lathery	Froth is absent from mouth and nostrils. If present, it is coarse
2.	Hands may be clenched due to cadaveric spasm with weeds, aquatic vegetation and mud present within the fists	Cadaveric spasm of hand is absent
3.	Mud, algae and froth are present in trachea and bronchioles	Mud, algae and froth are not present in trachea and bronchioles
4.	Mud, algae and froth are present in the stomach	Mud, algae and froth are not seen in the stomach
5.	Lungs are voluminous, ballooned and bulging with rib markings over the surface	No such finding is present
6.	Injuries, if present, could be correlated with drowning	Injuries could not be correlated with drowning.
7.	Gettler's and diatom test are positive	Gettler's and diatom test are negative
8.	Typical features of drowning death are present, e.g., cutis anserina, washerwoman's hand, retracted genitalia, water in the middle ear, etc.	These features of drowning are absent

The classical signs of drowning are:

- The presence of objects such as weeds, sand, mud and other debris firmly clenched in the hand.
- The presence of white fine lathery froth at the mouth and nostrils.
- The presence of fine froth in the air passages.
- Voluminous waterlogged lungs.
- The presence of sand, mud, etc. in the air passages.
- The presence of water, especially which contains mud, sand, etc. in the stomach and/or small intestines.

These classical signs are present only when the body is examined within a few hours of death. The signs are liable to be altered with a lapse of time and decomposition. The laboratory examination discussed previously may be helpful in diagnosis.

MANNER OF DEATH

Suicide

If the incident is witnessed and the witness's version is reliable, the diagnosis of suicidal manner in drowning is relatively easy. Possibility of the presence of a suicide note should also be explored. But in real practice, most of the cases of suicides are not witnessed. Scientific forensic examination of the scene of occurrence reveals some vital clues regarding the suicidal ideation, although not conclusive in many cases. In some cases, the victims tie their limbs together to avoid any possibility of change of mind and to ensure death. In some cases, they attach some heavy objects with tied limbs or with the trunk. Knots of these ties should be analyzed systematically to rule out any remote possibility of homicidal drowning or postmortem immersion (Figure 7.19). Findings of any other failed attempt of suicide or hesitation wounds may be present, and the same should be interpreted with caution. People committing suicide may tie their hands or feet together, or heavy articles such as stones may be attached to their body before jumping into the water. A murderer may also tie the hands and feet of his victim before

throwing him into the water. The examination of the knot or ligature as to whether the deceased could have tied it by himself/herself in the manner in which it was found will be useful in deciding between suicide and homicide.

In suicidal drowning, injuries are usually absent on the body. However, injuries due to contact with hard projecting objects during a fall may be seen. Besides, a suicidal person may inflict injuries with a cutting weapon or a firearm before jumping into the water.

A history of financial difficulties, mental depression, previous attempts at suicide or evidence of preparations for the act is a useful indicator of suicide. Women usually fasten their clothes before jumping into water for the fear of exposing nakedness.

Homicidal

Homicidal drowning is rare indeed. The question of homicide is raised when the signs of struggle are present on the banks of the pond, articles other than those of the deceased are found on the bank and fragments of cloth, hair, etc. are found firmly grasped in the hands of the deceased.

Infants and children may be robbed of expensive ornaments and thrown into the water. An adult person in possession of his senses cannot usually be pushed into the water unless he is taken unaware. However, when he is intoxicated or stupefied, he can be pushed into the water with relative ease. If resistance has been offered, marks of violence will be seen on the body. When the body is highly decomposed, great care should be taken before declaring that drowning was homicidal. All attending circumstances should be considered before giving an opinion. The examiner should be satisfied in that the death could not have occurred in any other way.

Case Report 3: An Un-Witnessed Drowning Case with Homicide Allegations

Two boys about 14 years of age went to Yamuna River without informing their parents. Both of them did not know how to swim. One of them went missing, and the second boy did not reveal anything with certainty. The next morning, the dead body of the missing boy was found floating in the river

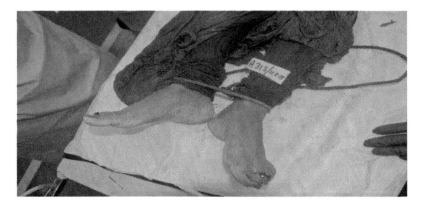

FIGURE 7.19   Tied lower limbs in case of suicidal drowning.

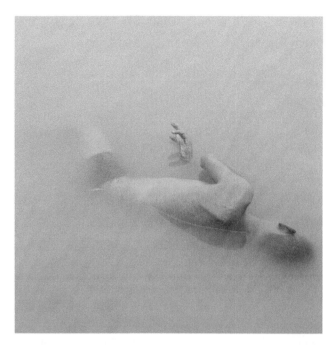

FIGURE 7.20 The dead body of the missing boy found floating in the river near the shore.

(Figure 7.20). In the nearby area along the shore, clothes and footwear of the boy was found untouched and intact. The boy was wearing only his undergarments. Autopsy was carried out in a nearby mortuary. Postmortem examination showed mud and silt particles in trachea. Lungs were boggy and pinkish froth was coming out. There were no external injuries present over the body. Viscera and diatoms were not preserved since there was no doubt in the cause of death and no allegations were made from the side of relatives.

Since the behavior of the boy who accompanied the victim to the river was suspicious on the day the victim went missing, the father of the victim approached the authorities for conducting an enquiry regarding the manner of death of his son. He alleged that there were injuries over the neck of his son citing some photographs captured during the

recovery of the body in a mobile phone. The boy who was present at the scene of incident was an eyewitness, and as per his narration, when the victim went deeper, he slipped and drowned. As per the direction of Honorable High Court, Sub Divisional Magistrate was directed to investigate the matter and report to the court. The AIIMS Forensic Department was contacted for expert medico-legal opinion with respect to the case.

The AIIMS Medical Board ruled out the possibility of external injuries by detailed analysis of photographs captured from different angles. The Medical Board interacted with the autopsy surgeon as well for a few clarifications, studied all the evidences kept on record and visited the alleged scene of crime (Figure 7.21) to study the alleged mechanism of death. The Medical Board got a chance to interact with the suspected boy at the scene of crime and discussed the sequence of events as per his version of the history.

The Medical Board concluded the case as 'cause of death in this case is ante-mortem drowning. Only based on the documents and facts in front of the Board for perusal, the possibility of homicidal drowning cannot be ruled out with certainty'.

Opining the manner of death in case of drowning in a deep water collection where the victim does not know swimming or if he is incapacitated is difficult to prove if the incident is not witnessed and no injury suggestive of the manner is present over the body.

Accidental

Accidental drowning is not uncommon and mostly occurs in people who do not know swimming. Children, the elderly and the intoxicated may drown accidentally while walking by the side of a well or a pond. A person may develop convulsions while drawing water from a well and fall into it. Occasionally, a boat or ship may capsize with several people on board. Accidents during swimming and bathing are common. When diving, the head may get embedded in the mud at the bottom of the pond. In these cases, the body will be almost naked with only a loin cloth or a swimming

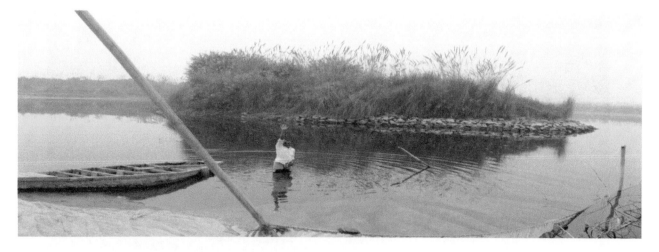

FIGURE 7.21 Feasibility study of the alleged mechanism of drowning conducted during the scene of crime visit. Person in the photograph indicates the water level present at the time of incident.

costume. Floods are also common causes of accidental drowning in India. The insane, epileptics and the intoxicated may drown accidentally in shallow water.

ASCERTAINING THE DURATION OF FLOATATION

The floatation of the body after drowning occurs after a variable period. Putrefactive gases play an all-important role in floatation. For this reason, the body floats early in still water, especially in water that contains plenty of decaying organic matter, which hastens putrefaction. On the other hand, putrefaction (and hence floatation) is delayed in clear running water. Salinity retards floatation. Floatation is relatively faster in summer than in winter. Because floatation of the body depends on many variables, it is not possible to estimate the time of death, based on floatation, with any certainty.

CASE REPORT 4: DROWNING

In January 2018, a boy and a girl who allegedly were lovers went missing from their respective homes. They were last seen alive on the bridge over a canal near their village (Figure 7.22). Three days later, the girl's body was recovered near a field almost 120 km away from where she was last seen, near a tributary to the same canal.

She was naked from waist down and the remaining clothes were torn. Also, multiple injuries were present on her face and body, including breasts and perineal area (Figure 7.23), thus raising a suspicion of sexual assault prior to her death, and the missing boy was considered a prime suspect and search for him continued. On the 7th day after the incident, the boy's body was recovered entangled in a barrage of the same canal about 25 km away from the bridge in a highly putrefied condition.

On postmortem examination of the girl's body, multiple injuries both internal and external were present along with

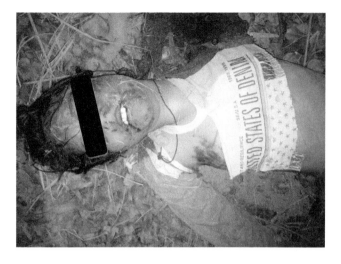

FIGURE 7.23   Deceased female was in semi-naked state with clothes torn and multiple injuries over the body.

classical internal findings of drowning like characteristic lung findings, white, fine, lathery froth in the air passages, etc.

The appearance of injuries over her face and body, especially those over the breasts, abdomen and extensive ones over the perineal area including vagina and anus, had raised the suspicion of violent sexual assault prior to death.

On postmortem examination of the male, his body was found to be highly putrefied and emitting foul smell. The body including face and genitals were bloated, reddish marbling was present over the limb and trunk and washerwoman hand and feet with degloving was seen. There was epidermal slippage over the body, scalp hair was pluckable, eyeballs were soft and protruding and tongue was clenched between teeth. Facial features were partly identifiable in spite of the bloating.

Two parallel superficial incised wounds were present over the right wrist suggestive of suicidal attempt. Internally lungs

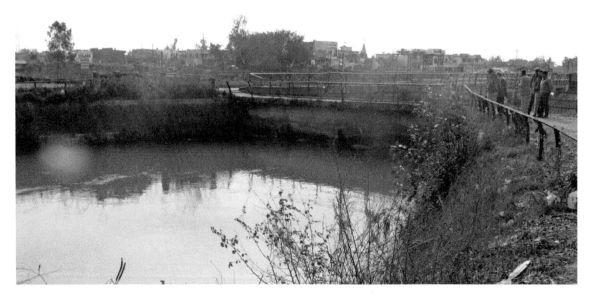

FIGURE 7.22   The bridge over the canal where the couple were last seen alive.

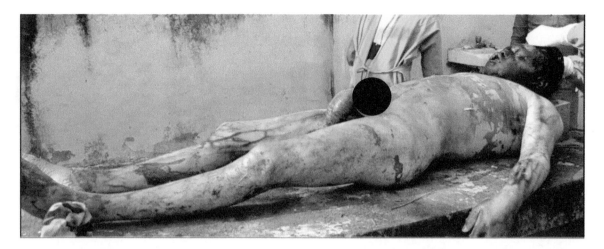

FIGURE 7.24 Dead body of the deceased male, which was in an advanced decomposition state with slippage of epidermal layer, bloating of face and genitals.

were voluminous, ballooned up and crepitant, consistent with emphysema aquosum. All other organs were in various stages of putrefaction, and no remarkable findings were seen.

Postmortem of both cases was done in different local hospitals, but the findings especially in case of the female body proved to be inconclusive and more so irregular to commission sexual assault. Both the cases were then referred to AIIMS for expert opinion by a board. After meticulous examination of all findings photographs, documents and site visit, it was opined that the cause of death in both cases was asphyxia as a result of ante-mortem drowning.

It was also concluded that most of her injuries were ante-mortem, which were produced during traveling of the body and impact with various blunt objects/surfaces or due to pressure of the water. These injuries were categorized as unintentional and accidental, and since there was no evidence of defense injures, homicide was ruled out. The second set of injuries over the private parts of the victim were concluded to be postmortem in nature and caused by decomposition and by bacterial and other microbial activity as well pressure of water or the impact of blunt objects since these parts consist of delicate and soft skin and mucosal lining. In the absence of any ante-mortem injuries in the private parts and lack of defense wounds, sexual assault was also ruled out.

In these types of cases, meticulous examination of injuries is required to distinguish between ante-mortem and postmortem injuries and if possible the manner in which it was inflicted. Sometimes, this effort is all that is required to recognize a crime or a simple death.

CASE REPORT 5: DROWNING OF A PERSON KNOWING HOW TO SWIM

On the night of May 2017, a 30-year-old Indian Foreign Service (IFS) officer was having a get-together with his friends and colleagues near a swimming pool within the premises of the Foreign Service Institute. All those present

were having a swim inside the pool. During this time, one of the ladies present who allegedly did not know how to swim was inside the pool. She accidentally slipped into the deeper end of the pool and started shouting for help. When the other guests helped her out of the pool, they noticed that the deceased was missing. On further search, his unconscious body was found floating in the middle of the pool. His body was removed from the pool, given CPR and taken to the hospital where he was declared brought dead.

Postmortem was done at AIIMS by a board of doctors. It revealed a few external injuries on his face, left leg and wrist. Internally, trachea (Figure 7.25) and bronchi (Figure 7.26)

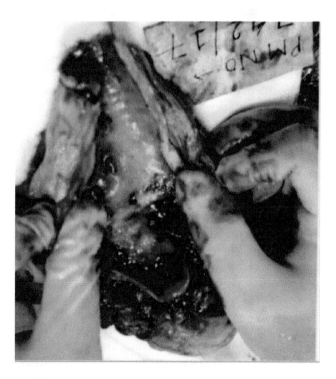

FIGURE 7.25 Fine froth seen in the trachea characteristic of drowning.

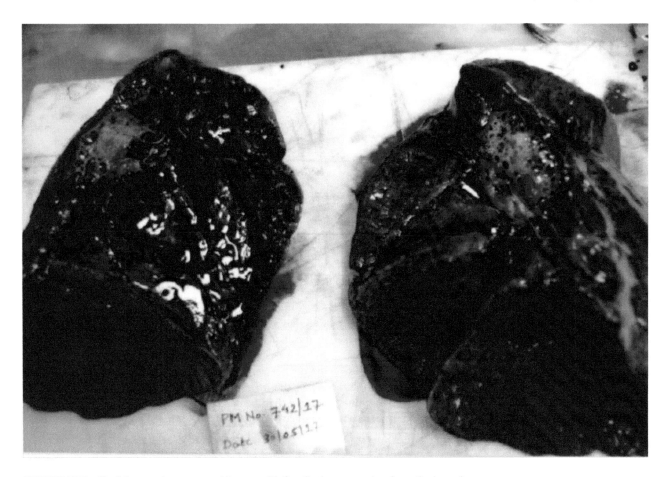

FIGURE 7.26 Both lungs edematous and boggy with fine froth seen oozing from the bronchus.

contained characteristic fine froth of drowning and both lungs were edematous and boggy with blood-mixed froth oozing out from lung parenchyma on cut section. They weighed 615 gms and 590 gms respectively. All other organs were congested and no abnormality was detected.

The issue in this case was that how a healthy, young man who apparently knew swimming could drown in a swimming pool while surrounded by his friends. The injuries found on his body further raised suspicion regarding the manner of his death.

Viscera examination report revealed a blood alcohol content of 165 mg/100 mL.

After meticulous examination of injuries and other findings of the body, the cause of death was given as asphyxia due to ante-mortem drowning. The injuries present over the body were concluded to be superficial and fresh and attributed to struggle at the time of drowning and also due to the resuscitation attempt.

The fact that a healthy young swimmer allegedly drowned in a swimming pool could be explained by the alcohol content in his blood, which in turn led to his inebriated state, resulting in accidental drowning in a swimming pool. So before giving any opinion in such cases, all circumstances should be considered and a thorough examination of injuries should mandatorily be done.

BIBLIOGRAPHY

1. DiMaio VJ, DiMaio D. Forensic Pathology, 2nd ed. Boca Raton: CRC Press; 2001.
2. Lunetta P, Modell JH, Sajantila A. What is the incidence and significance of 'dry-lungs' in bodies found in water? American Journal of Forensic Medicine and Pathology. 2004;25:291–301.
3. Modell JH, Bellefleur M, Davis JH. Drowning without aspiration: is this an appropriate diagnosis? Journal of Forensic Sciences. 1999;44:1119–23.
4. Bierens J, Lunetta P, Tipton M, Warner DS. Physiology of drowning: a review. Physiology. 2016;31:147–66.
5. Nishino T. The swallowing reflex and its significance as an airway defensive reflex. Frontiers in Physiology. 2013;3:489.
6. Giammona ST, Modell JH. Drowning by total immersion. Effects on pulmonary surfactant of distilled water, isotonic saline, and sea water. American Journal of Diseases of Children. 1967;114:612–6.
7. Swann HG. Editorial, mechanism of circulatory failure in fresh and sea water drowning. Circulation Research. 1956;4:241–3.
8. Tabeling BB, Modell JH. Fluid administration increases oxygen delivery during continuous positive pressure ventilation after freshwater near drowning. Critical Care Medicine. 1983;11:693–6.
9. Tadié JM, Heming N, Serve E, Weiss N, Day N, Imbert A, et al. Drowning associated pneumonia: a descriptive cohort. Resuscitation. 2012;83:399–401.

10. Kringsholm B, Filskov A, Kock K. Autopsied cases of drowning in Denmark 1987–1989. Forensic Science International. 1991;52:85–92.

11. Idris AH, Berg RA, Bierens J, Bossaert L, Branche CM, Gabrielli A, et al. Recommended guidelines for uniform reporting of data from drowning: the 'Utstein style'. Circulation. 2003;108:2565–74.

12. D'Ovidio C, Rosato E, Carnevale A. An unusual case of murder-suicide: the importance of studying knots. Journal of Forensic and Legal Medicine. 2017;45:17–20.

13. Vincenzi FF. Drug-induced long QT syndrome increases the risk of drowning. Medical Hypotheses. 2016;87: 11–13.

14. Hadleya JA, Fowler DR. Organ weight effects of drowning and asphyxiation on the lungs, liver, brain, heart, kidneys, and spleen. Forensic Science International. 2003;133: 190–6.

15. Kohlhase C, Maxeiner H. Morphometric investigation of emphysema aquosum in the elderly. Forensic Science International. 2003;134:93–8.

16. Peter TE, Matthew JD. Pneumonia associated with near-drowning. Clinical Infectious Diseases. 1997;25:896–907.

17. Haffner HT, Graw M, Erdelkamp J. Spleen findings in drowning. Forensic Science International. 1994;66:95–104.

18. Byard RW. Drowning and near drowning – definitions and terminology. Forensic Science, Medicine and Pathology. 2017;13:529–30.

19. Levy-Khademi F, Brooks R, Maayan C, Tenenbaum A, Wexler ID. Dead sea water intoxication. Pediatric Emergency Care. 2012 Aug;28(8):815–6.

20. Bortolotti F, Del Balzo G, Calza R, Valerio F, Tagliaro F. Testing the specificity of the diatom test. Medicine, Science and the Law. 2011;51:S7–S10.

21. Ahlm K, Saveman B-I, Björnstig U. Drowning deaths in Sweden with emphasis on the presence of alcohol and drugs – a retrospective study, 1992–2009. BMC Public Health. 2013;13:216.

22. Vernuccio F. Role of virtopsy in the postmortem diagnosis of drowning, C-1074, ECR 2014, European Society of Radiology.

23. Hayashi T, Ishida Y, Mizunuma S, Kimura A, Kondo T. Differential diagnosis between freshwater drowning and saltwater drowning based on intrapulmonary aquaporin-5 expression. International Journal of Legal Medicine. 2009;123:7–13.

24. Hürlimann J, Feer P, Elber F, Niederberger K, Dirnhofer R, Wyler D. Diatom detection in the diagnosis of death by drowning. International Journal of Legal Medicine. 2000;114:6–14.

25. Ludes B, Coste M, North N, Doray S, Tracqui A, Kintz P. Diatom analysis in victim's tissues as an indicator of the site of drowning. International Journal of Legal Medicine. 1999;112:163–6.

26. Clark DH. Post-mortem pink teeth. Medicine, Science and the Law. 1984;24(2):130–4.

27. Azparrena JE, Ortegaa A, Buenob H, Andreua M. Blood strontium concentration related to the length of the agonal period in seawater drowning cases. Forensic Science International. 2000;108:51–60.

28. Robert JE. Severe hypernatremia from sea water ingestion during near-drowning in a Hurricane. Western Journal of Medicine. 1997 Dec;167(6):430–3.

29. Duband S, Forest F, Gaillard Y, Dumollard JM, Debout M, Péoc'h M. Macroscopic, histological and toxicological aspects of early Gammarus pulex scavenging. Forensic Science International. 2011;209:e16–22.

8 Deaths Due to Asphyxiant Gases

CARBON MONOXIDE POISONING

Carbon monoxide (CO) also known as the "Invisible Silent Killer" causes asphyxia by replacing oxygen. It is a colorless, odorless, non-irritating and flammable gas which is lighter than air and often proves dangerous, especially when the victim is asleep. CO is a by-product of incomplete oxidation or combustion of carbonaceous materials e.g. biomass, fossil fuels and volatile organic compounds. According to NCRB statistics 2019, out of 21,318 deaths due to poisonous gases, only 35 were reported to be due to CO. Normal CO level in plasma is 1–5%. CO exposure may occur accidentally or intentionally and the signs and symptoms depend on the duration of exposure and level of carboxyhemoglobin (COHb).

SOURCE OF ORIGIN

It originates both from natural and anthropogenic source. Naturally, CO is emitted into the atmosphere through photo-oxidation. CO is also produced endogenously in animals and humans during the oxidative breakdown of heme by microsomal heme oxygenase (HOs) along with iron and biliverdin.

Anthropogenic or man-made sources include automobiles, boilers, room heater, geyser, oil-burning furnaces, portable generators, charcoal grills, tobacco smoking etc. The majority of anthropogenic or man-made CO is produced from fossil fuel powered automobiles.

1. **Hydrocarbons:** CO is produced due to incomplete burning of carbon containing compounds like coal, wood, petroleum, fertilizers, dried dung and natural gas. The concentration of CO in the atmosphere is more in urban regions than rural due to industrialization.
2. **Exhaust Gases:** Combustion of petroleum products in motor vehicles is the major source of CO. It can be fatal if the motor vehicles are kept with the running engine in a closed space/garage even for a small duration. The petrol-driven vehicles produce more CO than the diesel vehicles.
3. **Fire:** Burning of almost any material results in the formation of CO.
4. **Cigarette smoke:** About 4% CO is released from cigarette smoking. The level of CO detected in the blood of a smoker could be about 10% whereas that in a non-smoker could be about 2%.
5. **Endogenous production:** CO is also produced by the endogenous metabolic process of the human body in a range of 0–5% and there is about 0.5% of CO in the blood. The percentage of COHb is higher in smokers, infants and among the person with hemolytic anemia.[4]

MECHANISM OF ACTION OF CARBON MONOXIDE

CO has affinity for heme-containing proteins which leads to various hypoxic and non-hypoxic effects (Figure 8.1). CO after inhalation gets absorbed rapidly and extensively into the blood. The affinity of CO to bind with hemoglobin is 200 times greater than the oxygen which leads to the formation of COHb, and this decreases the oxygen carrying capacity of blood along with shift the O_2 dissociation curve toward left. This direct effect leads to anemic hypoxia and later on tissue hypoxia especially those with the highest oxygen demand, i.e., brain and heart. Apart from hemoglobin other hem containing protein affected by CO are myoglobin, cytochrome and guanyl cyclase which produces respective symptoms.[5] CO bind to myoglobin with affinity 60 times stronger than oxygen. Myoglobin binding of CO inhibits the transport of O_2 to the mitochondria that may lead to decrease oxygen storing capacity of muscles and causes myocardial and skeletal muscle hypoxia, direct cellular necrosis and rhabdomyolysis.[6]

As CO binds to cytochromes, it compromises energy production at mitochondrial level and produces disturbance in physiological regulatory systems like nitric oxide cell signaling pathway, prostaglandin cell signaling pathway, mitochondrial respiration and oxidative phosphorylation.[7]

The CNS is affected by CO release at neuronal level, which initiates over-release of glutamate (an excitatory amino acid), influx of calcium into the cells, free-radical-mediated injury and additional neutrophil activation, with final result lipid peroxidation, neuronal death and demyelination. CO-mediated brain injury is a type of post-ischemic reperfusion phenomenon caused by conversion of xanthine dehydrogenase to xanthine oxidase and leads to the formation of reactive oxygen species which are responsible for lipid peroxidation. It also affect CNS by the over release of glutamate, influx of calcium into the cells, and additional neutrophil activation, with final result in neuronal death and demyelination.[8]

DOI: 10.1201/9780429026317-8

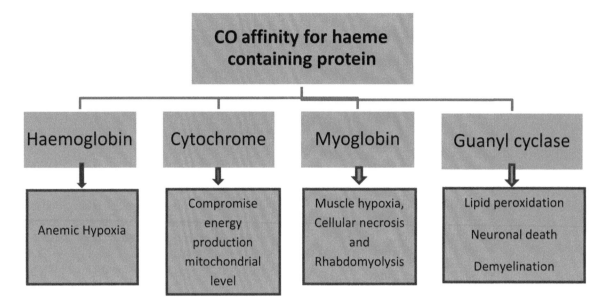

FIGURE 8.1   CO-affinity for heme-containing protein.

SIGNS AND SYMPTOMS OF POISONING

ACUTE POISONING

CO poisoning relatively common in temperate countries as compare to tropical countries where coal gas is used for heating and illumination. Signs and symptoms may vary according to the metabolic state and ability of a person to withstand the lack of oxygen. This is the reason why with the same level of exposure of CO some people recover and live while it became lethal to others. Patients with comorbid condition like anemia, cerebral sclerosis, coronary artery disease and pulmonary disease are less able to tolerate the compromise due to decreased oxygen carrying capacity of blood. Acute poisoning is mostly accidental in manner. Defective exhaust system of a motor may cause rapid acute poisoning by CO, especially when the window panes are closed. By preventing the combination of oxygen with hemoglobin CO is the perfect asphyxiant. Organ with high metabolic and oxygen demands are most sensitive to the effects of CO poisoning. Severity of CO poisoning (Table 8.1) depends on duration of exposure, amount of CO in the inhaled air, and general health of the affected individual. Although CO poisoning is harmful for all systems but most frequently CNS and cardiovascular systems are affected (Table 8.2).[4] Most common and first symptom appear is related to CNS, i.e., headache.[9]

Apart from neurological and respiratory symptoms, major cardiac manifestation are hypoxic damage to the myocardium leads to sinus tachycardia, atrial fibrillation, ST segment depression and T wave abnormalities on electrocardiogram and elevated level of CK-MB and Troponin I.[10]

Post-Interval Syndrome

Sadullah Saglam et al. described a case of 11-year boy brought to the Emergency Room with GCS 12, who was discharged with normal report and COHb level after 2 days but he report again with confusion on 3rd day with GCS 10. A symptom-free period is seen after acute phase. That period may be permanent or patient may enter the late phase characterized by encephalopathy symptoms.[11]

CHRONIC POISONING

Chronic symptoms are said to be occurred probably as a result of direct action on cytochrome oxidase and perhaps other oxidative systems and an effective reduction in oxygen availability.[9] After resolution of symptoms of acute poisoning or long-term slow exposure to toxic level, leads to neuropsychiatric sequelae which are seen within 3–240 days (frequently within first month). Delayed impairment may begin subtly with changes in behavior or cognitive ability,

TABLE 8.1

Severity of Symptoms of Poisoning is Categorized as Follows

Severity	Saturation of COHb (%)
Mild	10–30
Moderate	30–40
Severe	>40

TABLE 8.2
Clinical Features of Carbon Monoxide Poisoning on the Basis of COHb Level

Saturation of COHb (%)	Clinical features
0–10	No appreciable symptoms
10–20	Breathlessness, slight headache, lassitude, skin flushes
20–30	Throbbing headache, irritability, emotional instability, defective memory, buzzing in ears, breathlessness
30–40	Severe headache, nausea, vomiting, dizziness, visual impairment, breathlessness, mental confusion, muscular weakness and incoordination
40–50	All symptoms are intensified, increasing confusion, sometimes hallucinations, severe ataxia, rapid respiration and collapse
50–60	Syncope or coma with intermittent convulsion, tachycardia with weak pulse, rapid respiration, Cheyne–Stoke response, respiratory paralysis resulting in coma. Skin may show pink or red discoloration
>60%	Increasing depth of coma, rapidly fatal due to respiratory arrest.

personality and be more apparent with severe dementia, psychosis, Parkinsonism or gait disturbances.[12]

Apart from neuropsychiatric sequelae, rhabdomyolysis, non-cardiogenic pulmonary edema, multi-organ failure, disseminated intravascular coagulation, acute tubular necrosis can be seen during chronic exposure.

PREGNANCY AND CARBON MONOXIDE POISONING

CO poisoning in a pregnant women produces more fatal hypoxic effects on fetus. Placental diffusion of CO occurs and increases with gestational age. Acute CO toxicity in pregnant women will lead to fetal hypoxia due to decreased level of maternal oxygen and increased passage of CO through placenta.[13]

Fetal hemoglobin has a 10–15% higher affinity for CO than adult hemoglobinthat causes severe effect in fetus as compared to adults. The level of fetal morbidity and mortality in acute CO poisoning is significant, because of high affinity of CO and decreased rate of its elimination, which leads to severe fetal poisoning or death even when maternal survival may still occur.[14]

GUNSHOT WOUND AND CARBON MONOXIDE

CO along with other carbonaceous particles are expelled from the muzzle under high pressure. It leads to the formation of COHb, which stained the surrounding tissue with cherry-red discoloration, at the entrance wound. Depending on the distance traveled by the gunpowder, discoloration decreases and rarely seen over exit wound. It helps to differentiate the gunshot wound with stab injury, perforation of lungs. However, few case reports depict cherry discoloration over the exit wound and absent around the over entrance, where it would be expected. The explanation could be that hard contact of the muzzle with the skin, the large amount of projectile's kinetic energy cause massive tissue destruction at entrance and trajectory, which resulted in cherry-red muscle discoloration located at the exit wound.[15]

SCUBA AND CARBON MONOXIDE

Although CO poisoning is a rare event during a SCUBA diving but still some cases are reported. It occurs when SCUBA tanks are filled with faulty oil-contaminated air compressor. Even a small amount of COHb is fatal, as its effect increases as the pressure on the body rises. Symptoms deep down are the same as on the surface but due to increase pressure the symptoms are more severe and of early onset.[16]

DIAGNOSIS

Diagnosis of CO poisoning in forensic aspect is concluded on the basis of history, Hospital stay treatment record if (present), postmortem examination, radiological examination, laboratory estimation of CO level of blood and crime scene investigation. Cumulative effects of all the examination help us to reach to a diagnosis.

TREATMENT

- The person should be removed immediately from the place of incidence.
- Artificial respiration by manual methods or use of a respirator should be done if respiration has ceased or been impaired.
- Hyperbaric oxygen, i.e., 100% is the main stay treatment for CO poisoning, it shorten the half-life of COHb and accelerates the release of CO from hemoglobin along with increase oxygen uptake by tissues. Oxygen at a pressure of 2–2.5 atmosphere is considered ideal; pressures above 3 atmospheres may lead to oxygen toxicity. As per Lindell K. Weaver, treatment of patients with acute, symptomatic carbon monoxide poisoning with three hyperbaric-oxygen sessions within a 24-hr period appears to reduce the rate of cognitive sequelae 6 weeks and 12 months later.[17] Prolonged administration of hyperbaric oxygen, as used in non-human studies, is clearly teratogenic.[18]

- In order to prevent lung infection, antibiotics are given prophylactically. Prognosis should be guarded as the patient may die of complications at a later stage.

AUTOPSY

History and crime scene examination furnish a lot of information in determining the cause of death as carbon monoxide poisoning. But in some cases with an ambiguous history, high degree of suspicion is required to reach to a conclusion. CO poisoning should always be considered when a comatose person is found in a confined area with poor ventilation. Autopsy plays a crucial role in reaching to a conclusion of death due to CO.

EXTERNALLY

The characteristic external finding is the cherry-red color hypostasis (Figure 8.2). It is more evident if the level is >30%, below that level proper light is required for visualization or it may go unnoticed. If a person is dark skinned or anemic, it is difficult to appreciate but still it can be appreciated on the inner aspect of lips, tongue, nail beds and conjunctiva (Figure 8.3). Rigor mortis is usually delayed. Present of black color carbon particles present over the external nares and mouth if person was alive during the fire incidence and are not confirmatory but only suggestive to CO poisoning. Fine froth is seen at nostrils/mouth with features of pulmonary edema that occurs as a result of bronchial irritation due to smoke. If death is not immediate and patient survived for prolong time then skin lesion may develop that portray as discolored edematous area, bullae, necrosis or ulceration.

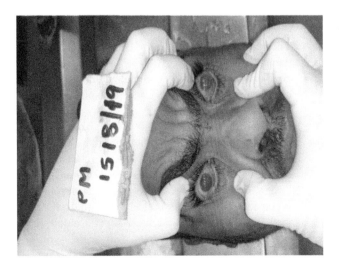

FIGURE 8.2 Cherry red color hypostasis in a case of CO poisoning.

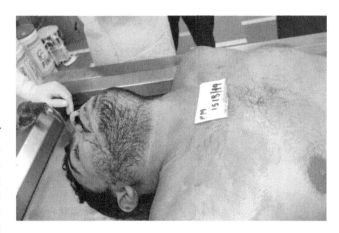

FIGURE 8.3 Congestion of conjunctiva.

INTERNALLY

Musculature and visceral organs show bright cherry-red color discoloration (Figure 8.4). Larynx, Trachea and bronchus shows black color soot particles.[19] As the organs with high metabolic rate will get more affected, i.e., heart and brain. The brain shows hyperemia, edema and petechial hemorrhages (Figure 8.5). Selective areas of brain are more prone to damage caused by COHb and the rate of damage increase with increase in exposure duration of the deadly gas. Lesions seen over the basal ganglia and periventricular white matter which are more clearly evident on CT scan. Bilateral necrosis with low density in globus pallidus is the most characteristic findings apart from other as seen more clearly on CT scan examination. Due of absence of postmortem clotting as in usual cases, fluidity of blood is a well appreciated sign in such cases.

If a person has inhaled superheated air then edema and swelling of airways present and cause reflex closure and prevent the entering of soot and damage below that level.

RADIOLOGICALLY

- **X-Ray:** Pulmonary infiltrates present with increase in alveolar and interstitial density.
- **Computed tomography:** Earliest changes in brain to be detectable in CT scan appeared after few days of exposure with the increased duration finding on the CT scan become more evident. So serial CT scanning may be a better guide for diagnosis of CO poisoning. The severity of the white matter change appears to provide the best clue to prognosis. The following are the CT scan finding:
  1. Ventricular dilation
  2. Low density in globus pallidus

3. Diffuse low density in periventricular white matter
4. Widening of sulci[20]
5. Bilateral globus pallidus calcifications
6. Hemorrhage at thalamus and basal ganglia[21]
- **Magnetic resonance imaging (MRI)**: Restricted diffusion in the bilateral globi pallidi and hippocampus seen. On T2-weighted gradient echo images petechial hemorrhage of the bilateral globi pallidi along with peripheral enhancement on T1-weighted images obtained after intravenous administration of a gadolinium chelate.[22]

Sample Collection

Blood sample should be collected from peripheral veins. In charred bodies where blood or visceral organ are not recovered than bone marrow should be collected for the estimation of COHb. Sample should be collected as early as possible as the half-life of COHb is 4–5 hr so with the passage of time its level reduces and then it is difficult to interpret the exact CO level and its concerned outcomes. So its preferred to collect the blood sample at the time of arrival of patient in the emergency. The decomposition of a body doesn't produce CO. COHb is relatively stable product and can be stored without any preservative. Being a stable product sometimes despite of embalming, presence of COHb is seen. Gary W. Kunsman et al., in his study of 2 years, stated that if sample collected during autopsy stored at 2 or 3 degree then repeated analysis can be done without much difference. The preservative, volume of headspace and initial percentage of COHb does not significantly affect the percentage of COHb level in postmortem blood specimens.[23]

Analysis of Carbon Monoxide in Blood

The determination of CO in blood can be done by an absolute quantity of CO per given quantity of blood, expressed in cc and it measures the CO after its liberation. It is a quantitative analysis. The relative content of CO in blood is expressed as percentage saturation of hemoglobin with CO. It is a qualitative analysis. Various methods to determine COHb are described as follows:

1. *Haldane's carmine method:* CO content is ascertained from the color of the greatly diluted blood solution, which is more or less pink, that depend on the percentage saturation of the hemoglobin with CO. This method is largely dependent upon subjective causes and is not very exact.

2. *Sayers and Yant's pyro tannic acid method or Kunkel's test:* Blood with COHb remains cherry

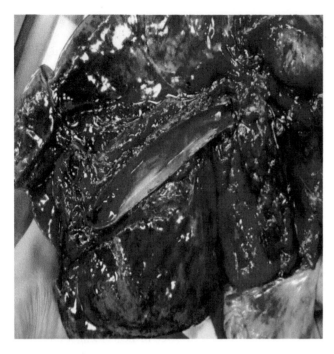

FIGURE 8.4 Intense congestion of visceral organs with cherry red discoloration.

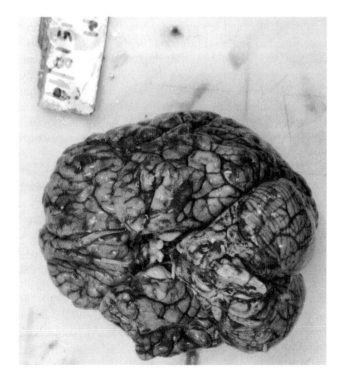

FIGURE 8.5 Edematous and hyperemic brain with cherry red discoloration.

red even after addition of tannic acid, when the oxygenated blood turns deep brown.[24]

3. *Hoppe-Seyler's test:* Few drops of blood are added to a solution of 10% of sodium hydroxide. Normal blood turns brownish-green, but if CO is present, the color will remain pink.[25]

4. *Gas chromatography:* It is widely used in clinical and toxicological laboratories. But blood containing MetHb also from exhaust fumes, is determined by gas chromatography, the measured value is higher than the actual value.

5. *Spectrophotometry:* It is quantitative analysis of a substance in a solution by measuring the difference in intensity of incident and transmitted light when the solution is placed in the path of a light source of defined wavelength; the difference is called the absorbed light or absorbance. It is very simple method and produces data of the same accuracy as gas chromatography. But it is a better option when the blood samples also contain Met-Hb from exhaust fumes along with COHb. [26]

Spectrophotometric analysis allows quantitative measurement of a substance in a solution by measuring the difference in intensity of incident and transmitted light when the solution is placed in the path of a light source of defined wavelength; the difference is called the absorbed light or absorbance.

DIFFERENTIAL DIAGNOSES

As the presentation of CO is highly variable and postmortem findings are nonspecific so high degree of suspicion is obligatory to rule out other condition which mimic it. The major conditions to be differentiated are alcohol intoxication for neurological symptoms, barbiturate poisoning for blister formation in chronic exposure, rupture of blister leaves red raw surface which can mimic second degree burn, cyanide poisoning and hypothermia for cherry-red discoloration. Other minor mimickers are drug overdose, encephalitis, meningitis, hypoxic encephalopathy, diabetic keto acidosis, intracranial pathologies etc.

CASE REPORT: TRAGEDY AT UPHAR CINEMA

On 13/06/97, a fire broke out in Uphaar Cinema Hall resulting in 59 deaths and injuries to many others. The fire occurred on the ground floor from a transformer oil leak, and involved the parking lot where a lot of cars were parked. The resulting smoke traveled up and reached the upper floors including the auditorium and as a result 59 people died allegedly due to smoke inhalation.

As per Government of Delhi, it was decided not to conduct postmortem on the body of the victims. Only one postmortem was conducted by the Army Hospital with respect to the deceased being one of their officers, who died in AIIMS.

Postmortem examination of the said victim revealed a 29 years old male, well-built and nourished, with rigor mortis and postmortem lividity present all over the body. Pupils were dilated and fixed with hazy cornea. Blood mixed frothy fluid was oozing out of the nostrils and mouth. No external injuries were present. On internal examination, frothy blood mixed fluid with blackish particles were present within the mouth, pharynx and esophagus and the mucosa was congested. Mucosa of nasopharynx, larynx, trachea and bronchi were parched and congested. Frothy blood mixed fluid with black particles were present within the lumen. The right and left lungs weighed 750 gm and 630 gm, respectively. Both lungs were subcrepitant and thin, pinkish fluid exuded on sectioning and compressing. Rest of the systems were within normal limits.

On histopathological examination, there was congestion and edema of all organs of upper and lower respiratory tract. The presence of foreign particles containing soot was found in the lumens upto the respiratory bronchioles. Pulmonary edema was present, and early tubular necrosis and interstitial edema was seen in both kidneys and fatty changes were seen in the liver.

With so many people involved in the incident, it was pointing to a stampede occurred while trying to escape the fire and smoke and also presence of burn injuries due to the fire of quite a large scale. But surprisingly, deaths occurred mostly due to only smoke inhalation and no external injuries including burns injuries were present on the body of the deceased.

MEDICO-LEGAL IMPORTANCE

Saturation of hemoglobin with CO help us to formulate a part of opinion and are quite decisive in cases of criminal investigations and civil litigation. Saturation level of >50% indicates CO poisoning as the primary cause of death. Level between 10% and 50% shows that smoke was inhaled, CO could have been a contributing factor and proves beyond doubt that the deceased was alive when the fire started and saturation level <10%, signifies that the individual was died shortly afterwards.[27] The presence of COHb is a sign of life when the fire started but its absence doesn't suggest that death has occurred before fire.

In CO poisoning there are various possibilities of death as acute asphyxiation and acute asphyxiation with delayed or secondary symptoms and chronic poisoning. In acute case, death remains usually suicidal or accidental and cause of death can be easily framed on the basis of symptoms and crime scene examination. But the problem arises when the patient recover and in few days to week he/she again develops acute symptoms of very high severity to brain and heart then it is very difficult to correlate it with the initial exposure to CO poisoning and controversy occurs in adjusting claims for disability.

Mostly the incidences of CO poisoning occur in closed spaces, garage or car with tightly closed windows. In a short interval, accumulation of gas becomes lethal. CO poisoning in open space is rare event. But few cases of poisoning using motor vehicle exhaust in an open space with suicidal tendency is also documented.[28]

CO poisoning is the most common accident in natural cooking gas leakage in kitchen at home. At times, mass deaths may occur in instances where a large building catches fire, the cause of death is by inhalation of smoke containing CO. Homicide by CO poisoning, though rare, is reported time to time. Victims are usually children, elderly and the persons who are intoxicated with drugs that incapacitate them to respond to the surrounding intoxication.

BIBLIOGRAPHY

1. National Crimes Record Bureau, Accidental Deaths & Suicides in India 2019, page 34. Available from: https://ncrb. gov.in/sites/default/files/ADSI-2019-FULL-REPORT.pdf.
2. Hanst PL, Spence JW, Edney EO. Carbon monoxide production in photooxidation of organic molecules in the air. Atmospheric Environment. 14:1077–88.
3. Coburn RF, Blakemore WS, Forster RE. Endogenous carbon monoxide production in man. Journal of Clinical Investigation. 1963;42:1172–8. 10.1172/JCI104802.
4. Gozubuyuk AA, Dag H, Kacar A, Karakurt Y, Arica V. Epidemiology, pathophysiology, clinical evaluation, and treatment of carbon monoxide poisoning in child, infant, and fetus. Northern Clinics of Istanbul. 2017;4(1):100–107.
5. Chavouzis N. Ioannis Pneumatikos, carbon monoxide inhalation poisoning. Pneumon Number 1, January—March 2014;27:21–4.
6. Finely J, VanBeck A, Glover JL. Myonecrosis complicating carbon monoxide poisoning. Journal of Trauma. 1977;17: 536–40.
7. Hardy KR, Thom SR. Pathophysiology and treatment of carbon monoxide poisoning. Journal of Toxicology Clinical Toxicology. 1994;32:613–29.
8. Thom SR. Dehydrogenase conversion to oxidase and lipid peroxidation in brain after carbon monoxide poisoning. Journal of Applied Physiology. 1992;73:1584–89.
9. Matthews G. Occupational medicine toxic gases. Postgraduate Medical Journal. 1989;65,224–32.
10. Satran D, Henry CR, Adkinson C,Nicholson CI, Bracha Y, Henry TD. Cardiovascular manifestations of moderate to severe carbon monoxide poisoning. Journal of the American College of Cardiology. 2005;45(9):1513–16.
11. Saglam S, Cortuk M, Gunes H, Colak S, Kandis H, Saritas A, Dikici S. Carbonmonoxide post-interval syndrome. Journal of the College of Physicians and Surgeons Pakistan. 2015;25(11):847–8.
12. Huzar TF, George T, Cross JM. Carbon monoxide and cyanide toxicity: etiology, pathophysiology and treatment in inhalation injury. Expert Review of Respiratory Medicine. 2013;7(2):159–70.
13. Greingor JL, Tosi JM, Ruhlmann S, Aussedat M. Acute carbon monoxide intoxication during pregnancy. One case report and review of the literature. Emergency Medicine Journal. September 2001;18(5):399–401.
14. Omaye ST. Metabolic modulation of carbon monoxide toxicity. Toxicology. Nov 2002;180(2):139–50.
15. Bogdanović M, Atanasijević T, Popović V, Durmić T, Radnić B. Gunshot Suicide: Cherry-red discoloration of the temporal muscle beneath the exit wound. The American Journal of Forensic Medicine and Pathology. 2019 Jun;40 (2):147–9.
16. Allen H. Carbon monoxide poisoning in a diver. Archives of Emergency Medicine. 1992;9:65–6.
17. Weaver LK, Hopkins RO, Chan KJ, Churchill S, Elliott CG, Clemmer TP, et al. Hyperbaric oxygen for acute carbon monoxide poisoning. New England Journal of Medicine. 2002;347:1057–67.
18. Miller PD, Telford IR, Haas GR. Effect of hyperbaric oxygen on cardiogenesis in the rat. Biology of Neonate. 1971;17:44–52.
19. Jorge Dinis-Oliveira R, Carvalho F, MagalhÃEs T, Santos A. Postmortem changes in carbon monoxide poisoning. Clinical Toxicology. 2010;48:762–3.
20. Chang KH, Suh CH, Choo IW. Magnetic resonance (MR) imaging in delayed encephalopathy of acute carbon monoxide poisoning-comparison with CT. Journal of the Korean Radiological Society. 1986 Jun 1;22(3):332–8.
21. Park YK, Won HS, Lee SR, Hahm CK. Computed tomographic findings of acute carbon monoxide poisoning. Journal of the Korean Radiology Society. 1983;190:498–505.
22. Kim DM, Lee IH, Park JY, Hwang SB, Yoo DS, Song CJ.. Acute carbon monoxide poisoning: MR imaging findings with clinical correlation. Diagnostic and Interventional Imaging. 2017;98:299–306.
23. Kunsman GW, Presses CL, Rodriguez P. Carbon monoxide stability in stored postmortem blood samples. Journal of Analytical Toxicology. 2000 October 1;24(7):572-8.24.
24. Pilaar WMM. Determination of carbon monoxide in blood. Journal of Biological Chemistry. 1929;83:43–50.
25. Sehrawat S, Khanna P. A review: On carbon monoxide poisoning. International Journal of Information and Computing Science. August 2018;5(8):131–5.
26. Sakata M, Yoshida A, Haga M. Simple determination of carboxyhemoglobin by double wavelength spectrophotometry of absorbance difference and the comparison with gas chromatographic method. Forensic Science International. March–April 1983;21(2):187–95.
27. Widdop B. Analysis of carbon monoxide. Annals of Clinical Biochemistry. 2002;39:378–91.
28. Żaba C et.al. Suicidal carbon monoxide poisoning using motor vehicle exhaust in an open space. Medical Principles and Practice. 2019;28:490–92.

CARBON DIOXIDE POISONING

Carbon dioxide (CO_2) is an odorless, colorless, and non-flammable gas. It is a normal constituent of air, i.e., 300 ppm or approximately 0.04% of atmospheric air. It is present in the atmosphere in gaseous form. It is transported in the form of liquefied compressed gas, and used in solid form as dry ice.[1]

SOURCES AND USES

Naturally, CO_2 is produced as a result of respiration process and is also found in atmospheric air. Various metals like aluminum, magnesium when suspended in CO_2, ignite and sometimes explode. In the atmosphere, CO_2 gets accumulated in the bottom of any closed space and displace much of the oxygen as it is heavier than air (molecular weight of CO_2 being 44). As CO_2 is odorless and non-irritant, it usually causes silent asphyxia.[2] When the gas is compressed at constant room temperature, it will eventually condense to liquid form. The liquid form is more compact than the gas form of CO_2 and thus it can be transported and stored in metal cylinders at normal room temperature.[3] The solid form, also known as dry ice, is made by liquefying CO_2 and transferring it into a container, where it is frozen at a temperature of $-109°$ F and compressed into solid ice. Dry ice is widely used to bring special fog effect in various public activities. It gets converted from solid to gaseous form by a process known as sublimation.

In day-to-day life, CO_2 is produced as a product of combustion, fermentation[4], geothermal emissions, automobile emission and during the formation of alcoholic beverages[5].

As mentioned earlier, CO_2 has the ability to displace oxygen from incendiary environment so it can be efficiently used as a fire extinguisher.[3] It is also used in hydrocracking and hydrotreating petroleum products and as a coolant. In food processing industry, it is used in refrigeration, carbonation of beverages and as a preservative.[6]

In medical field, it is used in gynecological and surgical laparoscopic procedures to insufflate the fallopian tube or the peritoneal cavity to allow visualization of the abdominal viscera.[7] However, its use also comes with a potentially lethal complication of gas embolism during insufflation process.[8]

There are various fetal malformations or disease states that can be treated with the help of partial amniotic carbon dioxide insufflation (PACI) technique in a wide range of gestational ages.[9]

MECHANISM OF ACTION

CO_2 is absorbed passively through the lungs by inhalation. Exposure can also occur through skin or eye contact. It is carried in the blood as bicarbonates and excreted via lungs and some part via kidney. Chemoreceptors in the carotid body, arch of the aorta, and the medulla oblongata are sensitive to small changes in the CO_2 concentration, compensating it immediately and keeping the homeostasis maintained. Increases in CO_2 concentration will alter the buffering capacity of CO_2 leading to an acidosis and increase in the potassium concentration. Peptides, proteins and amino acids are known to form N-carboxy derivatives (carbamates) in the presence of high concentration of CO_2 and are responsible for the neurological signs seen in carbon dioxide excess in the body.[10]

CO_2 has direct toxicological effect causing asphyxiation and at high concentration, it produces narcosis like effects.

The mechanism of CO_2 narcosis is closely related to fall of cerebrospinal fluid pH. Narcosis begins when pH falls below 7.10 and reaches to maximum when cerebrospinal pH reaches to 6.80. Narcosis of CO_2 inhalation is due to hydrogen ion only.[11]

CLINICAL FEATURES

The severity of the symptoms depend upon the concentration of CO_2 (as described in Table 8.3) and the duration of exposure. The Occupational Safety and Health Administration and the American Conference of Governmental Industrial Hygienists exposure limit to CO_2 is 5,000 parts per million (9,000 mg/m³), or 0.5% for an 8-hour time-weighted average.[1]

Increased CO_2 concentration will affect every system in one way or the other. The most affected common systems are cardiopulmonary and central nervous system (CNS) with minor effects on other systems (Table 8.3). With increasing CO_2 concentration, the pH of the blood starts falling. As acidity increases, the chemoreceptors located at the carotid body, arch of the aorta, and the medulla oblongata get stimulated, and compensation occurs to some extent. Further increase in level leads to hypoxia and dyspnea. With further increasing level, failure of buffer mechanism occurs and finally the respiratory rate increases and patient presents as hyperventilation.

After an initial increase in the level of CO_2, the respiratory rate declines slowly. Respiratory acclimatization, however, involves a continuous increase in tidal volume. Changes in respiratory pattern are associated with an increase in physiological and anatomical dead space.[12]

Constant elevation of pCO2 induces progressive increase in the resorptive capacity of the kidney to completely reabsorb bicarbonate.[13] It also leads to cerebral vasodilation which in turn causes severe headaches.[14] Acute hypercapnia causes repolarization abnormalities reflected by an increase in QT dispersion, which may provide an environment for arrhythmogenesis.[15]

TREATMENT

Rescuers should be employed with a positive-pressure self-contained breathing apparatus otherwise they may become secondary victims.[3] A room should be ventilated by opening doors and windows. The victim should be removed

---

TABLE 8.3

Clinical Features of Carbon Dioxide Poisoning on the Basis of CO_2 Level

Concentration (%)	Effects
2–5	Headaches, dizziness, sweating, dyspnea
6–10	Hyperventilation, tachycardia, worsening dizziness, visual and sensory discrimination decline
11–17	Drowsiness, muscle twitching, loss of consciousness
>17	Convulsions, coma, death

from the exposed environment to avoid further exposure. Rapid resuscitation should be started with high oxygen concentrations by non-rebreather masks to prevent irreversible neurological injury. Supportive care should be given.

AUTOPSY

Deaths due to asphyxia as a result of exposure to CO_2 have no pathognomonic autopsy findings. External examination of the body is mostly unremarkable. Internal examination sometimes shows nonspecific findings such as passive hyperemia of the internal organs, pleural petechia, and edema with a moderate congestion of the lungs and the brains[16].

In cases with a history of contact with dry ice, there may be intact or ruptured clear blisters at the contact site, apart from nonspecific generalized findings.[2]

SAMPLE TO BE PRESERVED

CO_2 can be produced as a result of putrefaction so exact level of CO_2 measurement is mostly unpredictable. All the viscera along with blood is collected to rule out alcohol, commonly abused drugs and psychiatric medications.

DIAGNOSIS

The diagnosis of asphyxia due to CO_2 intoxication is a diagnosis of exclusion and is based on the circumstances surrounding death, scene investigation, and exclusion of other causes of death.[17]

MEDICO-LEGAL IMPORTANCE

Sudden death is possible due to exposure to high concentration of CO_2 in collaboration with low oxygen concentration. Occupational disasters occur in the factories dealing with the use of CO_2. So, both the employers and employee must be aware about the working area. There should be continuous monitoring in the workplace, and proper handling and labeling of CO_2 containing containers.

CO_2, even though vital for living organisms, is extremely toxic in high concentrations. Most commonly, accidental occupational exposure occurs. There are some scenarios in which people can die suddenly in environments with abnormal composition. Analysis of environmental gases in crime scene investigation should be done, especially in cases of sudden death at industrial or workplace settings. There may be a prosecution related to health and labor safety laws or even under the criminal law.[18] Sometimes CO_2 may be a potent weapon in murder-suicide. Crime scene investigation plays an important role in such circumstances.

In 1986, potential toxicity of CO_2 was demonstrated by people in Cameroon, West Africa, when there was a natural release of carbon dioxide gas from Lake Nyos, a volcanic Crater Lake leads to deaths of around 1700 people. A similar incident in Lake Monoun had killed 37 people in 1984.[20]

BIBLIOGRAPHY

1. National Institute for Occupational Safety and Health. The registry of toxic effects of chemical substances: carbon dioxide RTECS FF6400000, CAS 124-38-9
2. Hsieh C-C, Shih C-L, Fang C-C, Chen W-J, Lee C-C. Carbon dioxide asphyxiation caused by special-effect dry ice in an election campaign. The American Journal of Emergency Medicine. 2005;23(4):567–568.
3. Halpern P, Raskin Y, Sorkine P, Oganezov A. Exposure to extremely high concentrations of carbon dioxide. Annals of Emergency Medicine. 2004;43(2):196–9.
4. Zaba C, Marcinkowski JT, Wojtyla A, Tezyk A, Tobolski J, Zaba Z. Acute collective gas poisoning at work in a manure storage tank. Annals of agricultural and environmental medicine. 2011;18(2):448–51.
5. Kettner M, Ramsthaler F, Juhnke C, Bux R, Schmidt P. A fatal case of CO_2 intoxication in a fermentation tank. Journal of Forensic Sciences. 2013;58(2):556–8.
6. Langford NJ. Carbon dioxide poisoning. Toxicological Reviews. 2005;24(4):229–35.
7. Gardner NHN. Death following tubal insufflation with carbon dioxide. Proceedings of the Royal Society of Medicine. 1966;59:833–4.
8. Yacoub OF, Cardona I, Coveler LA, Dodson MG. Carbon dioxide embolism during laparoscopy. Anesthesiology: The Journal of the American Society of Anesthesiologists. 1 December 1982;57(6):533–5.
9. Kohl T, Tchatcheva K, Weinbach J, Hering R, Kozlowski P, Stressig R, Gembruch U. Partial amniotic carbon dioxide insufflation (PACI) during minimally invasive fetoscopic surgery: Early clinical experience in humans. Surgical Endoscopy. 2009;24(2):432–44. doi:10.1007/s00464-009-0579.
10. Max B. This and that: the neurotoxicity of carbon dioxide. Trends in Pharmacological Sciences. 1991;12:408-11.
11. Eisele JH, Eger EI, Muallem M. Narcotic properties of carbon dioxide in the dog. Anesthesiology. 1967;28(5):856–65.
12. Schaefer KE, Hastings BJ, Carey CR, Nichols G. Respiratory acclimatization to carbon dioxide. Journal of Applied Physiology. 1963;18(6):1071–8.
13. Van Ypersele de Strihou C, Gulyassy PF, Schwartz WB. Effects of chronic hypercapnia on electrolyte and acid-base equilibrium. III. Characteristics of the adaptive and recovery process as evaluated by provision of alkali. Journal of Clinical Investigation. 1962;41(12):2246–53.
14. Patterson JL, Heyman A, Battey LL, et al. Threshold of response of the cerebral vessels of man to increase in blood carbon dioxide. Journal of Clinical Investment. 1955; 34:1857–64.
15. Kiely DG, Cargill RI, Lipworth BJ. Effects of hypercapnia on hemodynamic, inotropic, lusitropic, and electrophysiologic indices in humans. Chest. 1996;109(5):1215–21.
16. Srisont S, Chirachariyavej T, Peonim AVM. A carbon dioxide fatality from dry ice. Journal of Forensic Science. 2009;54(4):961–2.
17. Dunford JV. Asphyxiation due to dry ice in a walk-in freezer. The Journal of Emergency Medicine. 2009;36(4):353–6.
18. Milroy CM. Deaths from environmental hypoxia and raised carbon dioxide. Academic Forensic Pathology. 2018;8(1):2–7.
19. Sautter J, Gapert R, Tsokos M, Oesterhelweg L. Murder-suicide by carbon dioxide (CO_2) poisoning: a family case from Berlin, Germany. Forensic Science, Medicine, and Pathology. 2013;10(1):97–102. doi:10.1007/s12024-013-9495-6.

20. Baxter PJ, Kapila M, Mfonfu D. Lake Nyos disaster, Cameroon, 1986: the medical effects of large scale emission of carbon dioxide? British Medical Journal. 27 May 1989;298(6685):1437–41.

CYANIDE POISONING

Hydrogen cyanide (HCN) and its salts are potentially deadly and rapidly-acting chemical asphyxiants causing painless and quick death. HCN is a chemical compound of carbon and nitrogen having triple bond. Inorganic cyanides like sodium cyanide, potassium cyanide are potentially dangerous than organic cyanides and are usually called as nitrile-like acetonitrile as these nitriles don't release cyanide ion. It can exist as gas (HCN) as well as solid (salts of sodium and potassium cyanide-white, crystalline powder). When HCN is dissolved in water, hydrocyanic acid is formed which is a colorless volatile liquid and is extremely toxic. Cyanide has a peculiar bitter almond odor and is a cytotoxic poison. The ability to smell cyanide is genetically governed and is a sex-linked recessive trait. Therefore, not everybody can smell it.

SOURCES OF CYANIDE

Common sources of cyanide poisoning include smoke inhalation from residential and industrial fires, burning plastic furniture, burning silk or wool, especially in a closed space. Cyanide is also released during cigarette smoking.

Naturally, cyanides are found in bitter almonds; and fruits like apricot, peach, plum, and cherry. These contain cyanogenic glycoside (amygdalin), which is hydrolyzed during digestion to release hydrocyanic acid.[1] Laetrile (another name for amygdalin derived from apricot kernels), which was formerly used as an anticancer agent, releases cyanide upon metabolism.[2]

Many edible plants contain cyanogenic glycosides, including cassava (an edible tuberous root) which is one of the main sources of calories in Tropics. In order to prevent poisoning, it needs to be detoxified by soaking, drying and scraping them before consumption. Cyanogenic glycosides are converted to HCN following destruction of plant tissues during consumption, or by the gut microflora.

However, in a well-ventilated room, bitter almond odor from the victim and the crime scene may not always be detected.[3]

USES OF CYANIDE

Cyanide is used in electroplating, metal processing, photographic process, production of synthesis of rubber, manufacture of plastic, gold and silver industries, food industries as an anticaking agent. It is used in manufacturing insecticides and rodenticides. Occupational hazards due to cyanide occur to the persons who are working in such industries.

A safe regimen of 3.5 mg per kg of sodium nitroprusside should be used to the anticipated total dose for the period of hypotension. A dose more than that for required effect may get accumulated to toxic level. The lethal dose of sodium nitroprusside appears to be 7 mg per kg.[4]

MECHANISM OF ACTION, ROUTE AND DOSE

Cyanide ion is readily absorbed from various routes like lungs, GI tract, and even through the intact skin. Cyanide causes histotoxic anoxia as the tissue is not able to utilize the oxygen. It does this by inhibiting oxidative phosphorylation where oxygen is utilized to produce ATP (adenosine triphosphate), which is an essential form of cellular energy. One of the major parts of this process is the transfer of electrons from NADH (nicotinamide adenine dinucleotide) to oxygen via a chain of electron carriers. This reaction is catalyzed by cytochrome oxidase (cytochrome a3) enzyme system in the mitochondria and it is a terminal enzyme of mitochondrial electron transport chain. Cyanide combines with cytochrome oxidase and the combination forms a complex, i.e., cytochrome a3-CN which causes blockage of electron transfer from cytochrome a3 to molecular oxygen and the chain of cellular respiration is halted which leads to the decreased production of ATP. Due to this, energy production is diverted to the alternative anaerobic pathway leading to the formation of lactic acid, which further causes metabolic acidosis. HCN is metabolized in the liver by a mitochondrial enzyme, rhodanese (sulfotransferase) which catalyzes the transfer of sulfur from thiosulfate to cyanide to yield the relatively nontoxic thiocyanate which gets excreted in urine. Adequate amount of tissue rhodanese is available to deal with relatively large amounts of cyanide, but because of low endogenous supply of thiosulfate the reaction is limited leading to accumulation of deadly cytochrome a3-CN complex.[5]

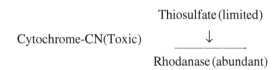

Thiosulfate (limited)

Cytochrome-CN (Toxic) $\xrightarrow{}$ Rhodanase (abundant)

Thiocynate (relatively non-toxic)

The active form of cyanide is HCN. When salts of cyanide are ingested, they react with the acid containing HCl or with water to release the toxic HCN. So, people having achlorhydria, are immune to cyanide poisoning. Cyanide also inhibits various enzymes like glutathione dehydrogenase, superoxide dismutase, carbonic anhydrase, catalase, superoxide dismutase etc. Apart from acting on the electron transport chain, it also acts as a corrosive on the mucosa. Cyanide metabolites are excreted primarily in the urine, and small parts through the lungs. Fatal dose of cyanide salts (of sodium, potassium, or calcium) is 100–200 mg. 20 ppm is maximum safe period for prolonged exposure.[6]

CLINICAL FEATURES

ACUTE POISONING BY CYANIDES

Acute intoxication in cyanide is fatal as it is rapidly acting and highly toxic. The onset of symptoms depends upon the route of exposure, dose intake, duration of exposure and availability of the antidote. The appearance of symptoms varies from few seconds in cases of inhalation to several minutes after ingestion of salts to many hours after skin absorption. Clinical manifestations are due to dysfunction of oxygen-sensitive organs, so it predominantly involves the CNS and cardiovascular system. On acute exposure, the patient develops CNS manifestations as headache, vertigo, agitation, confusion, generalized weakness, difficulty in swallowing, convulsions and coma. The patient experiences tachycardia and hypertension initially, followed by bradycardia and hypotension.[2]

Cutaneous manifestations occur due to diminished consumption of oxygen and the patient's external appearance might be misleading with rosy skin color even during cardiac arrest rather than typical cyanosis.[7]

Manifestations may include respiratory abnormalities (progressing from tachypnea and dyspnea to respiratory depression and apnea), hemodynamic instability, metabolic acidosis and possibly, local irritant effects after oral ingestion of cyanide.[8]

Gastrointestinal toxicity may occur following ingestion of inorganic cyanide and include nausea, vomiting and abdominal pain. These symptoms are caused by corrosive nature of cyanide salts and depict as hemorrhagic gastritis. Survivors of serious, acute poisoning may develop delayed neurologic sequelae later on. Inhibition of the terminal step of electron transport in cells of the brain results in loss of consciousness, respiratory arrest and ultimately, death.

Absence of cyanosis and bradycardia are the two important clinical features of late cyanides poisoning ("late" implying that the patient is already in coma, with hypotension and apparently inadequate ventilation) which are of cardinal importance.[9]

CHRONIC FEATURES

Chronic exposure occurs in people who are engaged in occupation like electroplating, extraction of gold, silver from ores, metallurgy and photographic procedures. As they are in continuous exposure of low dose of cyanide and its congeners. The chronic exposure involve almost affect each and every system. Cyanide-induced neurodegeneration is selective in nature related variable susceptibility to oxidative stress. [10]

Neurological symptoms include headache, weakness and objectionable changes in taste and smell, irritation of the throat, on exacerbation the patient became confused, hallucinated and have slurred speech. Gastrointestinal symptoms include vomiting, disturbance in salivation and abdominal colic. Hematologic ally patient depicts significantly higher hemoglobin and lymphocyte count and also

the presence of punctate basophilia. Enlarge thyroid gland is also seen in various cases.[11]High cyanide exposure with low protein and sulfur from a dietary source such as unprocessed cassava root causes optic neuropathy, often associated with sensory ataxia and pyramidal tract involvement.[12]

TREATMENT

DECONTAMINATION

Decontamination is the prime part of the treatment. Withdraw the patient from the site of exposure and remove the clothing and accessories and prevent the inhalation exposure. Dermal decontamination can be done by washing the exposed area with water. Gastrointestinal decontamination is helpful if some form of cyanide may have prolonged absorption kinetics. For patients presenting within 1 hr of ingestion, it is advisable to perform orogastric lavage and administering activated charcoal in attempt to retrieve any amount of the cyanide.[13] One gram of activated charcoal binds to only 35 milligram of cyanide.[14]

Antidote kit: The major three constituents of antidote kit are: amyl nitrite, sodium nitrite and sodium thiosulfate. Amyl nitrite has rapid onset of action and have short half-life and administered by inhalation to generate methemoglobin.

Sodium nitrite is given intravenously to increase the content of methemoglobin. Cyanide preferentially bind to the ferric iron of methemoglobin to form cyanmethemoglobin, i.e., methemoglobin prevents the cyanide to combine to the cytochrome and enabling the mitochondria to reactivate electron transport. Sodium thiosulfate, the third component of the cyanide antidote kit, has poor penetration into the mitochondria that leads to its slow onset of action. It act as sulfhydryl donor. Transfer of sulfur from thiosulfate to the cyanide ion is done by rhodanese (sulphtransferase), a mitochondrial enzyme that is present in abundance in our body.[15]

Thiosulfate reversibly combines with cyanide and with the help of rhodanese it get converted into a less toxic thiocyanate which got excreted in urine. The primary concerns in this administration of the cyanide antidote kit are, it's side effects, which include severe hypotension, methemoglobinemia and hypersensitivity reactions. However, the antidote for methemoglobinemia is methylene blue and this agent will counteract excess methemoglobin formation.

Apart from antidote kit nowadays hydroxocobalamin has been gradually expanding recognition in treatment because of its safety and effectiveness. Cyanide has a greater affinity to bind with hydroxocobalamin rather than cytochrome oxidase a_3 forming cyanocobalamin.[16] Hydroxocobalamin can decrease mortality with less severe associated side effects with no neurological sequelae. Its freeze-dried preparation available and named as Cyanokit.[17]

Combination of hydroxocobalamin as a first-line antidote followed by the continuous administration of sodium thiosulfate can have a positive effect on the survival without long-term neurological and visual sequelae in cases of massive cyanide poisonings.[18]

Dicobalt edetate is also used in management of cyanide as they act as a direct binding agents. It is given intravenously. 4-Dimethyl-aminopheno induces formation of methemoglobinemia that attract the cyanide to combine with it and leads the formation of cyanmethemoglobin. It is also given intravenously as an adjunct therapy.[19]

Internationally there are various difference of opinion regarding using of antidotes. In the United States, sodium nitrite is the drug of choice, whereas in UK dicobalt edetate is a preferred choice, Germany recommended dimethyl aminophenol and France is in the favor of newest drug, i.e., hydroxocobalamin. [20]

Supplemental oxygen will be a crucial part of supportive care and it has a synergistic effect with antidotes. Seizures resulting from cyanide poisoning may be refractory and require aggressive management. Hemodialysis particularly beneficial in the face of worsening acidosis and failing renal function.

AUTOPSY FINDINGS

EXTERNALLY

Rigor mortis was appreciated all over the body and sets early. The postmortem staining is brick red due to excess oxyhemoglobin (since tissue is prevented from using oxygen). The skin, mucous membranes, face and lips shows dark brick red color. The odor of HCN (smell of bitter almonds) can be detected and on opening the body bluish discoloration of extremities present.

INTERNALLY

The odor of HCN (smell of bitter almonds) can be detected on opening the body. Tracheal congestion and hemorrhages present. Stomach shows hemorrhagic gastritis (corrosive nature). Mucosa shows blackened and eroded surface with peculiar smell. Lungs are congested and edematous with subpleural or confluent alveolar hemorrhages are seen and on cut section exudes blood mixed with froth suggestive of pulmonary edema. Brain softened and edematous. [21] Congestion of lung liver kidney gastrointestinal tract is found. Disseminated petechia are present over the pleura, lungs, brain, meninges and pericardium.[22]

SAMPLES COLLECTED

The most appropriate fluids and tissues to remove for chemical analysis are blood, stomach contents, lung, liver, kidney, brain, heart and spleen. Lung should be sent intact, sealed in a nylon bag. Spleen is said to be the best specimen for cyanide analysis since it generally has the highest concentration of the poison owing to a strong presence of RBC. Samples for the cyanide should be examined as soon as possible.

As blood containing cyanide get instable with increased postmortem interval. Instability of the cyanide containing blood toward the bacteriological activity is reduced by adding 2% sodium fluoride.[23] Storage of blood sample is a concerned as blood with low content of cyanide should be stored at 4°C while blood with high concentration of cyanide is best to keep at −20°C.[24]

While interpreting the results, the possibility of spurious postmortem formation of cyanide in the decomposing tissues as a result of microbial action should be keep in mind during calculation of the amount. [25]

LAB ESTIMATION OF CYANIDE

On sport identification: Methods for identification of cyanide in the blood are too time-consuming to be of value in the management of acute poisoning, but examination of the gastric aspirate by the given method will be of utmost use as it can detect the presence of cyanide in 5 to 10 minutes. A total of 5 mL of gastric aspirate is taken and a few crystals of ferrous sulfate and 5 drops of 20% sodium hydroxide are added. The mixture is boiled, cooled and acidified with 10% hydrochloric acid (8–10 drops). If greenish-blue color is seen (due to the formation of Prussian blue), the presence of cyanide is confirmed (purplish color indicates salicylates). Since the reagent are stable and easy to use, this minimizes the time.[9]

Micro estimation of cyanides can be done using Coleman Universal spectrophotometer using 1% aqueous chloramine T solution initially followed by 6 mL of the pyridine-pyrazolone reagent. After 20 minutes the optical density is compared with that of a reagent blank. The amount of cyanide present in the unknown solution is determined from the standard curve. About 98–100% of cyanide in quantities ranging from 0.2 to 1.2 µg may be recovered by this method.[26]

Apart from them various analytical methods are present for the determination of cyanides nowadays. Researchers from diverse environmental, medical, forensic and clinical arena shows a great interest in this venture. The recent methods include naked eye visual detection, spectrophotometry/colorimetry, capillary electrophoresis fluorometry, chemiluminescence, atomic absorption spectrometry, electrochemical methods, mass spectrometry and gas chromatography.[27]

Serum cyanide level is confirmatory, but difficult to accomplish in practice. Analysis of blood for the presence of cyanide should be conducted as soon as possible, because it decomposes with time. The normal blood cyanide level is less than 0.2 µg/mL. A cyanide level above 2 µg/mL can produce severe toxicity, and a level above 5 µg/mL may be lethal if not treated immediately.[28]

DIAGNOSIS OF CYANIDE POISIONING

After considering all the facts about cyanide now the question come to summarize how to diagnose the case of cyanide poisoning. The most important clue to diagnosis is the circumstantial evidence, rather than the signs or symptoms.

Detection of source of cyanide at the crime scene is an important clue. Apart from that, on autopsy bitter almond smell, bright red color lividity and gastric chemical injury add on to the diagnosis. However, the odor of bitter almond from the crime scene may not always be detected in a well-ventilated area. Moreover, the ability to sense the "cyanide smell" is genetically related. Last but not the least, laboratory confirmation of elevated cyanide in blood confirms the diagnosis to a great extent. [29]

MEDICO-LEGAL ASPECTS

As the death due to cyanide is rapid and painless but suicide due to cyanide is relatively rare because of its restricted availability. Cyanide pills also known as suicide pill are used to avoid torture when get arrested or get interrogated.[30]

Occupational exposures increase the risk of suicide by cyanide ingestion. It is easily available for the persons who are working in the professions such as goldsmiths or textile industry workers.[31] Here ingestion of potassium cyanide sodium nitroprusside,[32] or a locally-purchased substance intended for cleaning metal, coins, or jewelry is frequently encountered.[33] Here workers can easily misuse it resulting in fatal incidences.

Accidental incidences occur occasionally, e.g., after fumigation, eating bitter almonds, apricot, peach, plum, pear and apple, may occasionally lead to fatalities. Fires involving polyurethane furniture (plastics), silk or woolen articles, can release cyanide and this may result in accidental deaths of people exposed to it. Due to its peculiar bitter almond smell and taste, it is rarely used as homicide. Cyanide along with carbon monoxide are used in gas chamber for capital punishment is considered to be the most dangerous, most complicated and most expensive method of administering the death penalty. Cyanide can be used in Chemical Warfare and Terrorism Agent, as it causes major morbidity and mortality to human to a great extent.[34]

Cyanide has both positive and negative aspects. In a positive sense, it is used in various industrial, agricultural and medical sectors but at the same time its negative impact cannot be ignored. So a variety of laws have been implicated to control its negative impacts. Various laws like *Poison Act, 1919, The Poison And Dangerous Substances Act, 1957 are relevant here. Along with that, laws* related to adulteration of food and drinks with cyanide, i.e., Sec 272 IPC, negligent conduct with respect to cyanide Sec 284 IPC and causing hurt by means of cyanide Sec 328 IPC are also applicable here.

BIBLIOGRAPHY

1. Sayre JW, Kaymakcalan S. Cyanide poisoning from apricot seeds among children in central Turkey. New England Journal of Medicine. 1964;270:1113–5.
2. Suchard JR, Wallace KL, Gerkin RD. Acute cyanide toxicity caused by apricot kernel ingestion. Annals of Emergency Medicine. December 1998;32:742–4.
3. Zacarias, CH, Esteban, C, Rodrigues, GL, Nascimento, EDS. Occupational exposure to hydrogen cyanide during large-scale cassava processing, in Alagoas State, Brazil. Cadernos de Saúde Pública. 2017;33(7).
4. Davies, et al. A sudden death associated with the use of sodium nitroprusside for induction of hypotension during anaesthesia. Canadian Anaesthesia Society of Journal. September 1975;22(5).
5. Egekeze JO, Oehme FW. Cyanides and their toxicity: A literature review. Veterinary Quarterly. 1980;2(2):104–14. DOI: 10.1080/01652176.1980.9693766.
6. Oke OL. The role of hydrocyanic acid in nutrition. World Review of Nutrition and Dietetics. 11:170–98.
7. Borron SW, Baud FJ. Acute cyanide poisoning: clinical spectrum, diagnosis, and treatment. Arhiv za higijenu rada i toksikologiju. September 1996;47(3):307–22.
8. Holland MA, Kozlowski LM. Clinical features and management of cyanide poisoning. Clinical Pharmacy. September 1986;5(9):737–41.
9. Lee-Jones M, Bennett MA, Sherwell JM. Cyanide Self-poisoning. British Medical Journal. 1970;4(5738):780–1. doi:10.1136/bmj.4.5738.780.
10. Mills EM, Gunasekar PG, Li L, Borowitz JL, Isom GE. Differential susceptibility of brain areas to cyanide involves different modes of cell death. Toxicology and applied pharmacology. 1999;156(1):6–16.
11. El Ghawabi SH, Gaafar MA, El-Saharti AA, Ahmed SH, Malash KK, Fares R. Chronic cyanide exposure: a clinical, radioisotope, and laboratory study. Occupational and Environmental Medicine. 1975;32(3):215–9.
12. Freeman AG. Optic neuropathy and chronic cyanide intoxication: a review. Journal of the Royal Society of Medicine. February 1988;81:103–6.
13. Gracia AR, Shepherd G. Cyanide poisoning and its treatment. Pharmacotherapy. 2004;24(10):1358–65.
14. Andersen A. Experimental studies on the pharmacology of activated charcoal. I. Adsorption power of charcoal in aqueous solutions. Acta Pharmacology. 1946;2:69–78.
15. Hall AH, Saiers J, Baud F. Which cyanide antidote? Critical Reviews in Toxicology. 2009;39(7):541–52.
16. Hamel J. A review of acute cyanide poisoning with a treatment update. Critical Care Nurse. 2011;31(1):72–82.
17. Meillier A, Helle C. Acute cyanide poisoning: hydroxocobalamin and sodium thiosulfate treatments with two outcomes following one exposure event. Case Reports in Medicine.2015:1–4.
18. Zakharov S. Successful use of hydroxocobalamin and sodium thiosulfate in acute cyanide poisoning: A case report with follow-up. Basic & Clinical Pharmacology & Toxicology. 2015;117:209–12.
19. Bhattacharya R. Antidotes to cyanide poisoning: present status. Indian Journal of Pharmacology. 2000;32:94–101.
20. Cummings TF. The treatment of cyanide poisoning. Occupational Medicine. 2004;54:82–5.
21. Yadukul S, Venkataraghava S, Fathima T, Gaonkar VB. Fatal suicidal case of cyanide poisoning—A case report. Journal of Forensic Toxicology and Pharmacology. 2014;3:3.
22. Ballantyne B. Artifacts in the definition of toxicity by cyanides and cyanogens. Fundamental and Applied Toxicology. 1983;3:400–408.
23. McAllister JL, et al. The effect of sodium fluoride on the stability of cyanide in postmortem blood samples from fire victims. Forensic Science International. 2011;209(1–3):29–33.
24. Ballantyne B. Changes in blood cyanide as a function of storage time and temperature. Journal of Forensic Science and Society. 1976;16(4):305–10.

25. Karhunen PJ, Lukkari I, Vuori E. High cyanide level in a homicide victim burned after death: evidence of post-mortem diffusion. Forensic Science International. 1991;49(2):179–83.

26. Epstein J. Estimation of microquantities of cyanide. Analytical Chemistry. 1947;19(4):272–274.

27. Ma J, Dasgupta PK. Recent developments in cyanide detection: A review. Analytica Chimica Acta. 19 July 2010;673(2):117–125.

28. Dasgupta A, Wahed A. Common poisonings including heavy metal poisoning. Clinical Chemistry, Immunology and Laboratory Quality Control. 2014:337–351.

29. Yu JC-C, Mozayani A. Medicolegal and forensic factors in cyanide poisoning. Toxicology of Cyanides and Cyanogens. 2016:276–282. doi:10.1002/9781118628966.ch20.

30. Frank M et.al. Cyanide fatalities: case studies of four suicides and one homicide. American Journal of Forensic Medicine and Pathology. December 2002;23(4):315–20.

31. Coentrão L, Moura D. Acute cyanide poisoning among jewelry and textile industry workers. American Journal Emergency Medicine. January 2011;29(1):78–81.

32. Froldi R, Cingolani M, Cacaci C. A case of suicide by ingestion of sodium nitroprusside. Journal of Forensic Science. November 2001;46(6):1504–6.

33. Garlich FM et.al. Poisoning and suicide by cyanide jewelry cleaner in the US Hmong community: a case series. Clinical Toxicology (Philadelphia). February 2012 ;50(2):136–40.

34. Greenfield RA, et al. Microbiological, biological, and chemical weapons of warfare and terrorism. American Journal of Medical Science. 2002;323(6):326–40.

SEWER GAS POISONING

Sewer gas is a complex mixture of gases that is toxic and nontoxic formed as a result of the decay of industrial wastes and domestic water waste. The major components of sewer gas include: hydrogen sulfide (H_2S), carbon dioxide (CO_2), methane (CH4), ammonia (NH_3), and sometimes also contain sulfur dioxide (SO_2), nitrous oxides (NOx). Inhalation of theses harmful substances usually concerned with the occupation related fatalities.

- *Hydrogen sulfide:* H_2S has been referred to as the "knock down gas" because inhalation of high concentrations can cause immediate loss of consciousness and death. It is the most common and fatal sewer gas.[1]

H_2S is a colorless, flammable gas and highly toxic having smell of rotten eggs. It is classified as both a chemical asphyxiant and irritant gas. It is also known as hydrosulfuric acid, sulfurated hydrogen or stink damp. It causes histotoxic hypoxemia. It is heavier than air so it tends to accumulate at ground level and in confined spaces which usually leads to sudden occupational fatalities.[2]

Other sewer gases include carbon dioxide and methane which have little or no odor characteristics and have a saturated gas density approximately 1.5 and 0.6 times that of air, respectively. Methane is extremely flammable, has a wide explosive range, and a low flash point. These characteristics result in a substantial fire and explosion hazard. Ammonia

has a distinct, strong odor with good warning characteristics which are present well before attaining toxic levels.

SOURCES OF H_2S-RELATED FATALITIES

Sewers, mining and drilling operations, fisheries, farms, tanneries, petroleum refining, natural gas industries, tanning, wood pulp processing, rayon manufacturing, sugarbeet processing, industries dealing with sulfur containing chemicals or occupation that require entry into confined spaces. Usually H_2S get accumulated in closed spaces as a result of bacterial breakdown of sulfur containing organic waste materials. Natural sources are volcanoes, caves, sulfur springs and subterranean emissions.[3,4]

In residential areas the sewer gas can enter into the indoor air through leaks in your plumbing system due to improperly placed pipes or vents, clogged drain, with degraded, cracked or broken sewer system pipes.[5]

FATAL DOSE

Prolonged exposure to lower concentrations, such as 10–500 ppm, can cause various respiratory symptoms that range from rhinitis to acute respiratory failure. H_2S is immediately fatal when concentrations are over 500–1000 ppm.

MECHANISM OF ACTION

H_2S causes histotoxic hypoxemia because of its toxic properties. It gets quickly absorbed through the lungs and gastrointestinal tract and get eliminated through the lungs or in feces and its metabolites are passed in urine. Metabolism of H_2S proceeds through three primary pathways which include oxidation, methylation and reaction with metalloproteins or disulfide-containing proteins.

At low concentration, oxidation of H_2S occurs in liver that rapidly oxidizes sulfide into a sulfate or thiosulfate by oxygen bound to hemoglobin in the blood. [6]

At high concentration, H_2S combines with metalloproteins or disulfide-containing proteins to suppress aerobic metabolism in the various tissues especially by combining to cytochrome C oxidase in complex IV of the mitochondrial electron transport chain, and causes cellular toxicity via reduced ATP production and/or generation of oxidative stress.[7]

H_2S produces a high degree of oxidative stress in cells and tissues. It serve as an endogenous cell signaling agent and acts as a DNA-damaging mutagen. The oxidation of H_2S, in the presence of protein thiols, has the potential to generate protein per sulfides which is a well-known DNA-damaging agents. Hoffman, M et al. indicate that H_2S undergoes trace metal-mediated autoxidation to generate reactive oxygen species which act as DNA-cleaving agent.[8]

CLINICAL FEATURES

H_2S acts both as irritant and asphyxiant depending upon the dose and duration of exposure. Exposure even for short duration but with large quantity produce mainly symptoms

TABLE 8.4

Effects of H₂S at Various Concentrations (ppm)⁹

H₂S Conc. in ppm	Effects
0.02	Odor threshold
10	Unpleasant odor
30	Intense odor
50	Conjunctival and upper respiratory irritation over time
100	Olfactory fatigue in minutes
150	Olfactory nerve paralysis
200	Intense immediate stinging, eyes and throat; smell disappears rapidly
300–500	Pulmonary edema, apnea in minutes
700–900	Rapid loss of consciousness, apnea (central respiratory paralysis)
>1000	Near-instant respiratory paralysis and com

of irritation of mucous membranes, peeling of skin, respiratory and visual symptoms with reduced memory and concentration and complete loss of the sense of smell.

ACUTE POISONING

At low concentrations (50 ppm), it can cause local effects (irritative action), acting mainly on the mucous membranes of the airways, lungs and eyes causing eyes conjunctival irritation, rhinorrhea, teary eyes or cough. At higher concentration, it act as central nervous system (CNS) depressant, particularly of the respiratory center preventing mitochondrial oxygen utilization by inhibiting cytochrome oxidase and there by blocking cellular respiration. With increasing concentration and CNS depression, disruption of memory and motor functions, personality changes and hallucinations appear followed by respiratory depression and unconsciousness (Table 8.4).[6]

SUBACUTE POISONING

It is a condition in which manifestations occur after symptoms free period, the deceased begins to show dyspnea, chest tightness and hemoptysis. This lateness consistent with a subacute lung disease that later on develop into chronic functional disability. Para et al. describe a case where mild fibrosis develops as a sequel to the toxic exposure and could explain the maintenance of exertion dyspnea, decrease in lung volumes and DLCO in patient after five months.[10]

Chronic exposure of a low dose for a long time is studied less as compare to the acute manifestation. It usually affect olfactory sense and may alter the threshold for odor detection or cause complete anomia. A lot of studies are done to study the result of exposure of low dose, most of them claims that chronic exposure to low levels of H₂S are not associated with significant or permanent injury.

LAB INVESTIGATION DIAGNOSIS

Blood, urine, CSF and pleural fluid are obtained by sterilized syringe needle and samples are stored at −80 degree till they are analyzed. Samples are analyzed by gas chromatography and mass spectrophotometry. Thiosulphate being a major metabolite of H₂S acts as the most important indicator of H₂S poisoning. Thiosulphate and sulfide are detected as bis(pentafluorobenzyl)disulfide and bis(pentafluorobenzyl) sulfide, respectively. Normal level of thiosulphate in urine is 0.03 μmol/mL in a healthy person.

Fatality of a case is decided by blood concentration of thiosulphate. Its presence in the blood together with the analysis of sulfide are suggestive of fatal cases. Thiosulfate in urine is the only indicator to prove H₂S poisoning in nonfatal cases[11]. And its nondetectability in urine is suggestive of acute death.[12] Radiologically on X-ray and CT scan, pleural effusion and consolidation can easily be appreciated.

TREATMENT

Decontamination is the primary modality to remove the subject from the site of exposure and immediately transferred to fresh air. Local areas of exposure like skin and eyes should be thoroughly washed. As there is no specific antidote is currently available for sulfide poisoning and so treatment is largely supportive and is under study.

Hydroxocobalamin may be effective as it has a higher affinity for sulfide and its metabolite, i.e., thiosulfate so it binds with sulfide and nitrite generates both methemoglobin, which binds sulfide and nitric oxide, which can displace sulfide from cytochrome C oxidase than for H₂S itself. It is more useful if administrated immediately after H₂S exposure.[13]

Hyperbaric oxygen (HBO) increases tissue oxygen concentration, which should allow oxygen to better compete with toxins for binding sites on the cytochrome system. Apart from this, HBO increases the levels of endogenous oxidants such as glutathione disulfide and, thus, help in "sulfide detoxification." It has vasoconstrictive effect, which aid in decreasing cerebral edema and intracranial pressure that improves the neurological outcome.[14]

In severe cases, it is probably best to administer hyperbaric oxygen therapy as early as possible. HBO has also reported toxicity, including barotrauma, oxygen toxicity.[1]

Cobinamide, a drug in the advanced stages of development reduces sulfide toxicity and sulfide-induced oxidative stress in cells and returned cell proliferation and DNA synthesis to normal. It promise as a novel and first specific therapy for sulfide poisoning. Its half-life is 10 hr in animals and mode of excretion is by renal route.[7]

Supportive treatment is a main stay. Vitals are to be monitored periodically. Symptomatic patients must be kept under observation for an average of 48 hr, and monitored closely.

AUTOPSY FINDINGS

External: Congestion of the head, neck and shoulders. Cyanosis of lips and fingernail beds ears and intraoral mucosa present. An white froth is present at the nose and mouth. The sclerae and conjunctivae appeared to be red. Mild contusions and abrasions are seen as a result of fall in sewer.

On internal examination: Trachea and bronchi contained white edematous froth. Lungs were heavy with edematous with congestion. On cut section, a large amounts of edema fluid exuded from the parenchyma.[3]

Generalized visceral congestion, scattered intrathoracic petechia present and greenish discoloration of skin, blood, viscera and bronchial secretions noted.[15] Decomposition is said to be faster in H$_2$S-related death. Histological examination revealed, in both cases, an evident passive congestion and edema in lungs. None others remarkable abnormalities were noted.

MEDICOLEGAL IMPORTANCE

Occupational exposure is more often potentially life threatening to the workers who are engaged in cleaning of sewers or concerned factories. Most cases of poisoning are accidental in nature but rarely can be intentional.

Although suicidal manner is not so common but a lot of cases are reported with the same. Maebashi et al. reported 17 cases in Japan who died due to inhalation of intentionally generated H$_2$S gas. It has been generated by mixing sulfur-based bath powders or pesticides and acidic detergents.[16]

During an investigation of a death occur in confined space especially in or around a sewer H$_2$S toxicity should be keep in mind. Crime scene investigation, along air sampling whenever possible, plays a crucial role in achieving a diagnosis. To prevent such accidents employer should be cautious about various aspects like, install gas detection systems connected directly to high-volume ventilation systems that automatically trigger alarms. Release of any potentially dangerous emissions are carried out in the absence of staff and install powered gas extractors that are linked directly to the exterior of the building for the emission of potentially dangerous fumes.[17]

BIBLIOGRAPHY

1. Belley R, Bernard N, Côté M, Paquet F, Poitras J Hyperbaric oxygen therapy in the management of two cases of hydrogen sulfide toxicity from liquid manure. Canadian Journal of Emergency Medicine. 2005;7(04):257–61.
2. Ballerino-Regan D, Longmire AW. Hydrogen sulfide exposure as a cause of sudden occupational death. Archives of Pathology & Laboratory Medicine. 2010;134:1105.
3. Knight LD, Erin Presnell S. Death by sewer gas case report of a double fatality and review of the literature. The American Journal of Forensic Medicine and Pathology. June 2005;26(2).
4. Doujaiji B, Al-Tawfiq J. Hydrogen sulfide exposure in an adult male. Annals of Saudi Medicine. 2010;30(1):76–80.
5. Sastre et.al. Fatal accidental hydrogen sulfide poisoning: A domestic case. Journal of Forensic Science. January 2013;58(S1).
6. Harbison SC, Bourgeois JR. Hydrogen sulfide. In Hamilton & Hardy's Industrial Toxicology. 16 March 2015:325–30.
7. Jiang J, Chan A, Ali S, Saha A, Haushalter KJ, Lam W-LM, … Boss GR. Hydrogen sulfide—mechanisms of toxicity and development of an antidote. Scientific Reports. 2016;6(1).
8. Hoffman M, Rajapakse A, Shen X, Gates KS. Generation of DNA-damaging reactive oxygen species via the autoxidation of hydrogen sulfide under physiologically relevant conditions: Chemistry relevant to both the genotoxic and cell signaling properties of H2S. Chemical Research in Toxicology. 2012;25(8):1609–15.
9. Beauchamp RO, Bus JS, Popp JA, et al. A critical review of the literature on hydrogen sulfide toxicity. CRC Critical Review in Toxicology. 1984;13:25–97.
10. Parra O, Monso E, Gallego M, Morera J. Inhalation of hydrogen sulphide: a case of subacute manifestations and long term sequelae. Occupational and Environmental Medicine. 1991;48(4):286–7.
11. Kage S. et al. The usefulness of thiosulfate as an indicator of hydrogen sulfide poisoning: three cases. International Journal of Legal Medicine. 1997;110(4):220–2.
12. Kage S et al. Fatal hydrogen sulfide poisoning at a dye works. Legal Medicine. 2004;6:182–6.
13. Fujita Y et al. A fatal case of acute hydrogen sulfide poisoning caused by hydrogen sulfide: Hydroxocobalamin therapy for acute hydrogen sulfide poisoning. Journal of Analytical Toxicology. March 2011;35.
14. Smilkstein MJ, Bronstein AC, Manning Pickett H, Rumack BH. Hyperbaric oxygen therapy for severe hydrogen sulfide poisoning. The Journal of Emergency Medicine. 1985;3(1):27–30. doi:10.1016/0736-4679(85)90216-1.
15. Adelson L, Sunshine I. Fatal hydrogen sulfide intoxication. Archives of Pathology. 1966;81:375–80.
16. Maebashi K. et al. Toxicological analysis of 17 autopsy cases of hydrogen sulfide poisoning resulting from the inhalation of intentionally generated hydrogen sulfide gas. Forensic Science International. 15 April 2011;207(1–3):91–5.
17. Nogue S, Pou R, Fernandez J, Sanz-Gallen P. Fatal hydrogen sulphide poisoning in unconfined spaces. Occupational Medicine. 2011;61(3):212–4.

Index

Note: Locators in *italics* represent figures and **bold** indicate tables in the text.

Printed and bound by CPI Group (UK) Ltd, Croydon, CR0 4YY

17/10/2024

01775663-0012